# HANDBUCH DER NEUROCHIRURGIE

HERAUSGEGEBEN VON

H. OLIVECRONA
STOCKHOLM

W. TÖNNIS
KÖLN/RH.

SECHSTER BAND

## CHIRURGIE DER HIRNNERVEN UND HIRNBAHNEN

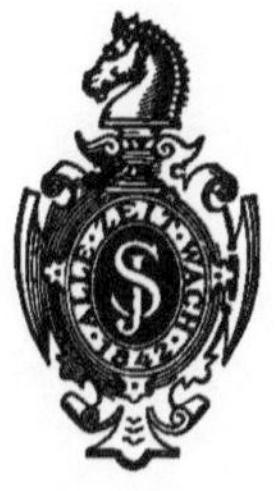

SPRINGER-VERLAG BERLIN HEIDELBERG GMBH
1957

# CHIRURGIE DER HIRNNERVEN UND HIRNBAHNEN

BEARBEITET VON

E. BUSCH · C. H. HERTZ · K. KETTEL · L. LEKSELL
K. LIDÉN · K. SCHÜRMANN · O. SJÖQVIST †

MIT 127 ZUM TEIL FARBIGEN ABBILDUNGEN

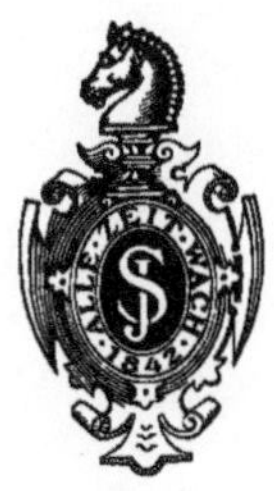

SPRINGER-VERLAG BERLIN HEIDELBERG GMBH
1957

URSPRÜNGLICH ERSCHIENEN BEI SPRINGER-VERLAG OHG. BERLIN · GÖTTINGEN · HEIDELBERG 1957
SOFTCOVER REPRINT OF THE HARDCOVER 1ST EDITION 1957

ISBN 978-3-642-85904-5 ISBN 978-3-642-85903-8 (eBook)
DOI 10.1007/978-3-642-85903-8

# Inhaltsverzeichnis.

**Surgery of the Cranial Nerves.**

By Docent Dr. Olof Sjöqvist †, with a chapter by Dr. Karsten Kettel-Hillerød/Dänemark.
With 38 Figures.

**Die Chirurgie der extrapyramidalen Hyperkinesen.**

Von Privatdozent Dr. K. SCHÜRMANN-Mainz. Mit 52 Abbildungen.

**Psychosurgery.**

By Professor Dr. EDUARD BUSCH-Kopenhagen. With 13 figures.



**Gezielte Hirnoperationen.**

Von Dozent LARS LEKSELL-Lund, mit Abschnitten von Dozent KURT LIDÉN-Lund und Dozent CARL HELLMUTH HERTZ-Lund. Mit 24 Abbildungen.

Olof Sjöqvist died December 4, 1954. Up to his death he worked on his chapter for this book and when he died it was nearly finished — the last part as notes, not unmarked by his sickness. The notes were assembled by one of his friends and very little changed. These pages will be a last greeting to the numerous friends of Olof Sjöqvist — a good and conscientious neurosurgeon, an untiring investigator, an ardent promotor of friendship in international neurosurgery — a gentleman gallant and debonair. A steadfast friend.

E. B.

# Surgery of the Cranial Nerves*.

By

**Olof Sjöqvist †.**

With 38 figures.

## A. Introduction.

Exact knowledge of the descriptive and functional anatomy of the cranial nerves was aquired at a comparatively late stage in the evolution of medical sciences. Galen described seven pairs of which the trigeminal branches formed three. Vesalius's description in the Tabulae sex and the Fabrica were even less accurate. The first to describe the trigeminal nerve as one single nerve was Fallopio. The difference in function between the facial and the trigeminal nerve was not understood until the appearance of the epoch-making studies of Charles Bell (1821). From the middle of the nineteenth century on the gaps still remaining in our knowledge of the gross anatomy of the cranial nerves were gradually filled by careful investigations of a row of important neuroanatomists (Kölliker, Meynert, G. Retzius, Cunningham, Hovelaque and many others). To our present knowledge of the gross anatomy of the cranial nerves probably very little can be added. For a detailed description of the macroscopic anatomy of the cranial nerves the reader is referred to the monograph of Hovelaque.

It should be borne in mind that two of the cranial nerves are no "nerves" in a strict sense since they contain no Schwann cells and are not covered by an ordinary neural sheath. The olfactory nerve—the bulbus olfactorius—is part of the brain. The optic tracts, the chiasm and the optic nerves form an extracerebral commissure and the retinae are parts of the brain. The nerve fibers of both the olfactory and optic "nerves" are lined by glia, not by Schwann cells.

A complete monographic description of the surgery of the cranial nerves should properly cover the surgical treatment of injuries, inflammations, dysfunctions, tumors etc. of all of the twelve pairs. This is, however, not practical. The traumatic injuries of the cranial nerves will be described in the chapter on closed head injuries (Vol. V). The tumors of the peripheral parts of the optic nerves belong to the surgery of the orbit and its contents (Vol. IV) whereas the tumors of the optic chiasm are so closely related to the pituitary and parapituitary tumors that they will be described in this connection (Vol. IV ,,Allgemeine Operationslehre", ,,Diagnostik intrakranieller Geschwülste", ,,Operative Behandlung der einzelnen Geschwulstarten"). Among the tumors of the remaining cranial nerves the neurinomas of the acoustic nerve play a predominant rôle. These are dealt within Vol. III (Zülch) and the chapters ,,Diagnostik intrakranieller Geschwülste" and ,,Operative Behandlung der einzelnen Geschwulstarten (Vol. IV). Surgery of painful disorders or other motor or sensory dysfunctions of the trigeminal, facial, acoustic and glossopharyngeal nerves will thus form the bulk of the present chapter.

* Herausgeber und Verlag sind Herrn Professor Dr. **E. Busch** zu besonderem Dank verpflichtet. Er hat es übernommen, das von Herrn Dr. **Sjöqvist** hinterlassene Manuskript druckfertig zu machen. In diesem Zusammenhang wurde die Abfassung des Kapitels "Operations on the Nerve within the Facial Canal" (Seite 37—46) Herrn Dr. **Karsten Kettel** übertragen.

# B. The Trigeminal Nerve.

*(Nervus trigeminus. Fifth Cranial Nerve.)*

## I. Surgical Anatomy.

The sensory trigeminal root leaves the brachium pontis in the shape of a solid cylinder, not as previously believed a bundle of fine filaments. The solid part of the root is pyramid-shaped and diminishes gradually in diameter giving off tiny rootlets in a similar way as does the cauda equina of the spinal cord. The total length of this so-called glial cone (Hulles) varies from 5 to 10 mm. The number of bundles close to the tip of the glial cone was found in one specimen to be 65 (Sjöqvist). These bundles are subject to additional branching and close to the Gasserian ganglion the number of bundles is more than a hundred. Close to the root there is a frequent intermingling and crossing over of bundles forming the *plexus triangularis* of Krause. In peripheral direction the sensory root flattens from side to side to rest on the impressio trigemini of the petrous bone. Also the motor root which leaves the pons a few millimeters more cranially has a small glial cone which splits into a number of root bundles. These, however, very soon fuse to form one, sometimes two, trunks situated on the medial side of the sensory root and easily distinguishable from the latter in the living by its whiter colour and more glistening appearance which no doubt is caused by the larger diameter and correspondingly greater content of myeline of its fibers. Even close to the ganglion the motor root is found behind the upper portion of the sensory root. but from there on it takes an oblique course to join the third trigeminal division. The solid character of the root is easily felt when the root is transected close to the pons according to Dandy's technique. There is a distinctly different "feeling" when the surgeon collects the rootlets on a blunt hook close to the ganglion in order to divide them. The Gasserian ganglion has the shape of a half-moon. Its superior horn is often drawn out to a long peak which is covered by the upper sensory rootlets. The ganglion itself may thus occasionally be damaged when the root section is performed very close to the ganglion.

The pontine end of the sensory root has close topographic relations to the petrosal vein. The vein is situated in immediate vicinity to the root, either running parallel to it or crossing over it before emptying into the superior petrosal sinus. This may cause a troublesome venous hemorrhage when the root is approached from behind in the Dandy operation. The main part of the fifth nerve root is situated within the cavum of Meckel which is a subarachnoidal pouch communicating with the lateral cistern. The roof of the cavum of Meckel is formed by the dura. The ringshaped ostium of the cavum is often of a markedly fibrous consistency which can be distinctly felt when the cavum is spilt open in the Taarnhøj operation. Within the roof of the cavum runs the superior petrosal sinus more or less at right angles to the root. It empties into the cavernous sinus. The anatomy of these veins can apparently vary a great deal. The trochlear and abducent nerves are situated medially and rather close to the root before entering the cavernous sinus.

The most distal part of the root, the Gasserian ganglion and the proximal parts of the second and third peripheral fifth nerve divisions are covered by the dura of the floor of the temporal fossa. In this place the dura can easily be split by blunt dissection in two layers and the inner layer elevated. Between these two layers but usually more firmly adherent to the outer leaf lies the greater superior petrosal nerve in its bony groove passing from the geniculate ganglion to the third trigeminal division. If this nerve is exposed, either in an operation for trigeminal neuralgia or for the purpose of transecting the nerve in unilateral migraine (Gardner's operation) tugging or pulling the nerve should be carefully avoided. This may cause a small hemorrhage within the facial canal which without doubt is the most common cause of the transcient facial nerve paralysis occasionally following these operations.

By elevating the dura from the floor of the temporal fossa in the direction forward and medially the second and third fifth nerve branches—the maxillary and mandibular divisions—can be exposed all the way to their exit from the cranial cavity via the foramen

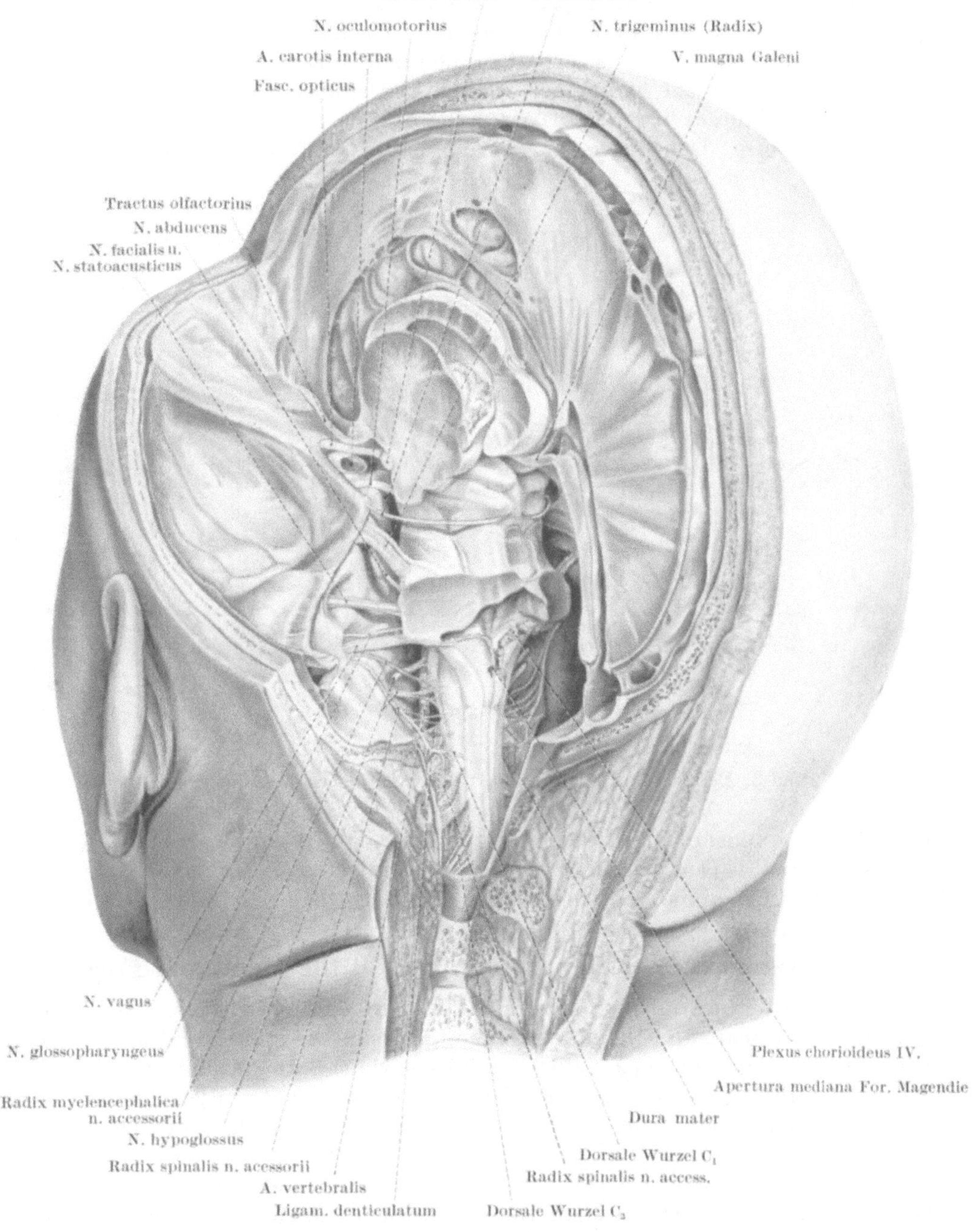


Fig. 1. The base of the skull with the cranial nerves. (After H. FERNER.)

rotundum and the foramen ovale. The first branch—the ophthalmic division—cannot be brought into view since it is entirely embedded in the cavernous sinus. If the cavernous sinus is more widely opened the ensuing hemorrhage can be copious. Even the risk of air embolism is present. This type of hemorrhage can, however, always be readily controlled by pressing a piece of muscle or fibrin foam against the bleeding spot.

The anatomy of the peripheral fifth nerve divisions is of a somewhat lesser interest than the more central parts of the nerve from a mere surgical point of view. It should be borne in mind that the mandibular nerve is situated in close vicinity to the Eustachian tube, which may be subject to damage in attempts to inject alcohol into the third division. This can result in a severe middle ear infection. The maxillary nerve runs through the orbit for a short distance and is situated only 1 centimeter from the optic nerve, a fact worth remembering when the second branch is injected. Alcohol may spread in the orbit causing damage to the eye-muscle nerves, the ciliary ganglion and even the optic nerve. The ophthalmic division also passes the orbit after having entered through the superior orbital fissure. Damage to this nerve must be carefully avoided when the orbit is

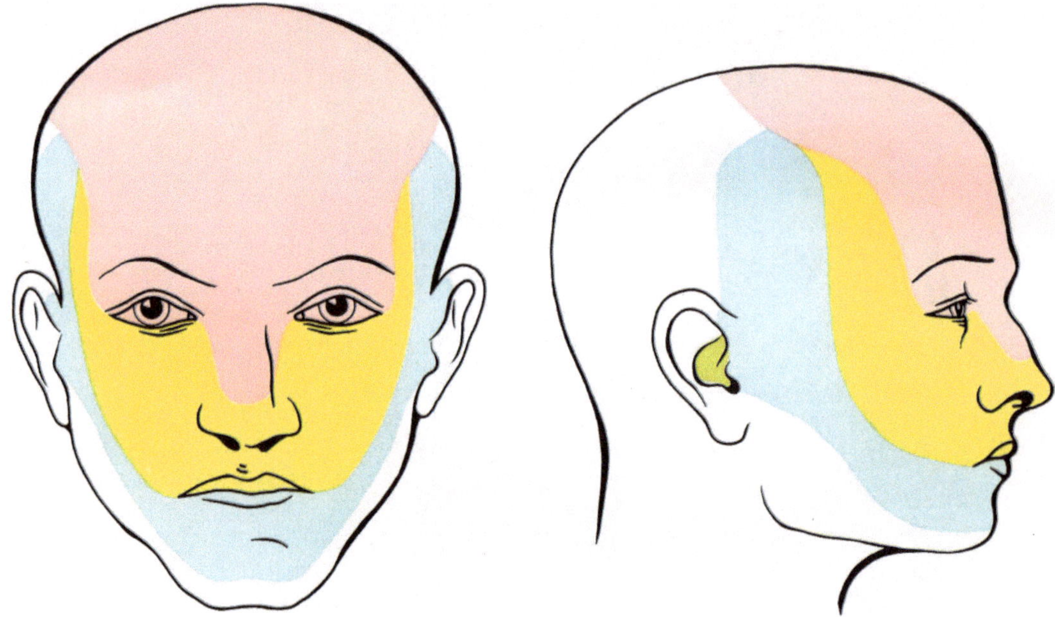

Fig. 2 and 3. Peripheral distribution of the three branches of the trigeminal nerve.

unroofed for the exposure of intraorbital tumors. The inferior alveolar nerve which runs in a bony canal is easily accessible for alcohol injection or avulsion after chiseling a small opening 10 mms. above the angulus mandibulae.

## II. Physiology. Sensory Innervation of the Head and Face.

The trigeminal nerve transmits superficial sensation from the face, the forehead, the anterior part of the scalp and the mucous membranes of the mouth and nose. An outline of the trigeminal area and the participation of its various branches is seen in Fig. 2 and 3. In the scalp the fifth nerve area borders upon the area innervated by the greater occipital nerve which mainly derives from the first and second cervical segment. On the chin the fifth nerve area borders upon the area innervated from the cervical plexus corresponding to the second cervical segment. The tongue which is equipped with a very highly developed sensory apparatus is innervated from the third trigeminal division with the exception of the sense of taste. The cornea and the conjuctiva bulbi are entirely innervated from the first trigeminal division. These structures do not possess tactile sensation. Proprioception from the masticatory muscles is also transmitted via the trigeminal nerve. The so-called "deep pressure pain" sensation of the face has aroused a considerable discussion. After the investigations of Davis (1923) it was believed that "deep pressure pain" was transmitted by the facial nerve and that this type of pain would remain even after sectioning of the fifth nerve root. This in turn might explain some of the failures of relieving pain in certain types of facial neuralgia by fifth nerve root section. In the light of later clinical experience this explanation, however, seems less probable. The type of pain which can be elicited by hard pressure against the periosteum of the frontal or maxillary bones is with all probability conveyed by the fifth nerve. It is true that proprioception from the facial muscles is transmitted via the seventh nerve but even an intense proprioceptive impulse can never be painful.

Within the mouth the trigeminal area borders upon areas innervated by the glossopharyngeal and vagus nerves. A description of the small but important glossopharyngeal area will be found later. Within the external auditory meatus and its surroundings (tragus, antitragus, anthelix) a small skin area is innervated by the sensory portion of the seventh nerve—the nervus intermedius or WRISBERG's nerve—which was conclusively proved by RAMSAY HUNT (1909). The sensory ganglion belonging to this nerve is the ganglion geniculi. This ganglion can be the seat of herpes zoster and the zoster eruption in these cases is strictly limited to the area mentioned above. The ear drum itself is at least mainly innervated by the tenth nerve.

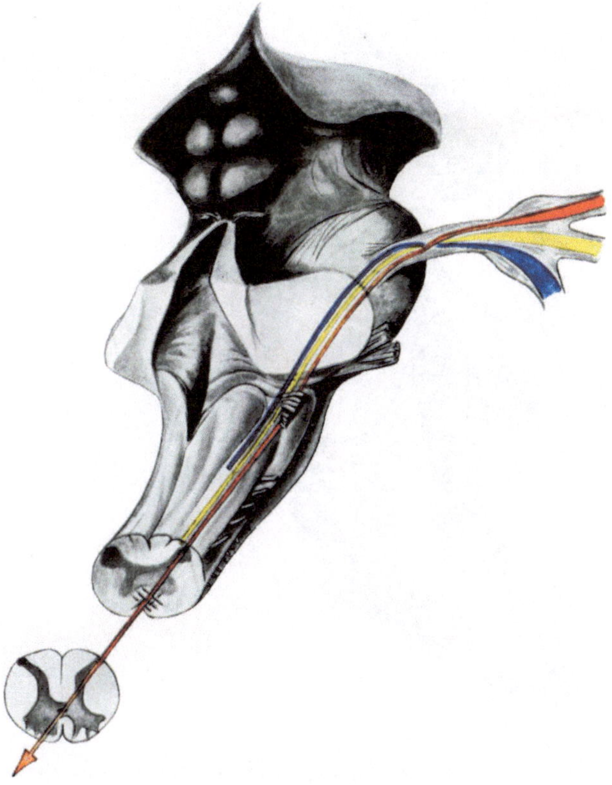

Fig. 4. Central distribution of the three branches of the trigeminal nerve.

The internal structure of the main trigeminal division and the sensory root was studed by SJÖQVIST in 1938. By *fiber analysis*, i.e by studying the distribution of fibers of different calibre in numerous transverse sections of the nerve the investigator is able to make conclusions concerning the transmission of various modalities of sensation within nerves. The pain-transmitting fibres are characterized by their minute diameter. Within the peripheral divisions the small pain-conducting fibres are irregulary intermingled with fibers transmitting other qualities of sensation. A similar, completely irregular intermingling of fibers of various calibre was found also in the sensory trigeminal root. A somewhat higher content of pain fibers was found in the upper portion of the root corresponding to the first division, a higher content of tactile and proprioceptive fibers was found in the lower portion corresponding to the third, i.e. mandibular division. This is doubtlessly accounted for by the different type of external sensation in the eye and the tongue (cfr. above). It was shown already in 1926 by FRAZIER and WHITEHEAD that at least close to the ganglion the fibers from the three different trigeminal divisions kept their place also within the root, i.e. the first division fibers are situated in the upper portion of the root, the second division fibers are situated in the centre and the third division fibers are situated within the lower portion of the root. It was previouly believed on account of older anatomic investigations and more recent ones by FRAZIER and WHITEHEAD that a rotation of the fifth nerve root amounting to almost 180 degrees took place during embryonic life. This would imply that the fibers belonging to the three different trigeminal divisions would take an almost reversed position within the pontine end of the root, the ophthalmic fibers thus being situated ventrally and the mandibular fibers dorsally. This has been claimed as an objection to the Dandy operation in which the root is sectioned closed to the pons. It could easily be seen already by the naked eye that such a rotation has not taken place in the adult human. The bundles run more or less parallel throughout the root. Neither did the microscopic studies of Sjöqvist support this opinion. A screw-like rotation of the fifth nerve fibers, however, does take place but not until the root has entered the pons.

The sensory fibers from the entire trigeminal area end in the pontine and spinal fifth nerve nuclei. The proprioceptive fibers from the masticatory muscles form the tiny mesencephalic tract ending in the mesencephalic nucleus (Wohlfart). The tactile fibers end in the so-called main sensory nucleus situated within the pons and bordering immediately upon the cranial part of the spinal nucleus. There is probably no sharp limit between these two nuclei. The spinal nucleus can be traced down at least to the third cervical segment in humans. It fuses without sharp limit with the substantia gelatinosa of Rolando. To reach the spinal nucleus the fifth nerve fibers pass downwards along the spinal trigeminal tract. As shown by Sjöqvist in 1938 the fibers within this tract are almost exclusively pain and temperature fibers. The transection of the tract (trigeminal tractotomy) results in thermal anesthesia and analgesia of half of the face. From experience gained in this operation (Sjöqvist, Grant and Weinberger, Walker and others) a rather detailed picture of the internal and functional structure of the spinal trigeminal tract can be given (cfr. Fig. 4 and 5).

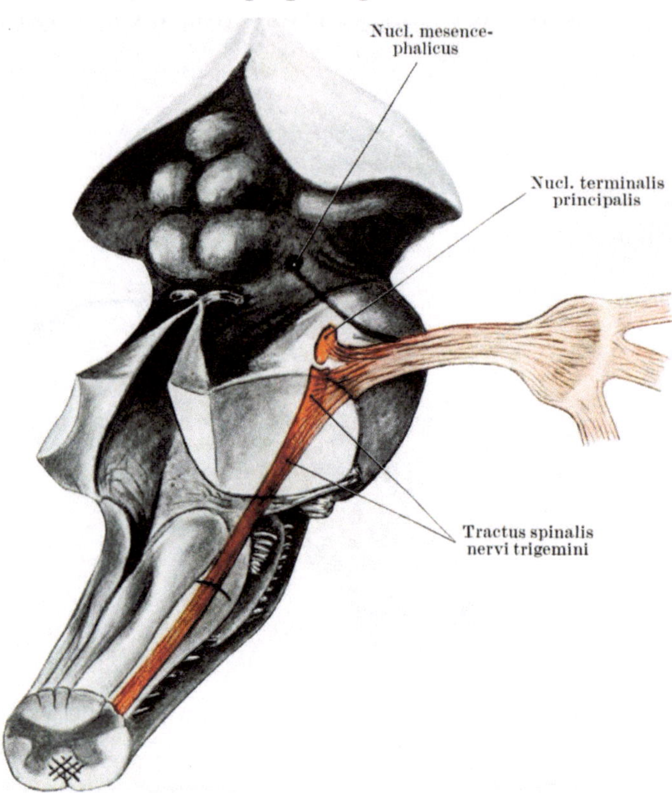

Fig. 5. Central distribution of the pain fibres of the trigeminal nerve.

Due to the rotation of the root within the pons which has been already mentioned the pain and temperature fibers lie dorsally in the tract and probably also laterally and more superficially than the mandibular fibers, since these are harder to reach in the tractotomy operation and more difficult to stimulate electrically during the operation. The bulk of pain fibers from all of the three divisions is still maintained at a level 3 to 4 mm. below the obex since it is possible to obtain an almost complete analgesia of half of the face by transecting the tract at this level (Grant). In the neighbourhood of this level the mandibular fibers begin to dive into the nucleus. A little further down also the maxillary fibers bend mesially to enter the nucleus, whereas the ophthalmic fibers run still further in a caudal direction until they reach their end station. This internal arrangement of the spinal tract fibers gives a clue to the clinical application of the tractotomy operation which will be dealt with later.

The secondary trigeminal fibers running from the pontine and spinal nuclei to the thalamus are still insufficiently known. In the collicular level they seemingly run within the most lateral part of the medial lemniscus, even partly within the lateral lemniscus (DOGLIOTTI, WALKER). The transsection of these parts of the lemnisci gives at least a partial blunting of pain sensation within the face, neck, arm and upper trunk.

The sympathetic nerves innervating blood vessels and sweat glands of the face derive from the cervical sympathetic chain. In the periphery they accompany the branches of the trigeminal nerve which they have joined peripherally to the GASSERian ganglion. There is, however, also a form of sweating, the *gustatory perspiration*, which has been proven to be of parasympathetic origin. The sweating seen in the so-called *auriculotemporal syndrome,* usually taking place after traumatic injury to the auriculotemporal nerve is also parasympathetic. No proof has been provided that autonomic nerves of the face—or elsewhere in the body—could transmit painful impulses. The so-called *sphenopalatine ganglion neuralgia* (SLUDER) is probably no clinical entity.

# III. Major Trigeminal Neuralgia.

*(Tic Douloureux. Typische Trigeminusneuralgie.)*

## 1. Early Descriptions.

Major trigeminal neuralgia presents a striking clinical picture and was, accordingly, early recognized and described in medical literature. According to FEDOR KRAUSE, whose careful historical survey in his monograph „Die Neuralgie des Trigeminus“ deserves special attention, *Avicenna* (9'century) gave a good description of the paroxysmal nature of pain in the face. The Englishman JOHN FOTHERGILL (1776) described this type of painful disease so accurately that only little has been added later to the clinical description of its symptoms and course. The following quotation from FOTHERGILL is a sample of his literary style and accuracy in observations:

*"This affection seems to be peculiar to persons advancing in years, and to women more than to men. I never met with it in anyone much under forty, but after this period no age is exempt to it . . . From imperceptible beginnings, a pain attacks some part or other of the face, or the side of the head; sometimes about the orbit of the eye, sometimes the ossa malarum, sometimes the temporal bones, are the parts complained of. The pain comes suddenly and is excruciating; it lasts but a short time, perhaps a quarter or half a minute, and then goes off; it returms at irregular intervals, sometimes in half an hour, sometimes there are two or three repetitions in a few minutes.*

*The kind of pain is described differently by different persons, as may be reasonably expected; but one sees enough to excite one's compassion if present during the paroxysm.*

*Eating will bring it on some persons. Talking, or the least motion of the muscles of the face affects others; the gentlest touch of a hand or a handkerchief will sometimes bring on the pain, whilst a strong pressure on the part has no effect.*

*It differs from the toothache essentially in many respects. It affects some who, from age, have few or no teeth remaining."*

In English medical literature major trigeminal neuralgia is often and for good reasons called FOTHERGILL's disease. The term "tic douloureux" was introduced by ANDRE in 1756. That the trigeminal and no other cranial nerve was the transmitter of pain in tic douloureux became evident when surgical attempts were made to relieve the symptoms by nerve sections (VON LANGENBECK). The general trend in the evolution of surgery in major trigeminal neuralgia has been to attack more and more central parts of the fifth nerve pathways. All surgical therapy has been symptomatic in nature with the important exception of the recently introduced and most promising method of TAARNHØJ.

## 2. Clinical Picture.

Pain in trigeminal neuralgia is paroxysmal in nature and elicited by external stimuli. In the very earliest stages it may be of a mild and more tickling character but very soon it becomes extremely intense. It is of course always difficult to evaluate the severity of a subjective sensation like pain, but from the writer's experience there is hardly any painful condition affecting the human body which is more excruciating than pain in trigeminal neuralgia. In earlier days when no relief could be offered to the sufferers suicide was not infrequent. Pain is described as "burning" or "flashing". Sometimes it is compared with an electric shock. It lasts from a few seconds up to about half a minute and subsides gradually, often with a series of minor paroxysms. This has been termed "afterdischarge" of pain. Immediately after pain has ceased there is a "refractory period" in which a new paroxysm cannot be elicited. This is something that many patients find out by their own experience and utilize for taking food. On occasion the patients may complain of a dull aching pain also between the paroxysms, but this type of pain is not severe and often missing. Very often the paroxysms appear in volleys in the course of one or several hours with pain-free intervals. Very characteristic is the way in which pain is elicited by external tactile or thermal stimulation. A slight touch of the face with the finger or with cotton-wool or a breeze of wind is sufficient to induce an attack of typical pain with a longer or shorter after-discharge. The taking of food is always difficult. The introduction of food or drink into the mouth and the chewing movements are usually accompanied by severe pain. In long-standing cases the patient may become emaciated and dehydrated. Washing the face or shaving may become difficult or impossible. Talking or mimic movements in general may provoke an attack and these patients have often a blank and motionless expression. Even slight facial weakness can sometimes be simulated in this way.

Pain is always unilateral and does never pass the midline. This fact is very important and a good guide when the patient is questioned concerning his subjective symptoms. It is true that trigeminal neuralgia on rare occasions can become bilateral but it always starts on one side. Usually there is a certain area of the skin or the mucous membrane of the mouth which cannot be touched without the appearance of paroxysmal pain. This has been called the "trigger zone". Pain always starts in one trigeminal division, usually the second or third, perhaps with a slight predominance of the second division. This means that pain is felt at first in the chin, the cheek, the tongue, the teeth or gums. It rapidly spreads to one whole division, i.e. to the entire lower jaw and the tongue and temple or to the whole upper jaw. Primary first division neuralgia is comparatively rare. In these cases pain almost never starts in the frontal region but in the neighbourhood of the inner corner of the eye and the bridge of the nose. In untreated cases pain may spread from one division to another and affect the entire half of the face.

A characteristic feature of major trigeminal neuralgia is its course drawn out for years or tens of years with long painfree intervals. The first painful period lasting perhaps for a few weeks only may be followed by a free interval of a year's duration or more. Sooner or later pain recurs and usually lasts for a longer period than the first time, the pain usually being more intense and widespread. Recurrences and free intervals alternate in the course of the years but invariably the free intervals tend to become shorter, the painful periods longer and more severe until the condition finally is completely unbearable to the patient. Trigeminal neuralgia is in itself not a mortal disease but the sufferer may succumb to intercurrent disease brought about by malnutrition or dehydration or he may shorten his own life. Such cases were still seen in the writer's country 20 or 25 years ago, but have almost completely disappeared with the introduction of modern neurosurgery.

Major trigeminal neuralgia is a disease belonging to old age. The vast majority of patients are 55 years old or more at the onset of symptoms. When the typical clinical picture is found in younger individuals a cholesteatoma of the cerebellopontine angle should always be suspected (cfr. p. 9). Disseminated sclerosis, also, seems to be a predisposing factor, tic douloureux being 4–5 times more common among patients suffering from disseminated sclerosis than among people in general. Within this group the onset of symptoms may come early in life. There is, however, a small group of patients who aquire the disease early without any detectable releasing factor.

As already mentioned the disease is unilateral in the vast majority of cases. The right side prevails somewhat to the left. According to the writer's experience bilateral neuralgia is seen in about 1 % of the cases. Even in this small group the onset is always unilateral. Usually the appearance of pain on the second side will take place years after it has been relieved on the first side by surgical methods. This small group of bilateral neuralgia is a special therapeutic problem.

Spontaneous complete relief of major trigeminal neuralgia has so far not been observed by the present author. Patients afraid of surgery and of surgeons often express the hope that the last free interval will became lasting. This hope is invariably in vain.

## 3. Considerations of Etiology.

The problem of the origin of major trigeminal neuralgia is still unsolved. In the vast majority of cases no gross anatomic changes are found which could give a clue to the etiology. In the nineties when FEDOR KRAUSE treated a great number of cases by excision of the ganglion of GASSER the excised specimens were examined microscopically. Blood extravasates, round cell infiltration and other chronic inflammatory changes were found in a certain number of the specimens which led KRAUSE to believe that the etiologic factors were situated in the ganglion. The findings of KRAUSE are, however, difficult to evaluate, since his specimens always were considerably traumatized at operation.

On account of the localization the patients themselves almost invariably believe pain to derive from some dental disorder. The majority of them see a dentist before they see a doctor. In bygone days the clinical picture of trigeminal neuralgia, unfortunately, was less well known to the dental profession and ten or twenty years ago it was the rule that no patient suffering from this disease had the true nature of his pain recognized until several teeth had been extracted, often so many as to impair masticatory function considerably. This is much less common nowadays. No convincing proof that dental disease could produce a typical paroxysmal neuralgia has to the writer's knowledge been presented.

The only gross anatomic lesions which are known occasionally to produce a typical tic douloureux are the cholesteatomas of the cerebellopontine angle (DANDY, FINDEISEN and TÖNNIS). A number of cases have been described in which a cholesteatoma of the angle was found on exposing the root by the cerebellar approach in trigeminal neuralgia and also cases in which removal of the tumor without interference with the root resulted in a lasting cure. One such case was seen by the author. On the other hand not all cholesteatomas of the angle produce paroxysmal pain and the typical picture of trigeminal neuralgia is rarely seen in other types of cerebello-pontine angle tumors (acoustic neurinomas, meningiomas). DANDY also describes a case in which an anomalous artery had caused a groove in the root, the patient suffering from major neuralgia. It seems thus that only a *slight* pressure on the root might be able to produce paroxysmal pain whereas a more heavy compression will result in painless hypoesthesia.

If the ganglion is interfered with by means of alcohol injection or electrocoagulation (cfr. later) in order to relieve trigeminal pain, a very complete anesthesia must be induced for a good result. On the other hand lasting relief is not unfrequently seen even after sectioning only moderate portions of the root, resulting in a very small anesthetic area not even covering the division to which the neuralgia was primary. OLIVECRONA believes in an abnormal tension of the root brough forth by the sinking of the brain due to compression of the intervertebral discs and consequent shortering of the spinelin elderly people. The interesting experiences gained in the TAARNHØJ operation also suggest the root to be the "guilty" portion of the trigeminal pathways. Further experience with this operation will probably throw more light on the problem of etiology.

Pain in trigeminal neuralgia is a sort of dysesthesia, an abnormal—painful—response to an inadequate—tactile—stimulation and has a marked afterdischarge. In this respect it has certain features in common with causalgic pain seen as a sequel to peripheral nerve injuries. There should be little doubt that causalgia is due to an artificial synapse within the nerve allowing centrifugal vasomotor impulses to bridge over to the afferent sensory components of the nerve and to be reflected backwards as a painful sensation. The presence of an artificial synapse in experimental injuries to peripheral nerves have been conlusively proven by electrophysiological methods by GRANIT, SKOGLUND and LEKSELL. It is very tempting to assume the existence of a similar artificial synapse within the trigeminal root in major neuralgia, a sort of short-circuiting allowing tactile impulses to bridge over first to the pain (and temperature) fibers of the same division, later to the entire fifth nerve root and to assume this artificial synapse or irritable focus to be produced by slight compression or abnormal tension of the root. The clinical features of trigeminal neuralgia could easily be explained and also the difference in effect between surgical interventions on the peripheral branches and the ganglion on the one hand and the fifth nerve root on the other. An "irritable focus" was believed by SJÖQVIST (1939) to exist in trigeminal neuralgia somewhere more peripherally or more centrally within the fifth nerve pathways. Increasing experience would seem to induce one to discard other levels than the root itself. On the other hand it is immediately evident that mere compression of the trigeminal root cannot produce the picture of tic douloureux. There is no resemblance whatsoever between this paroxysmal pain and the type of pain seen in nerve root compression for instance in protruded discs or spinal cord tumors or malignancies of the spinal column or the base of the skull.

As already mentioned disseminated sclerosis in one way or another predisposes to major trigeminal neuralgia. Whether or not a sclerotic plaque can produce a similar artificial synapse within the intrapontine part of the root is open to question.

## 4. Diagnosis.

From the description given above it should be evident that major trigeminal neuralgia gives a very striking clinical picture which can hardly be confused with any other type of facial pain. As in all painful conditions a careful history and a detailed analysis of the patient's symptoms is essential to make a correct diagnosis, the more so since objective signs as a rule are entirely missing. Stress should be laid on the paroxysmal character of the pain, of its strictly unilateral localization, never surpassing the midline, and the painfree intervals. These patients are often easily recognized as soon as they enter the consulting room. They have a suffering appearance and often a rigid mimic. When talking they may stop in the midst of a sentence with a grimace. Even if the patient is free of symptoms when seeing the doctor, the diagnosis is still as a rule easy by interrogating him carefully. It has been said that the painful paroxysms often are accompanied by tear-flow, flushing, salivation and other signs of autonomic hyperfunction. This may happen but is by no means common. It has also been said that the points of emergence of the trigeminal end branches, i.e. foramen supra- and infraorbitale and foramen mentale should be tender to pressure. This is certainly not the case in the majority of cases. On the contrary—tenderness over the foramina is frequently seen in atypical neuralgia and in disorders of the paranasal sinuses, not in major neuralgia. If the patient complains of a continuous aching pain day and night major neuralgia can be ruled out immediately. In all cases of facial pain X-ray examination of the paranasal sinuses should not be omitted and the sensation of the face and the corneal reflex carefully tested. Signs of disseminated sclerosis should be asked for and looked for (nystagmus, abdominal reflexes). If the case is by any means obscure, examination of the ears,nose and throat and a dental examination should not be omitted.

It should be borne in mind that the only painful condition of the face—excepting pain caused by spread of malignant disease—that can be successfully dealt with surgically is major trigeminal neuralgia. But this disease in turn can be relieved by surgery—and by surgery only.

## 5. Treatment.

The various types of medical treatment which have been tried in major paroxysmal neuralgia of the face have never given convincingly good results. In evaluating the results of treatment the tendency towards spontaneous remissions should be remembered.

Vitamine B has been tried and also nicotinic acid without any convincing effect. Analgetic drugs, especially morphia and its derivates, should never be given. In the first place they do not arrest the painful paroxysms, in the second place they may cause addiction. Drug addiction is, however, rarely seen in major trigeminal neuralgia.

Whether or not X-ray treatment can precipitate a remission is doubtful. It could come into question in cases where the diagnosis is unsettled, e.g. when pain has been present only for a very short time. The best way of establishing the diagnosis is, however, to block one of the peripheral fifth nerve branches with novocaine in order to render that part of the face anesthetic from which pain is elicited. If novocaine block is followed by prompt cessation of pain there is no reason to postpone a more radical type of surgical treatment.

The history of trigeminal nerve surgery dates back to the early 19th century. The very first attempts were directed toward the seventh nerve and a few unhappy individuals were left with pain persisting and a facial paralysis added. The first to operate on the fifth nerve branches was BERNHARD VON LANGENBECK. From peripheral nerve sections and avulsions which practically always were followed by recurrencies, the surgical procedures were directed towards more and more central parts of the fifth nerve pathways. After the intracranial section of the main peripheral branches performed by HARTLEY came the method of KRAUSE (1896), an excision of the GASSERian ganglion, which meant a great progress, since patients suffering from trigeminal neuralgia could now gain what they could not have gained before—lasting relief. The operative technique of KRAUSE was modified and improved by CUSHING who also very carefully studied the sensory disturbances following this operation. The next great step was the retrogasserian root section of SPILLER and FRAZIER, "physiologic exstirpation of the GASSERian ganglion", as they themselves called it, because the effect on facial sensation is the same as the exstirpation of the ganglion. It is the merit of SPILLER and FRAZIER to have thoroughly studied the consequenses of postganglionary root section in experiments on dogs and to have demonstrated that regeneration does not take place, before they adviced this procedure in man. The fact that HORSLEY had cut the fifth nerve root behind the ganglion in trigeminal neuralgia several years earlier does not lessen the merit of SPILLER and FRAZIER. The success of the SPILLER-FRAZIER operation—postganglionic section of the trigeminal root by extradural subtemporal approach—was complete, and it may well be said that major trigeminal neuralgia since the introduction of this technique lost most of its terror. Improvements in the technical performance of the operation were introduced by FRAZIER himself and by ADSON, who used a straight incision instead of the previously used curved one. In 1919 FRAZIER showed that it was possible to save the motor root and in 1925 he reported a series of cases in which he had performed subtotal section of the root with preservation of the upper rotlets corresponding to the first division. In this way corneal sensation was maintained and the risk of postoperative keratitis greatly diminished.

In 1925 DANDY published his method of sectioning the root at the pons after exposing it by a cerebellar approach: The posterior inferior half or two thirds of the root are divided with a blunt hook after elevating one cerebellar hemisphere and emptying the lateral cistern. The advantages of this method are that the motor root never is severed, that keratitis never occurs and that the sensory loss is small, disadvantages being that the operation is a major procedure, that complications in the form of hemorrhage during or after the operation is more frequent than in the subtemporal operation, and the number of recurrences higher.

Section of the spinal trigeminal tract—medullary trigeminal tractotomy—was introduced in 1938 by SJÖQVIST. This operation results in anesthesia for pain and temperature in half of the face with preservation of tactile sensation. In successful cases the paroxysms of pain are completely relieved and the patient has no dificulties in eating. The sensory loss is hardly even noticed by many patients. Keratitis does not occur and a motor paralysis is not to be feared. The drawbacks of this operation are the somewhat increased risk of a recurrence and the occurrence of unwanted side-effects—in the first place ataxia of the ipsilateral arm. As the Dandy procedure this operation carries a somewhat higher operative risk.

In the last two decades several surgeons have recommended intradural root section by a temporal approach (Dogliotti, Ribe Portugal).

The latest step in the evolution of surgery in tic douloureux is the splitting of the roof of the cavum of Meckel—decompression of the trigeminal root—which procedure was introduced by Taarnhøj in 1952. This operation is a completely new departure, since the fifth nerve pathways are not interfered with at all and no sensory loss produced. It sets out from the assumption, that the origin of pain lies in the nerve root and is brought about by some sort of pressure on the root. It is in fact the first real attempt of a causative therapy in trigeminal neuralgia. The experiences with this operation gained by Taarnhøj himself and by others are highly encouraging, but the operation has not been practiced long enough to allow judgement of its final value.

The method of injecting alcohol in the peripheral branches of the nerve for the relief of trigeminal pain was introduced in 1902 by Pitres and Verger, and further elaborated by Schloesser and by Horrax and Poppen. Its value lies mainly in giving the surgeon a chance of ascertaining the diagnosis and also to accustom the patient to the loss of sensation which will follow a more radical intervention on the nerve root. It cannot be expected to give a permanent relief. Alcohol injection in the ganglion of Gasser has been recommended by Härtel and by Harris. Although this procedure can offer a number of patients permanent relief of pain it has nowadays been mostly abandoned in favour of operations performed under the control of the eye. Alcohol injection in the ganglion is technically difficult and carries not inconsiderable risks of recurrencies and of injuries to other cranial nerves even if it is true that this method has given good results in large series (Harris).

Electrocoagulation of the Gasserian ganglion by means of a stereotaxic instrument was introduced in 1931 by Kirschner. Due to the ingenious design of Kirschner's apparatus it is as a rule not difficult to reach the ganglion via the foramen ovale and to destroy it completely or partly by the aid of the coagulating diathermy current, the drawbacks of the method being that it is not without mortality and carries a considerable risk both of recurrencies, of keratitis and of damage to other cranial nerves. Kirschner's method has found its place mainly in the hands of general surgeons without training in intracranial surgery.

Of all the different procedures mentioned above some few are now obsolete. The methods still practised which will be described in this chapter are

α) Extradural root section by the temporal approach
β) Section of the root close to the pons by the cerebellar route
γ) Intradural root section by the temporal or temporooccipital approach
δ) Medullary trigeminal tractotomy
ε) Decompression of the trigeminal root
ζ) Alcohol injection in the peripheral branches and the main divisions
η) Electrocoagulation of the Gasserian ganglion.

## a) Technique.

### *α) Extradural Root Section by the Temporal Approach* (Fig. 6–13).

This operation is done with the patient in a sitting position. Some surgeons prefer a special chair with a head rest, like a dentist's chair, others prefer to tilt the operating table. If the patient's legs are pulled up high ortostatic reactions are diminished. The operation can be undertaken under local anesthesia with a short intravenously induced general anesthesia during the later phases of the operation. This is a good form of anesthesia in elderly patients. Some surgeons prefer intratracheal anesthesia. If local anesthesia is chosen, morphia is not given shortly before the operation, as this will increase the risk of fainting, which is always present, when the patient is operated on in an upright position. The head shall be well supported to prevent its falling backwards. The skin incision is laid from the center of the zygoma upwards and is about 10 cm. in length. The incision shall not pass the arch of the zygomatic bone in order to avoid lesion to the upper rami of the facial nerve. After the skin has been incised the soft parts are bluntly dissected from the temporal fascia, which is incised. The temporal muscle is divided along the course of the fibers with cutting diathermy current and kept apart with a selfretaining retractor. The temporal bone is perforated with a burr and the bony defect enlarged with rongeurs. The defect should be circular with a diameter of 3–3,5 cm. The more experienced surgeon can get away with a smaller opening. Under all circumstances the bone should be removed down to the base of the skull. The dura is then dissected from the floor of the temporal fossa and elevated with a curved brain spatula. Oozing from the middle meningeal artery in this stage is controlled by the pressure of the spatula. The elevation of the dura proceeds in medial direction following the groove of the middle meningeal artery, until the foramen spinosum comes into view. Sometimes the foramen is hidden by a small bony elevation which may have to be chiselled away. When the foramen is clearly in view, the field is cleared by the sucker. A small piece of firmly twisted cotton-wool, the size of a rice-grain is introduced in the foramen with a blunt hook and pressed down in to the foramen to be left. This immediately arrests hemorrhage from the middle meningeal artery and its branches. With a straight long-handled knife with a narrow blade the middle meningeal vessels are cut and the elevation of the dura continued. The third trigeminal division is found a few millimetres medial to the foramen spinosum and 4–5 mm. anteriorly. It is always expedient to have an X-ray picture of the base of the scull (axial picture according to LYSHOLM'S terminology) in order to visualize the topography of the foramen spinosum and its surroundings preoperatively. The third division is then uncovered by pressing a blunt dissector against the dura immediately above the third division. By blunt dissection upwards and forwards the whole intracranial part of the third division and the lower margin of the second division comes into view. If the operation is done under local anesthesia the intravenous anesthesia is started at this juncture. As soon as the third division has been identified a few drops of 2% novocaine is injected in it. If the patient is of a calm temperament, the operation can be done entirely under local anesthesia if a further few drops (not more than $^1/_2$ cc.) is injected into the cavum of MECKEL between the root filaments. In the direction backwards the dura is more firmly adherent to the petrous bone. The dural adhesions

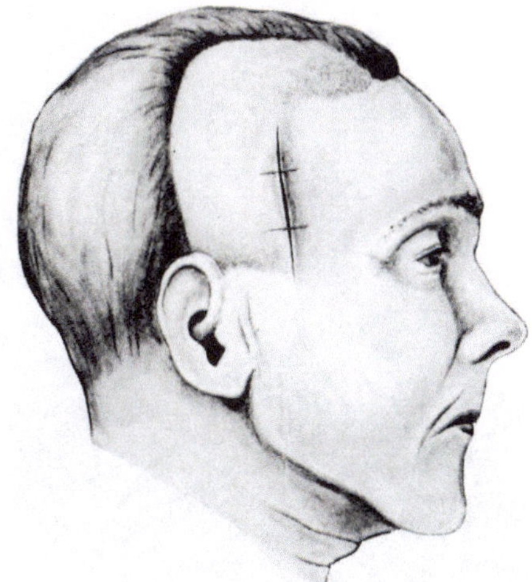

Fig. 6. Temporal trigeminotomy—skin incision.

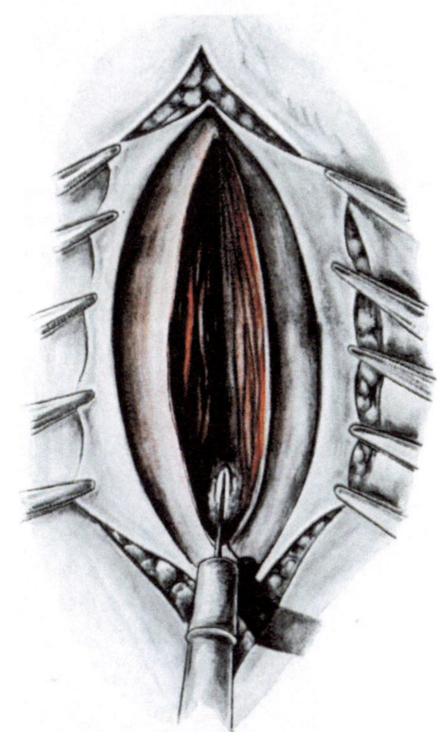

Fig. 7. Temporal trigeminotomy—muscle incision.

are here divided with a long narrow-bladed knife. The major superior petrosal nerve here comes into view running obliquely from behind to join the third division at the posterior margin of the foramen ovale. It should not be touched or pulled at. It is often possible to leave a thin layer of dura over this nerve. When the dissection upwards and medially has been carried sufficiently far, the most lateral part of the arachnoidal pouch which forms the cavum of Meckel will be seen bulging and pulsating. The ganglion itself is not seen, only outlined, since it is covered by the inner sheath of the dura. At this stage an illuminated retractor is introduced and held in place by an assistant. If venous oozing from the dura, especially from the region around the second division, obscures the field a small cotton pledget soaked in hydrogene peroxide, or fibrine foam with or without thrombine, can be introduced toward the foramen rotundum and left temporarily. Otherwise the field is easily kept clear by the sucker. The cavum of Meckel is now opened by an incision parallel to the edge of the dura. Cerebrospinal fluid immediately escapes and the trigeminal rootlets come into view. The opening in the cavum is widened by blunt dissection with a long narrow dissector or with the knife. The surgeon

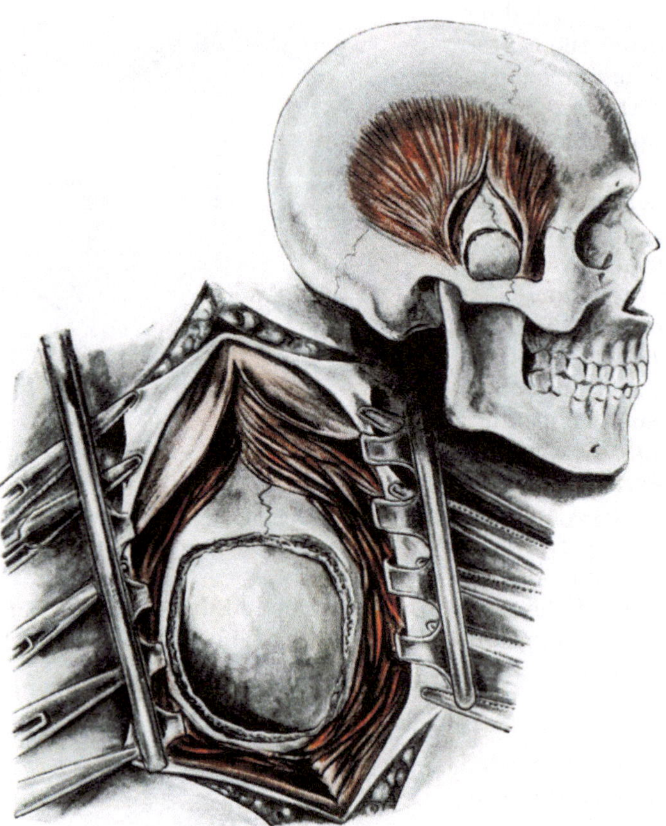

Fig. 8. Temporal trigeminotomy—bone defect.

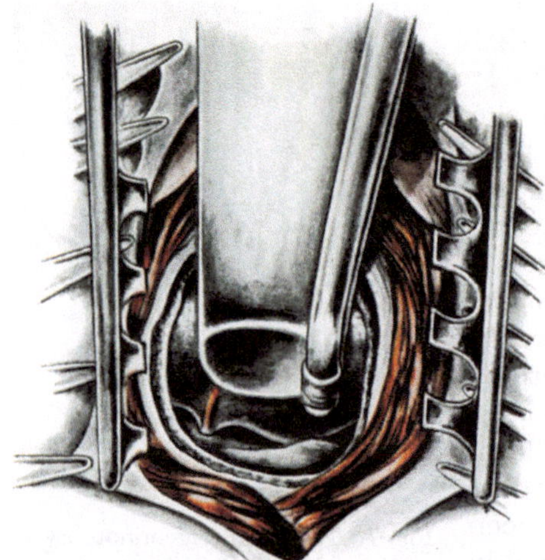

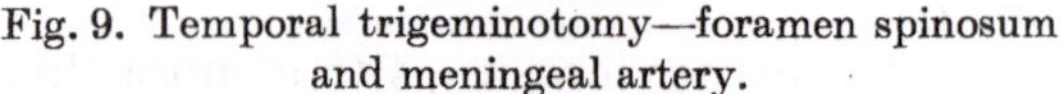

Fig. 9. Temporal trigeminotomy—foramen spinosum and meningeal artery.

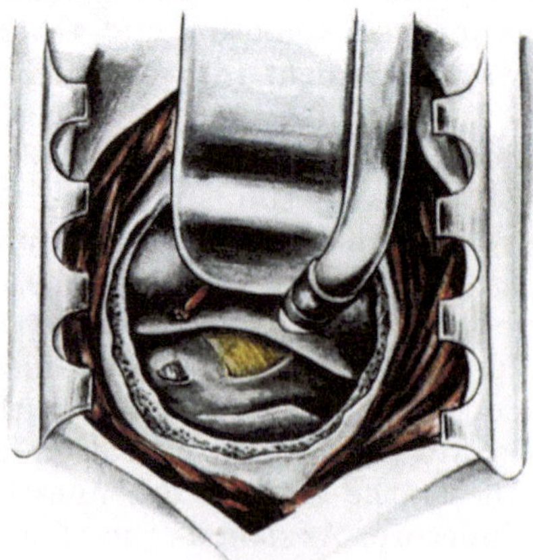

Fig. 10. Temporal trigeminotomy—meningeal artery divided, the third branch seen at the foramen ovale.

now sees most of the triangular plexus excepting its uppermost portion. The steps which now follow are the most important in the operation. Only by proceeding slowly and keeping a good orientation it is possible to divide the root partially and to save the motor root. A few of the lowermost rootlets are picked up on a blunt hook and torn gently or cut with a long-handled and angulated pair of scissors. The root section is carried on upwards, only a few rootlets at a time being picked up and cut or torn until the motor root comes into view. It lies behind the upper portion of the sensory root and is readily identified in most cases. Involuntary transection of the motor root is no catastrophe—the impairment of masticatory function is astonisingly small—but the ensuing temporal muscle atrophy will be disfiguring. When about $^3/_4$ of the sensory root is transected the operation is finished and only control of hemorrhage and closure of the wound remains. If the operation is done for pain from spread of malignant disease it is safer to divide the entire root. In other cases it is preferable to section rather too little than too much of the root. A moderate section very often will give lasting relief. Should a recurrence take place later, a second operation offers no difficulties. It is even easier than the first one, as the bony defect is already present and the middle meningeal artery is occluded. In recurrencies it is recommended to do a complete root section. — Cotton pledgets which have been left in the wound in the course of the operation are now removed and all bleeding points—from dural veins or from the peripheral end of the cut middle meningeal artery—are covered with fibrin foam or pieces of muscle. When all oozing is controlled the wound is irrigated with saline solution. The wound must not be closed until the irrigation fluid is crystal-clear. The temporal muscle and fascia are subsequently closed in layers with interrupted sutures around a thin drain of folded rubber cloth which is inserted down to the base of the scull to drain cerebrospinal fluid leaking out extradurally from the opening in the cavum of MECKEL. The galea and skin are finally closed with isolated sutures. The present author prefers thin catgut as suture material since silk and especially linen thread have a tendency of sequestrating later. The patient is immediately transferred to his bed and—provided there is no significant drop in the blood pressure—his head is supported by pillows in a somewhat elevated position for the first hours.

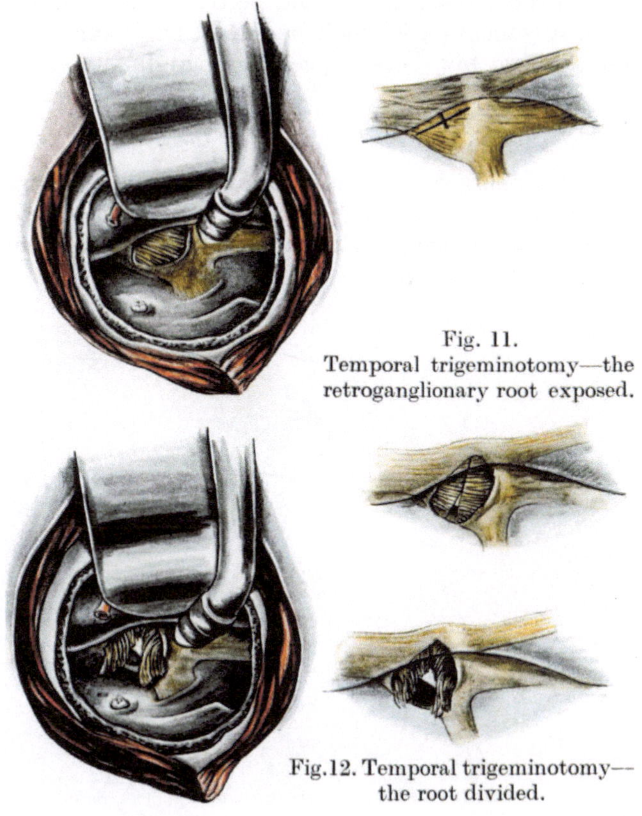

Fig. 11. Temporal trigeminotomy—the retroganglionary root exposed.

Fig. 12. Temporal trigeminotomy—the root divided.

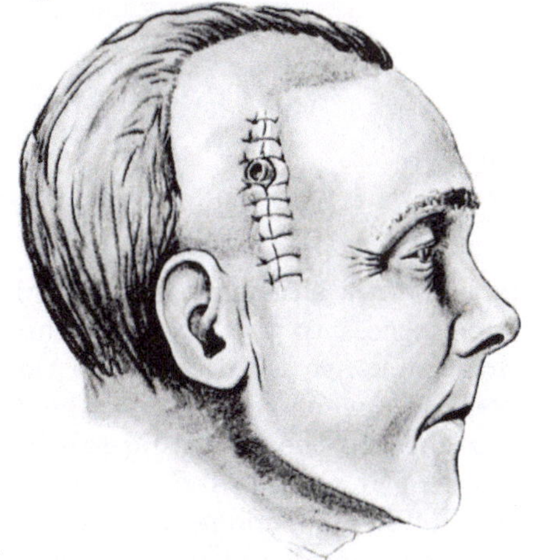

Fig. 13. Temporal trigeminotomy—skin suture.

The postoperative course is as a rule undisturbed. A rather severe headache, nausea and vomiting is often seen in the first 24–48 hours. They are accounted for by the entrance of air into the subarachnoidal space and are easily controlled with routine medical treatment. The dressings are changed after 24 hours and the drain removed. The stitches are cut after two and removed after three days. On the third or fourth postoperative day the patient may sit up in his bed and may be allowed to get up after one or two more days. The corneal sensation should be tested as soon as the patient is out of the anesthesia. If corneal sensation is abolished a BULLER shield or similar device is applied over the eye for the first few days, especially at night.

*β) Root Section Close to the Pons by the Cerebellar Approach* (Fig. 14).

This operation is preferably done under general intracheal anesthesia. The patient is premedicated in the usual way with luminal the night before and morphia and atropine an hour befor the start of the anesthesia. Many surgeons perform this operation with the

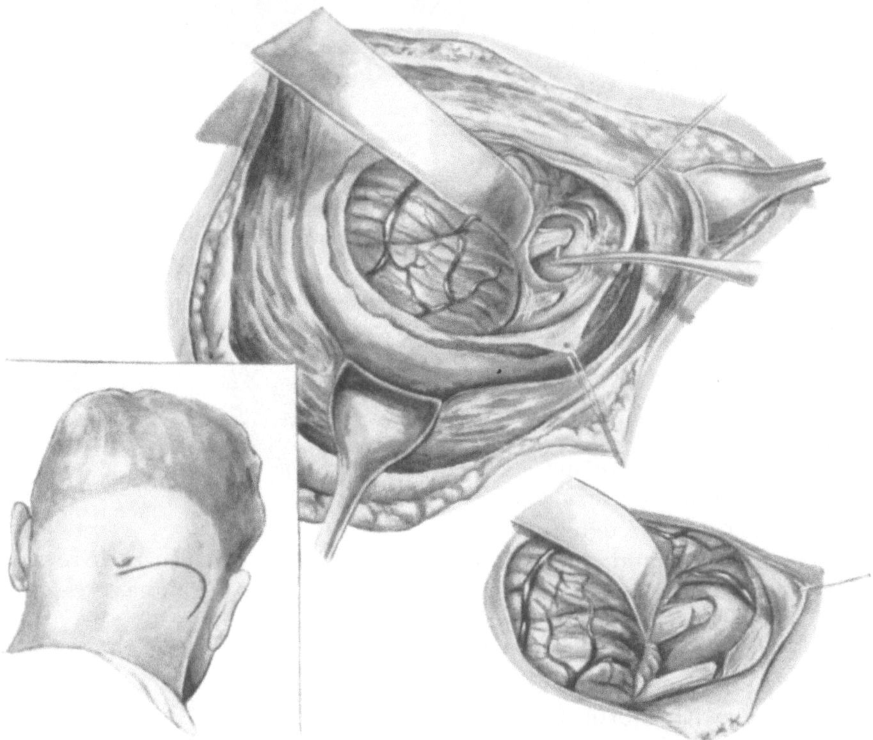

Fig. 14. Trigeminotomy by the cerebellar approach.

patient in a sitting position. This doubtlessly gives certain advantages in the form of a good access to the posterior fossa and a bloodless field. It has, however, also certain drawbacks, in the first place the risk of low blood pressure and of air embolism. The present author still prefers the prone position with the head supported by a head rest attached to the operating table. A lateral support should also be attached to the table allowing it to be tilted toward the opposite side. A curved incision is outlined over one cerebellar hemisphere and skin and muscles are infiltrated with 1% novocaine solution. The incision should pass down almost to the tip of the mastoid process. The extent of pneumatization of the mastoid bone should have been checked by X-ray examination before the operation. Opening the mastoid cells should be avoided. The skin and galea are incised and the muscles dissected from the occipital bone by cutting diathermy current. The bone is perforated and removed over the lateral part of the cerebellar hemisphere. The opening should extend as far laterally and upwards as the mastoidal cells and the sigmoid and lateral sinuses will permit. The dura is opened in T-shaped fashion and the edges held apart with sutures. If the intratracheal anesthesia is running smoothly, intracranial tension is not increased. The operating table is now elevated and tilted toward the unaffected side and the surgeon changes his position to stand beside the patient's head opposite to the field of operation. In this way he is able to look straight into the cerebellopontine angle. A middle-sized brain spatula in introduced toward the angle and the cerebellar hemisphere gently elevated. The pressure on the hemisphere must not be firmer than "just to counteract its weight" (DANDY). The slightest application of force will result in edema and hemorrhage within the cerebellum. As soon as the lateral cistern is encountered it is torn or incised with a knife. A gush of cerebrospinal fluid immediately follows. This will give the room necessary for further manipulations. The opening in the arachnoid is widened in all directions and the basal cisterns carefully emptied by the sucker. The surgeon should take plenty of time for this stage. Only by proceeding slowly, the room needed for a precise orientation will be gained and brain edema avoided. The exposed part of the cerebellum should be kept covered by a thin layer of moist cotton. When the cerebellum is retracted the acoustic nerve is readily identified. Still deeper in the wound the petrosal vein is seen passing obliquely upwards and laterally. The origin of the fifth nerve root is sometimes seen in the angle formed by the eigth nerve and the petrosal vein. Sometimes the root is more or less entirely covered by the vein. In the former case the vein can be held aside, in the latter it has to be carefully elevated with a tiny nasal forceps, coagulated with cutting current and divided with a long curved pair of scissors. When the pontine part of the trigeminal root is clearly in view a blunt hook is introduced from the side into the glial cone (cfr. above) and the posterior half or two-thirds of the root gently torn. In spite of all possible care it can on occasion not be avoided that the petrosal vein is torn, either during the exposure of the root or when it is transected. This will always be followed by a troublesome hemorrhage. If the bleeding is allowed to leak out into the basal cisterns a dangerous increase in the intracranial pressure will soon follow which may disturb or even block the access to the deeper parts of the cerebellopontine angle and cause disturbances in respiration. This is the intrinsic danger in this operation. Should a hemorrhage from the petrosal vein take place one had better cover the bleeding spot with a small pledget of cotton-wool soaked in hydrogene peroxide or with fibrine foam soaked in thrombine, pack the wound loosely with moistcotton and wait for a couple of minutes. After removal of the packing—not too early—the hemorrhage often has stopped and one is able to coagulate the vein or cover it with a piece of muscle or fibrine foam. If the vein entirely blocks the access to the root it may be feasible to apply a silverclip both to the vein and to the root, which will be partly crushed by the clip, as suggested by OLIVECRONA. This procedure is, however, followed by recurrencies even more often than the original DANDY procedure.

When all oozing is completely under control and the field has been repeatedly irrigated with saline solution the cerebellum is allowed to sink back, the dura is closed with interrupted silk and covered with a film of fibrine foam or oxycel. The muscles are approximated with isolated stainless steel sutures and the galea and skin closed with catgut and silk. A "cerebellar dressing" of gauze and adhesive plaster is applied and the patient brought in bed to lie on the unaffected side.

A careful postoperative control of blood pressure, pulse rate, respiration and consciousness must be kept up for at least two days. The cerebellar root section affects the general condition of the patients considerably more than the temporal extradural technique. The first days the patients must be frequently turned and have to be kept in bed for 8 or 10 days. After this interval the dressing is changed and the sutures removed.

### *γ) Intradural Root Section by the Temporal or Temporo-occipital Approach.*

Various methods to transect the fifth nerve root intradurally after it has been exposed by making an incision in the dural roof of the cavum of MECKEL have been suggested (DOGLIOTTI, PORTUGAL a.o.). This was, indeed, the technique used by SIR VICTOR HORSLEY in the first case in which a root section was done in tic douloureux in 1891. DOGLIOTTI

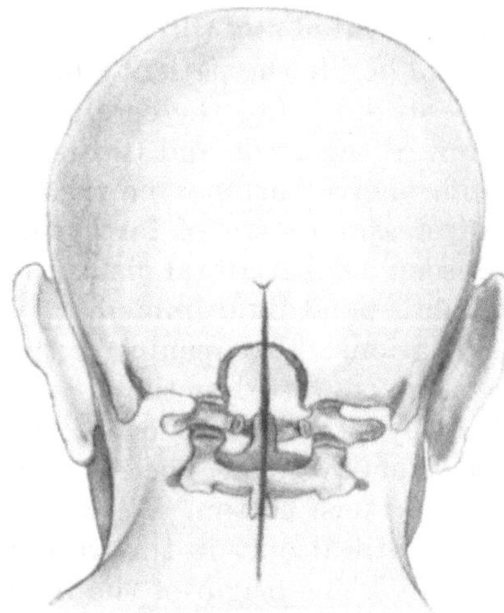

Fig. 15. Trigeminal tractotomy—skin incision and bone defect.

turns down a temporo-occipital flap, opens the dura and retracts the temporal lobe. The dura is incised over the cavum of Meckel and the root exposed near the middle of its course. It is then divided entirely or partially. The motor root is said to be easy to spare by this approach. Portugal's approach is similar but no flap is turned down. The sensory loss in this type of operations will be very much the same as in the approach of Spiller and Frazier. None of these procedures seem to offer any advantage over the Spiller-Frazier technique.

*δ) Medullary Trigeminal Tractotomy* (Fig. 15–20).

Tractotomy is also a major operation compared to the temporal root section, but is doubtlessly less difficult and less risky than the Dandy procedure. The patient is premedicated with luminal and morphia-atrophine. The author prefers a prone position also in this operation whereas other surgeons prefer to have the patient upright. A unilateral cerebellar exposure extending down to the foramen magnum and including a total or partial resection of the arch of the atlas is used only in the cases in which one wants to explore also the cerebello-pontine angle. In other cases the straight midline incision of Olivecrona is preferred. It is extended from the external occipital protuberance down to the third cervical vertebral. The author prefers intratracheal anesthesia combined with local infiltration. Some surgeons consider it an advantage to do the whole operation under local anesthesia, which will enable one to localize the tract from the patient's subjective sensations when the lateral part of the medulla is touched by a blunt hook or stimulated with a weak electric current (Olivecrona, Falconer). The incision is carried down to the occipital bone and held apart with a selfretaining retractor. Two burr holes are made on each side of the midline and the occipital bone is removed with rongeur forceps down to the foramen

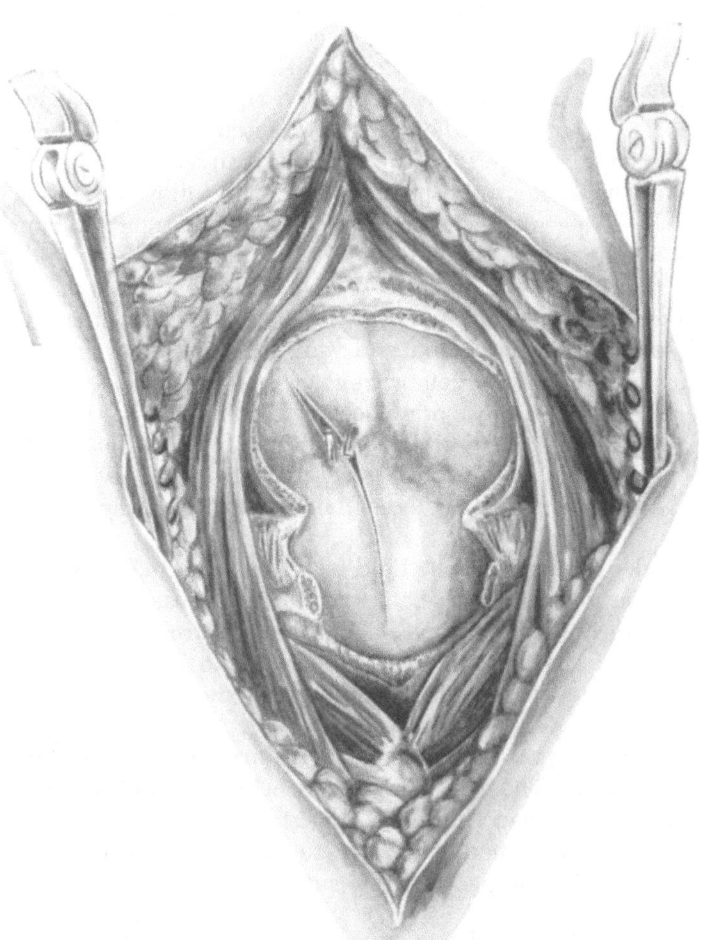

Fig. 16. Trigeminal tractotomy—incision of dura.

magnum leaving an almost circular defect with a diameter of about 3 cms. The author prefers to remove the arch of the atlas also. This is easily done and improves the access to the field. After hemostasis of oozing from the bone or from extradural veins which may be numerous over the atlanto-occipital membrane, the dura is opened by a curved incision with the convexity facing the side of operation and held apart with sutures. The arachnoid of the cisterna magna is torn and the posterior cisterns emptied by the sucker. One cerebellar tonsil is now gently elevated by a narrow brain spatula, bringing the dorsomedial part of the medulla oblongata in view. The posterior inferior cerebellar artery runs in a loop around the tonsil. In the majority of cases it can be elevated together with the tonsils. Sometimes it is expedient to leave it in place. The field is now exposed. One sees the rootlets of the vagus and spinal accessory nerves, the posterior columns, the obex and lowermost part of calamus scriptorius and also the vertebral artery which runs obliquely from its entrance in the skull to disappear underneath the medulla. The difficult step of the operation is to choose the point of incision to transect the spinal fifth tract completely. To do the incision as high up as several millimetres cranially to the obex and immediately underneath the lowermost vagus rootlets is not advisable since this involves risks to the restiform body and the spinocerebellar tracts. The point of incision is the tuberculum trigemini—also called tuberculum cinereum—where the tract lies superficially and immediately underneath the surface of the medulla. As evidenced by JIMINEZ GONZALES the site of this little eminence can vary considerably. It is a small triangular field bordering on the lateral edge of the uppermost part of the posterior columns and the lowermost part of the restiform body. If the tuberculum trigemini is carefully looked for it can be identified in about $^2/_3$ of the cases. It is usually situated at the level of the obex or a few millimetres caudally to this structure. This little eminence should be transected transversely to a depth of 2–$2^1/_2$ mm. The lenght of the incision should measure $2^1/_2$–3 mm. Sometimes a tiny pial vessel runs across the tuberculum. It can be transected without hesitation. The oozing soon stops after application of a hydrogene peroxide pledget. When the tract fibers are transected by the knife the patient usually will show some pain reaction if the anesthesia is not too deep. This is

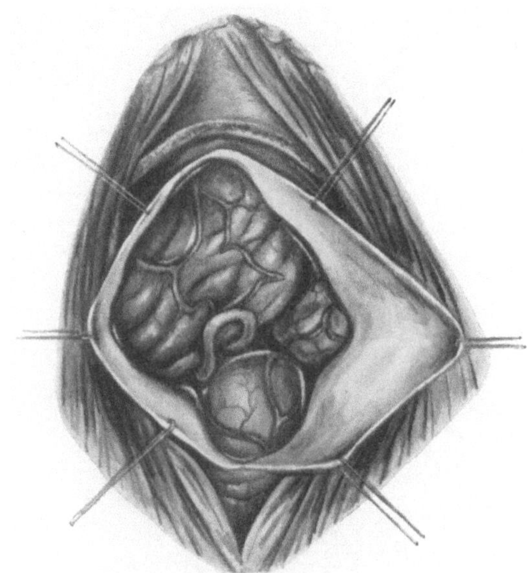

Fig. 17. Trigeminal tractotomy—dura opened. The medulla and cerebellar tonsil is seen.

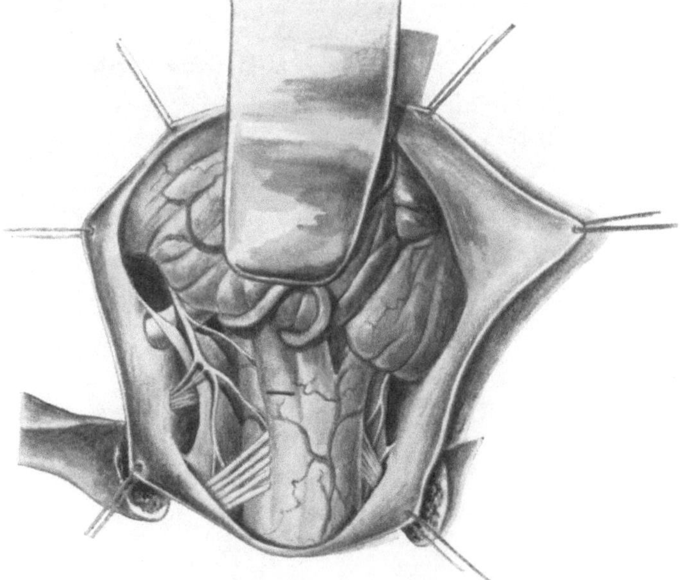

Fig. 18. Trigeminal tractotomy—incision of tract.

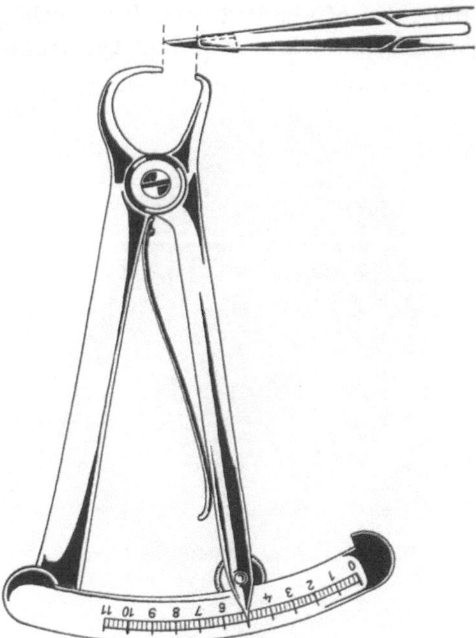

Fig. 19. Trigeminal tractotomy—broken razor blade fitted and measured.

a check that the incision has been made in the right place. A practical instrument for the in cision in the medulla is the broken edge of a razor blade held between the locked branches of a long straight artery forceps. If the tuberculum trigemini cannot be identified the incision is started immediately lateral to the eminence formed by the nuclei of Goll and Burdach at the level of the obex or a few millimetres caudally and is carried on to a depth of $2^1/_2$ mm. and to a length of 3 mm. If pain reaction in the form of accelerated respiration or body movements follow one can be fairly certain to have transected the tract. It is of importance not to start the incision too far dorsally in order not to injure the dorsal columns which will result in ataxia but also not to carry it too far ventrally when the spinothalamic tract may be involved resulting in contralateral hemianalgesia. The incision should not surpass 3 mm in depth. If it is made deeper the motor tenth nucleus may be involved which may give a recurrent nerve paresis.

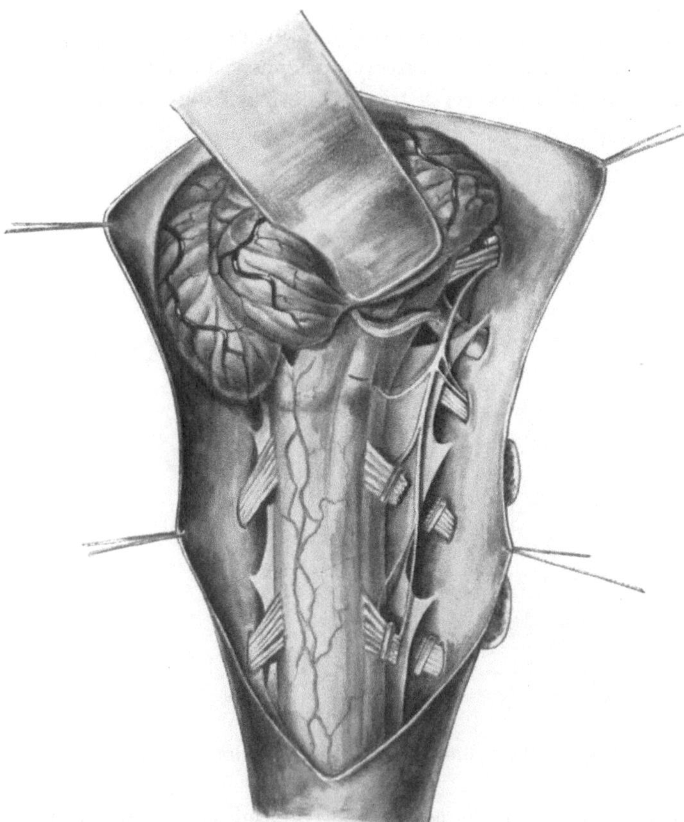

Abb. 20. Trigeminal tractotomy with section of superior cervical roots performed in pain surgery for carcinoma of face, neck and jaws.

There is usually no bleeding after the incision has been completed. The field is irrigated and the dura closed with interrupted silk sutures. It may sometimes be difficult to close the dura entirely. If a small gap remains this is covered with gel foam or oxycel. Oozing veins around the edges of the bony defect are also best covered with oxycel. The self-retaining retractor is now removed and after careful hemostasis the muscles are approximated with catgut, silk or stainless steel sutures or a combination of the three. Galea and skin are sutured in the usual way. A cerebellar dressing is applied and the patient laid in bed on his side. A test that the tractotomy has been successful is that the corneal reflex is absent on the side of the operation as soon as the patient comes out of the anesthesia. The postoperative care is the same as in the Dandy operation or, in fact, any major brain operation.

### ε) *Decompression of the Trigeminal Root* (Fig. 21–24).

In 1952 the Danish neurosurgeon TAARNHØJ published an operative method in trigeminal neuralgia which was founded upon entirely new principles since the operation did not aim at the interruption of any sensory conduction from the face. Setting out from experiences in a case of cholesteatoma of the cerebello-pontine angle suffering from tic douloureux which had been relieved by removal of the tumor without interference with the root, he assumed major trigeminal neuralgia to be caused by some sort of pressure on the root exerted in the cavum of MECKEL itself from the dura or from the superior petrosal sinus. TAARNHØJ, therefore, undertook to split the roof of the cavum in its full length from the ganglion to the incisura tentorii in a number of patients suffering from paroxysmal tic. His first operation was performed in July 1951 and at the appearance of his paper

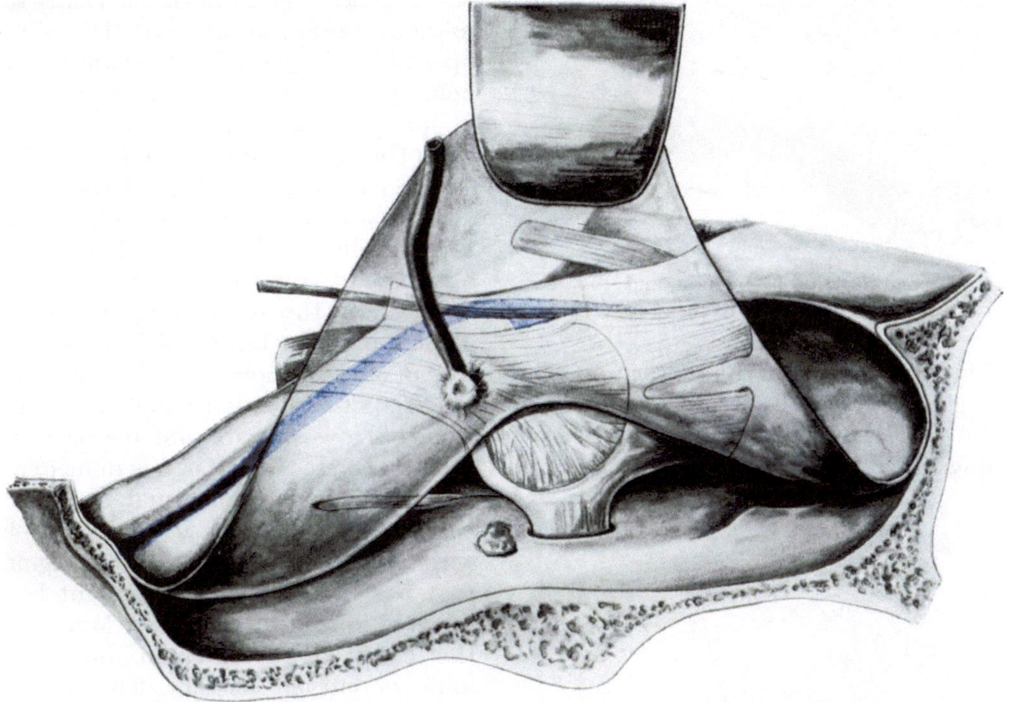

Fig. 21. Decompression of ganglion and root a.m. TAARNHØJ—general view extradural approach.

12 cases had been operated on with a postoperative observation time of up to 8 months. No recurrencies had occurred. TAARNHØJ's technique was immediately taken up by a number of other neurosurgeons. The present writer has until the end of 1952 operated on 10 patients. It seems likely that TAARNHØJ's experiences will be confirmed, namely, that lasting relief can be given in this way without any loss of sensation. If this comes true TAARNHØJ's operation will mark a new epoch in the surgery of major trigeminal neuralgia.

There are, however, some dangers and technical difficulties in this operation which have to be overcome. In the first place it may be difficult to avoid trauma to the trigeminal nerve itself. Damage to the upper rootlets will cause sensory disturbances of the first division including the cornea. One of the writer's cases developed a severe keratitis. There is also risk to the eye muscle nerves, in the first place the trochlear but also the abducens nerve. Trochlear nerve palsies was seen in several of TAARNHØJ's cases; fortunately they seem to be transient. There are also certain difficulties in dealing with the superior petrosal sinus. The hemorrhage from this sinus may become considerable and difficult to control since diathermy cannot be used for fear of damage to the root.

TAARNHØJ performed the operation with the patient in a recumbent position and exposed the roof of the cavum of MECKEL entirely intradurally. His technique was modified by several neurosurgeons who used a sitting position and exposed the root extradurally. Both techniques shall be described.

**Intradural approach.** General anesthesia is preferred. The patient is placed in a re-recumbent position with his head rotated to the opposite side. A similar skin incision is made as in temporal root section. The muscles and periosteum are incised and held apart by a self-retraining retractor. An opening is made in the bone somewhat larger than in the SPILLER-FRAZIER operation. The dura is elevated from the base and the foramen spinosum plugged in order to control bleeding from the branches of the middle meningeal artery. The dura is opened in a T-shaped fashion and the edges held apart by sutures. The temporal lobe is gently elevated and retracted medially until the basal cisterns can be opened and covered with moist cotton. In elderly individuals with some brain atrophy sufficient cerebrospinal fluid can be allowed to leak out so as to give ample room. In younger individuals the field is more restricted. The floor of the temporal fossa is exposed and the adjacent part of the tentorium. The cavum of MECKEL now has to be located. By touching the dura with a probe or a blunt hook a soft spot can be felt which is the roof of the cavum of MECKEL. The roof is incised with a long narrow-bladed knife in a place corresponding to the most lateral part of the cavum of MECKEL. If the incision is done over the medial part the incision may land into the cavernous sinus which is followed by brisk venous hemorrhage. When the trigeminal root has come into view a blunt hook is inserted into the cavum of MECKEL and the roof gradually elevated and split with knife or curved scissors. The incision is carried on in the lateral direction until the GASSERian ganglion is seen, in the medial direction all the way to the incisura tentorii. After this has been done the trigeminal root lies bare in the whole of its course from the cerebellopontine angle to the ganglion. The cerebral peduncle is easily identified. Running across the peduncle from the collicular region comes the tiny trochlear nerve to enter the cavernous sinus closely underneath and somewhat medial to the trigeminal root. This nerve can apparently be functionally damaged by the lightest touch and should be kept away from. Also the abducent nerve is sometimes seen. The roof of the cavum of MECKEL should preferably be split between silver clips applied by a long curved clip-holder (OLIVECRONA's tentorium clip-holder). This is, however, not always possible and once applied the clips have a great tendency to slip away. The superior petrosal sinus is usually seen more or less clearly. It crosses the root 4–6 mm. from the edge of the tentorium. Clips should be

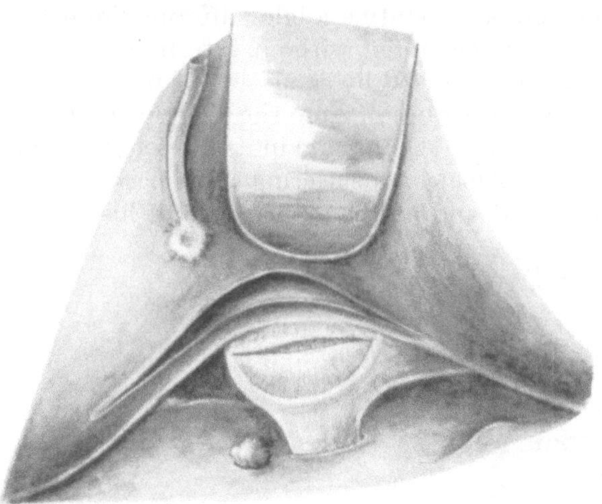

Fig. 22. Decompression of ganglion and root a.m. TAARNHØJ—transverse splitting of sheath.

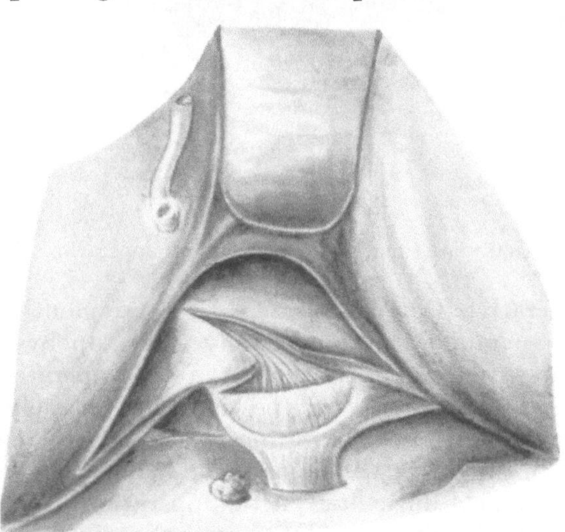

Fig. 23. Decompression of ganglion and root a.m. TAARNHØJ—longitudinal splitting of sheath.

applied to the sinus before it is divided but this is not always easy to accomplish. If veinous oozing continues after the splitting of the roof oxycel or gel foam is applied in a thin layer over the bleeding spots. This may, however, irritate the root and cause trigeminal pain during the first postoperative days. After all bleeding has been controlled the incision in the dura is closed with interrupted silk and the wound sutured in layers without drainage. A close postoperative control must be kept up for two or three days.

**Extradural approach.** The operation is most conveniently performed with the patient sitting with his head in an upright position. Local anesthesia with a short intravenous sleep or general anesthesia can both be used. The operation is started exactly as for a temporal root section (p. 12). The foramen spinosum is plugged, the middle meningeal vessels cut and the third division and the ganglion exposed. The arachnoid of the cavum of MECKEL is incised and cerebrospinal fluid allowed to escape. Immediately above the ganglion and a few millimetres lateral to it a 2 cm. long horizontal incision is made in the dura. A brain spatula is introduced through the opening and the lowermost and medial part of the temporal lobe is retracted and elevated giving access to the roof of the cavum of MECKEL and the tentorium. From the opening an incision is made at a straight angle toward the peripheral end of the sensory root, exposing the triangular plexus and the peripheral part of the root. A canulated probe is inserted into the cavum of MECKEL and the roof split parallel to the probe. The roof should be cut open as far laterally as possible in order to avoid venous bleeding from the dural sinuses. Now the superior petrosal sinus is seen, doubly clipped and divided with curved scissors and the incision is carried on to the in cisura tentorii until the root is exposed in its whole length. The trochlear nerve is more difficult to see in this approach and may be contused. Venous oozing is best controlled by gel foam or oxycel, while diathermy is avoided because of potential damage to the fourth nerve. When hemostasis is complete the wound is closed in the usual manner, a cigarette drain being left for 24 hours. Ordinary postoperative control.

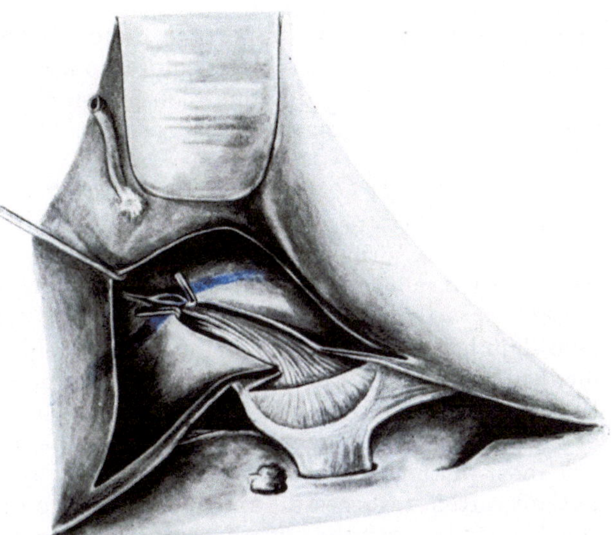

Fig. 24. Decompression of ganglion and root a.m. TAARNHØJ—division of superior petrosal sinus.

This approach and similar techniques have been used by GRAFTON LOVE, NORLÉN and in Copenhagen, where it gradually has supplanted the intradural approach as being quicker and safer. In about half of the cases the superior petrosal sinus can be left undivided. LOVE does not open the dura propria in order to prevent possible adhesions between the sensory fibres and motor root. In the extradural as in the intradural approach it is most important actually to see the root decompressed.

After the operation—whether it was done by the intradural or by the extradural approach—the patient usually complains of headache and nausea and sometimes also of slight or even more severe pain in half of the face, probably caused by irritation of the nerve root. This subsides within the course of three or four days. If the operation has been succesfully performed there should be no sensory disturbances of the face and the corneal reflex should be brisk. If this reflex is sluggish or absent one had better cover the eye with a BULLER shield or similar device.

*Addendum.* In 1954 STENDER described a "gangliolysis" of the Gasserian ganglion: Through the usual temporal extradural approach the dura propria covering the ganglion is excised and the *cavum* MECKELII wiedely opened. The method was tried in 16 patients with typical tic douleureux with good results over a period of observation of up to 13 months.

SHELDEN, PUDENZ, FRESHWATER and CRUE in 1955 published an interesting paper in which they reported 29 patients treated by means of what they call a "compression" technic. They think that compression of the trigeminal fibres during operation is the factor affording relief of pain in the decompression operation of TAARNHØJ. After exposing the posterior part of the ganglion and the posterior root in the usual manner, the dura propria was opened and the root fibres gently compressed by means of a dental roll or the back of a blunt dissector. All patients were relieved of pain and only some few had sensory disturbance. It would seem to be extremely difficult to say whether compression or decompression is the important factor in these operations as the "compressionists" avowedly decompress the root before compressing it and the "decompressionists" undoubtedly unwillingly do some compression. Electrophysiological studies should have possibilities of deciding the issue (E.B.).

### ζ) *Alcohol Injections in the Peripheral Branches and the Main Divisions.*

Alcohol injections played a considerable part in the treatment of trigeminal neuralgia in the preneurosurgical era. Surgeons without training in neurological surgery did not wish to perform intracranial operations, not even to recommend them. KRAUSE's operation doubtlessly carried a fairly high mortality and for tens of years operations for trigeminal neuralgia had a bad reputation among laymen and—what is more important—also in the medical profession. No wonder then, that many patients gratefully accepted the relief that could be give by injections, even if it was only a temporary one. With the evolution of surgical methods to relieve pain in trigeminal neuralgia definitely, alcohol injections have lost most of their former importance. They are difficult to perform, very painful to the patient, often unsuccessful and the relief given is only temporary. Alcohol injection into the GASSERian ganglion itself may secure definite relief but is not without mortality and the incidence of unwanted side effects (injuries to other cranial nerves, corneal complications) is comparatively high. In the modern neurosurgical clinic injections have thus only a moderate place in the therapeutic repertory. Excepting to very old or feeble patients or patients definitely refusing an operation, they are given in the first place to secure the diagnosis in cases with a very short history and secondly to let the patient become accustomed to the numbness of the face that will result from an intervention on the fifth nerve root. In the latter cases only a short-lasting anesthesia is aimed at. This in turn can be accomplished as well by peripheral injections as by central ones close to the base of the skull, which forms the reason why deeper injections, being more difficult, are being more and more rarely performed in neurosurgical centres. Absolute alcohol destroys the tissues by coagulation and gives a smaller or larger tissue necrosis. This should always be born in mind and alcohol should never be injected in large amounts and never before the surgeon has ascertained that the nerve to be injected has been reached by the needle. The branches of the fifth nerve which come in question for alcohol injections are the infraorbital nerve, the inferior alveolar nerve, the second and third main divisions and, much more rarely, the supraorbital nerve which is very seldom affected by paroxysmal neuralgia.

**Injection of the infraorbital nerve.** The patient is lying on his back, the head being supported by a not too soft pillow. The upper lip is gently pricked by a pin and the patient is instructed that after a successful injection pin-pricking should no more be felt. He is warned that when the nerve is hit by the needle point he will feel a strong burning sensation irradiating into the upper lip and in the nose. A quaddle of novocain is made in the skin at the border between the upper and middle third of the nasolabial furrow. The surgeon's left index finger is pressed against the margo infraorbitalis to protect the bulb and to give him a "stereotactic feeling". A 3–4 cm. long needle attached to a syringe is introduced through the "quaddle" obliquely upwards until it reaches the maxillary bone. The infraorbital foramen is situated 6–7 mm. underneath the medial part of the infraorbital rim and is searched for with the point of the needle. When the needle slides into the infraorbital canal it is introduced further 3 or 4 mm. and 0·5, maximum 1·0 cc. of absolute alcohol is injected. If the needle fails to slide into the infraorbital canal one has to be guided by the patient's subjective sensation. When burning pain is felt in the upper lip 0·5–1·0 cc. of alcohol is injected and the upper lip tested for anesthesia.

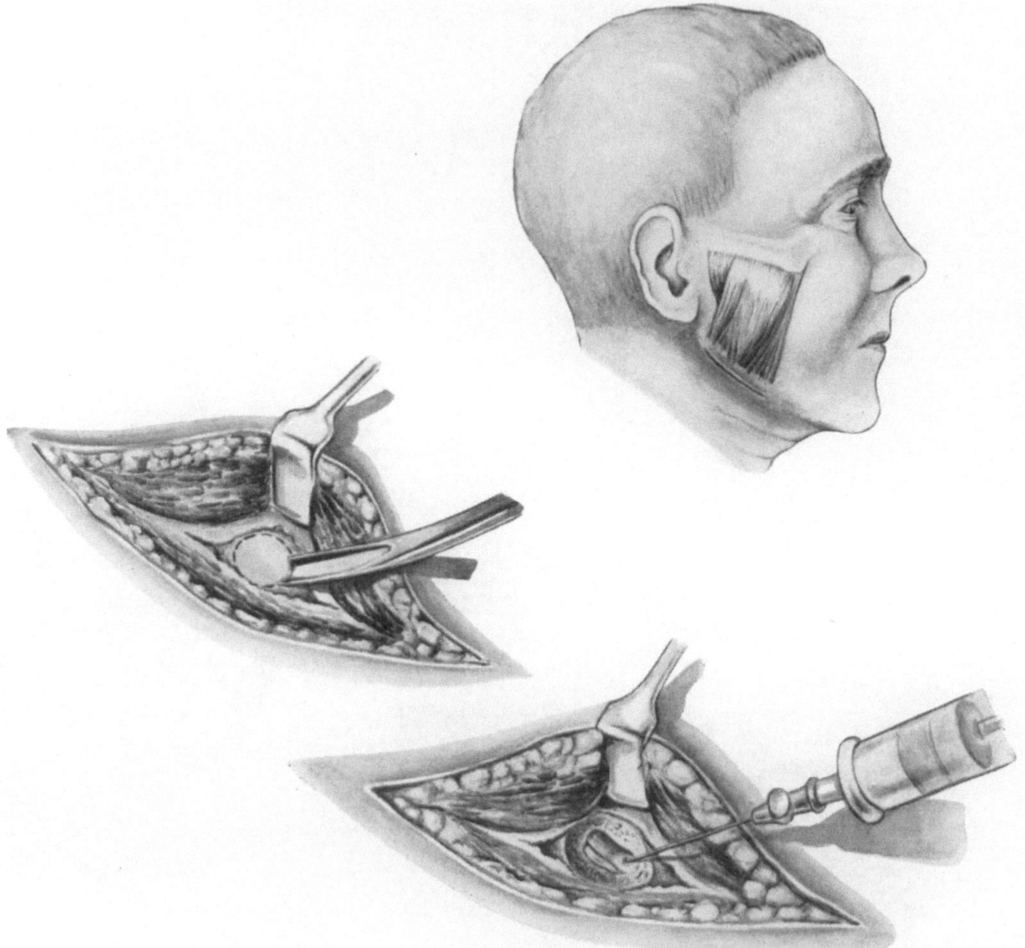

Fig. 25. Alcohol injection in mandibular canal by open method.

**Injection of the inferior alveolar nerve** (Fig. 25). This is best done under control of the eye after chiseling a small opening on the lateral aspect of the mandible into the canalis mandibulae. Under local anesthesia a 2 cm. long incision is made immediately under the angulus mandibulae, transecting the soft parts and the periosteum which is separated from the bone by an elevator together with the insertion of the masseter muscle. 10 or 11 mm. above the rim of the mandible a small opening is chiseled in the bone until the canalis mandibulae is unroofed. A fine needle is inserted in central direction as far as one can reach—usually 5–10 mm. and 0·5–1·0 cc. of alcohol is slowly injected. This will render the teeth of the lower jaw and the medial part of the lower lip anesthetic. The wound is closed with a few catgut and silk sutures.

**Injection of the supraorbital nerve.** A quaddle is made 1 cm. above the most medial part of the supraorbital margin. The supraorbital foramen is searched for with a needle in the same way as when injecting the infraorbital nerve. When burning pain is felt in the forehead irradiating toward the vertex of the skull 0·5–1·0 cc. of alcohol is injected. The supraorbital foramen is difficult to find and it is seldom possible to introduce the needle into the canal. The results are often unsatisfactory since the nerves spread out in a fan-like fashion immediately after they have left the foramen.

**Injection of the main second and third division** (Fig. 26). This can be done either close to the base of the skull in the immediate neighbourhood of the foramen rotundum and

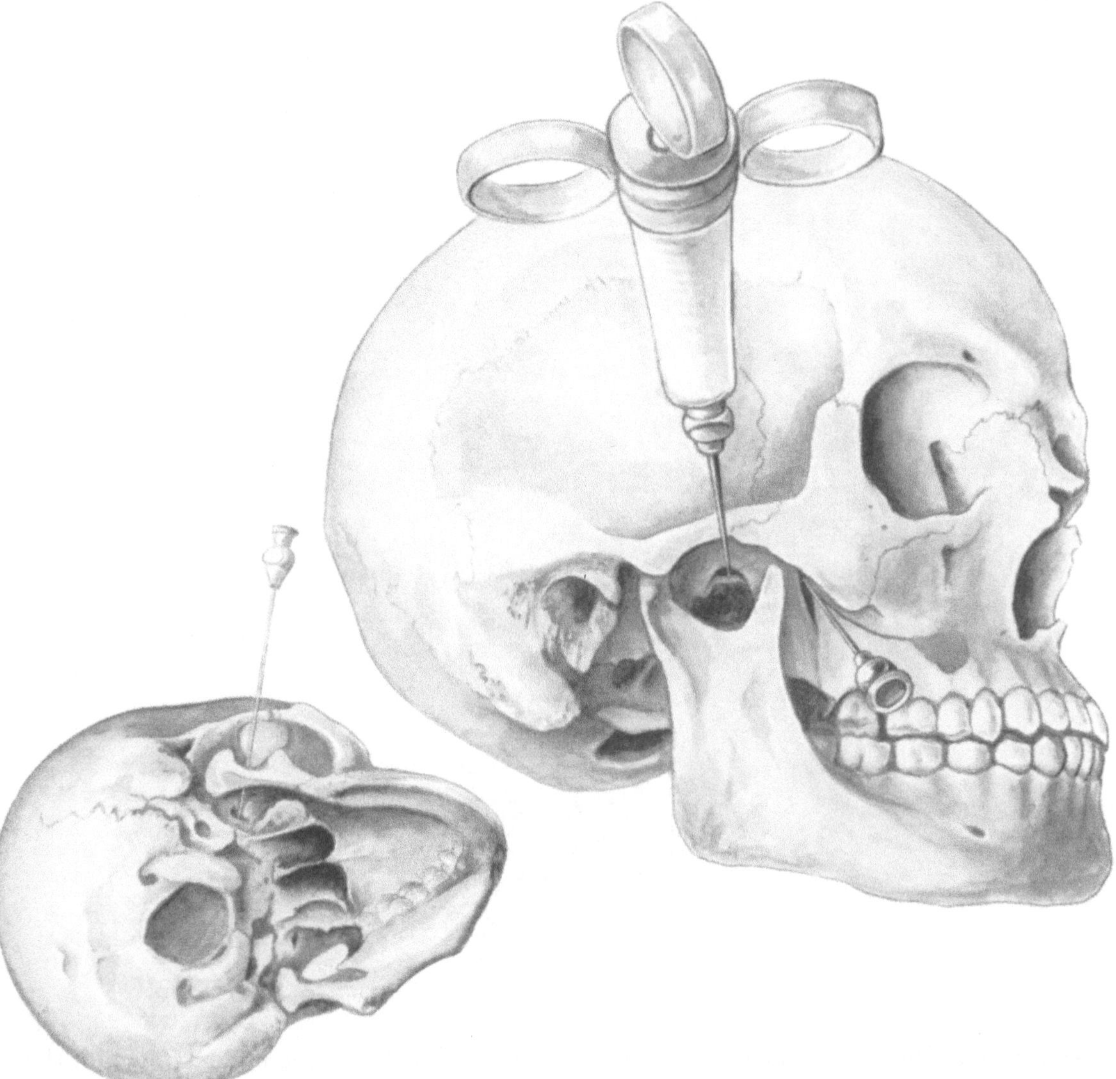

Fig. 26. Alcohol injection in main second and third divison (after Horrax and Poppen).

ovale or intracranially by an open method. In the rare occasions when these injections are necessary the writer prefers the open method.

*Direct injection of the third branch.* A thin needle 10 cm. long is fitted with a small piece of rubber 5 cm. from the point. On the skin is marked the highest point of the lower border of the zygomatic process. The needle attached with a syringe containing 1 cc. alcohol is inserted at this point in a slightly upwards and backwards direction. The third branch will be found at a depth varying between 4–5 cm. and one has a characteristic feeling when the needle enters the nerve, the patient usually experiencing a stab of pain irradiating into the third branch. 0·1 cc. of alcohol is injected and if the patient gets a severe stab of pain followed by numbness in the course of the nerve 0·2–0·3 cc. are injected and the needle withdrawn.

If pain is felt in the ear the needle may have entered the Eustachian tube. If pain is felt in the temporal region it may lie in juxtaposition to the meningeal artery. Before injection the plunger should, as usual, be withdrawn to be quite sure that the needle has not entered any of the numerous blood vessels in this region.

*Direct injection of the second branch* is considerably more difficult than of the third branch. The needle enters at a point just anterior to the coronoid process and just beneath the anterior part of the zygoma. HORRAX and POPPEN state that the needle should pass medially at a 40° angle entering the pterygo-maxillary fissure. The nerve should be entered somewhere between 5–6 cm. from the skin. It is recommended *never* to go deeper than 6 cm. because of the optic nerve. It is a wise rule *never* to inject even the smallest amount of alcohol if no stab of characteristical irradiating pain is felt by the patient.

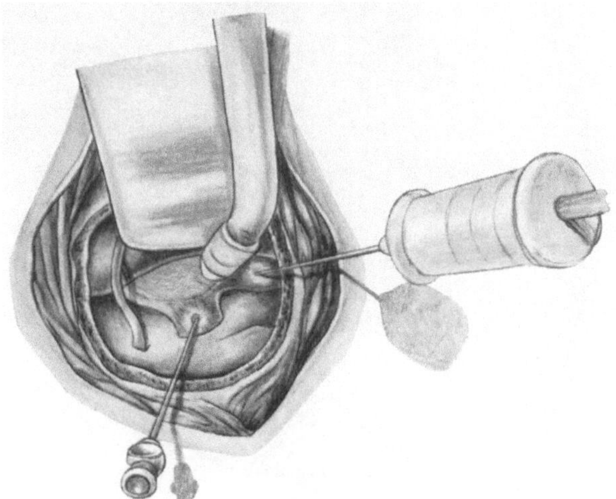

Fig. 27. Intracranial alcohol injection of second and third branch (SJÖQVIST).

The nerve may according to HORRAX and POPPEN be reached also posterior to the coronoid process, but this approach is considerably more difficult.

*Intracranial injection of the main branches* by the open technique (Fig. 27) is performed in the following way:

The patient is placed on the operating table in a sitting position. The intervention which is done under local anesthesia, is begun exactly as the temporal root section. The opening in the bone can be made smaller but must extend down to the base of the skull. The dura is elevated from the floor of the middle fossa along the groove of the middle meningeal artery until the foramen spinosum comes into view. With a narrow brain spatula the elevation of the dura is continued in medial direction anterior to the foramen spinosum until the outer rim of the foramen ovale and the lowermost part of the third division is seen. A few drops of 2% novocaine is injected in the third division. The remainder of the procedure can be done without any pain since the dura of the temporal fossa is innervated from the third division. By means of a broad dissector the third division is denuded a few millimetres upwards until it can be identified with certainty and if this is the branch to be injected 0·5 cc. of alcohol is slowly injected in the nerve trunk under control of the eye. If the second branch is to be injected the dura is freed still a little bit further forward until the maxillary nerve is encountered. It runs almost horisontally. Some venous bleeding is usually encountered at this stage and the field has to be kept clear by the sucker. The same amount of alcohol is injected in the nerve. Before closure of the wound the foramen spinosum is plugged with cotton-wool but the middle meningeal vessels need not to be transected. Gel foam or oxycel is placed on bleeding spots, the wound is irrigated and closed in layers after insertion of a thin rubber drain. Injection of the third division does not take more than 15 or 20 minutes, injection of the second division a few more minutes.

The main advantages of this technique are that the injection can be carried out with a minimum of pain, that the injection never fails and the effect will last at least 3–6 months and that there is no risk of damage to neighbouring structures; the disadvantages being that it cannot be carried out in the consulting room; the patient must be in a hospital and kept in bed for two or three days. The risk of an extradural clot is not entirely absent and the patient must be kept under routine control for 24 hours.

Alcohol injection into the Gasserian ganglion cannot be recommended and will not be described in this chapter.

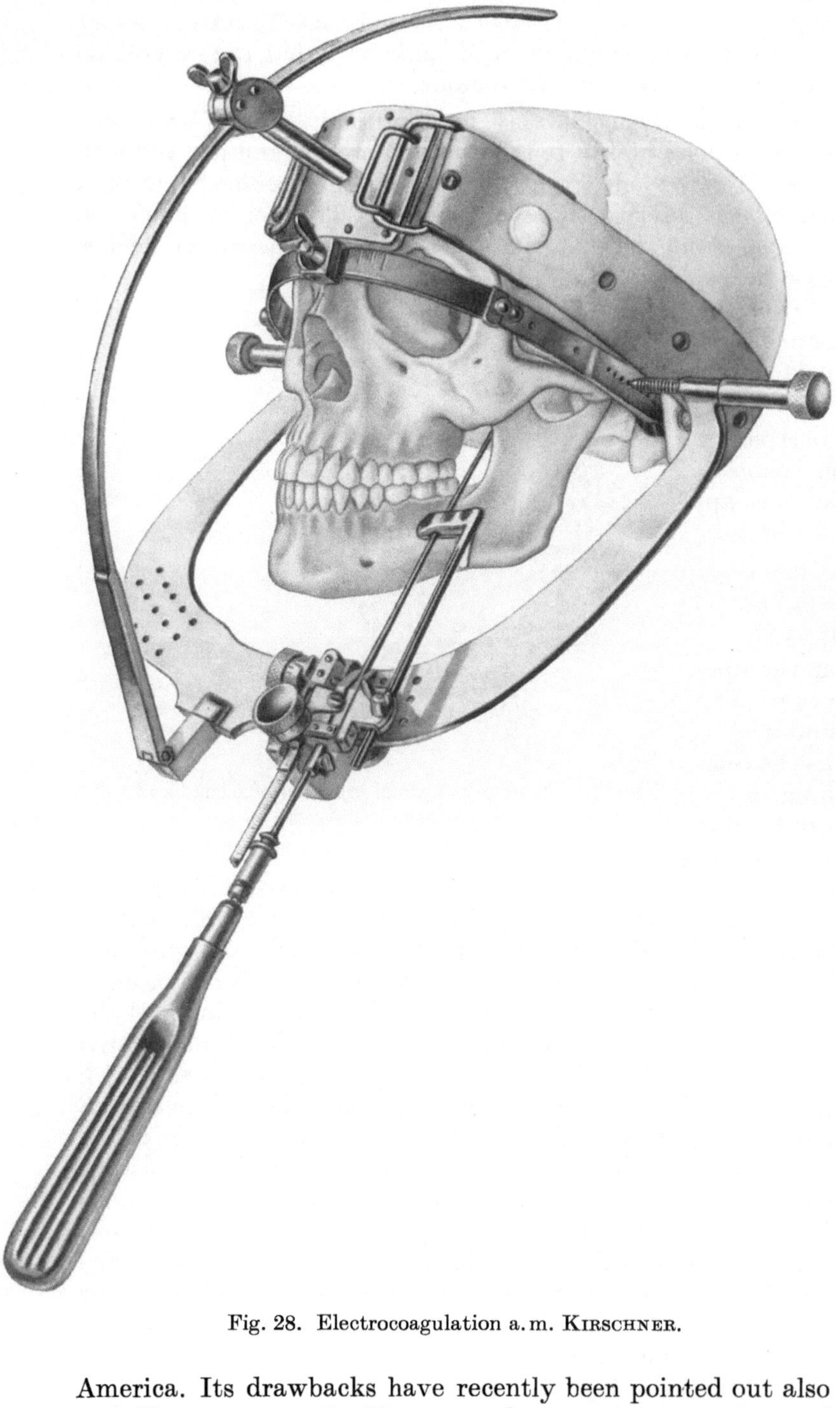

### *η) Electrocoagulation of the* Gasser*ian Ganglion.*

Kirschner's instrument, invented in 1931, is an ingenious stereotactic apparatus by means of which the foramen ovale can be punctured with a high degree of accuracy. Since the needle is inserted into the foramen ovale almost at right angles to the base of the skull it can be pushed forward into the middle fossa to reach also the ganglion of Gasser. Since the needle is electrically isolated except at its tip, a coagulating electric current can be led through it and the ganglion destroyed (Fig. 28). In this way a lasting relief can be given to sufferers of tic douloureux. With increasing experience it has yet become evident that this method is not without mortality and that the number of failures and of unwanted sideeffects is considerably higher than in intracranial root-sections performed by the open technique. The method was never generally adopted in the Scandinavian countries, in England or in America. Its drawbacks have recently been pointed out also from German side (Tönnis and Kreissel 1950). Kirschner's apparatus can be used also as an aid for alcohol injection in the third branch close to the foramen ovale. The technic will be evident from Fig. 28 while the reader for detailed description is referred to Kirschner's paper of 1936. Nowadays electrocoagulation a.m. Kirschner is rarely performed by competent neurological surgeons.

Fig. 28. Electrocoagulation a.m. Kirschner.

## b) Postoperative Complications and Sequelae. Unwanted Side-effects. Postoperative Paresthesias. Anaesthesia dolorosa.

The occurrence and frequency of postoperative complications vary considerably in the different procedures which have been described above. Differing is also the effect on the sensibility of the face as is the type and frequency of unintended injury to neighbouring structures leading to unwanted side-effects. The temporal root section of SPILLER and FRAZIER carries a low mortality and immediate postoperative complications are few. When larger series of cases operated on with this technique were available, it became however, very evident, that disagreeable numbness and paresthesias were frequent after this operation. With increasing experience we have also become familiar with the disagreeable sensation of numbness and the paresthesias which culminate in the distressing clinical picture of *painful anesthesia—anaesthesia dolorosa.* This was the main reason why other methods—the DANDY procedure, the tractotomy of SJÖQVIST and lately, the TAARNHØJ operation—were introduced. Even if these various procedures give very different late sequels which have to be dealt with separately, the immediate complications are very much of the same type.

### *Early Postoperative Complications.*

**1. Postoperative hematoma.** Extradural hemorrhage following temporal root section is extremely rare. The present writer has only seen this complication twice in a series of over 400 root sections. It developed early, i.e. within 6 hours, in both cases. If the patient becomes unduly drowsy, if the pupil of the side of operation becomes dilated or if the patient develops a facial weakness or hemiplegia an extradural clot should be suspected and the wound opened up, especially if blood pressure increases and the pulse rate goes down. Postoperative hemorrhage in the intradural procedures of DANDY and SJÖQVIST are more difficult to recognize. The bleeding usually comes from muscle-vessels and rarely gives symptoms until on the second or third postoperative day. Symptoms are often obscure and misleading. Disorientation, restlessness, followed by drowsiness and coma is seen, while a systemic deviation of pulse rate and blood pressure often is missing. FALCONER describes a case of postoperative clot after tractotomy which gave symptoms on the seventh postoperative day and was not recognized. In cases of doubt it is better to open up the wound at once.

**2. Facial nerve paralysis.** This is practically only seen after temporal root section by the extradural approach. Its relative frequency differs widely in various statistics—from 1—5%. The paralysis is seldom visible immediately after the operation, but appears on the first, second or even third postoperative day. The onset is slow and the paralysis is often incomplete, but always of the peripheral type. Usually the paralysis dissappears within 6 weeks to 3 months, but may end in slight but lasting disfigurement. The paralysis is presumably caused by a small hemorrhage in the facial canal, i.e. in the facial nerve itself or in the *ganglion geniculi* and brought about by pulling on the greater superior petrosal nerve. In order to avoid traction on this nerve the present author used to transect it as soon as it was exposed. This, however, gives inhibition of tear flow in one eye and cannot be recommended. The best way to avoid this complication is to leave a thin layer of dura on top of the nerve at exposure. Once the paralysis has developed nothing much but electrical stimulation can be done. The patient may well be reassured that the disfiguration is only temporary.

**3. Paralysis of other cranial nerves.** The eigth, ninth and tenth cranial nerves may be damaged in the DANDY operation if control of bleeding is difficult. Under such circumstances the seventh nerve also may be damaged. The fourth and sixth nerves are as already mentioned very vulnerable and may be functionally injured in the TAARNHØJ procedure. Abducent nerve paresis was seen once by the author after a temporal root section. In this case the bony roof of the carotid canal was partly missing. Injuries to one or more of the adjacent cranial nerves have repeatedly been described after alcohol injection of the Gasserian ganglion, as alcohol may leak into the subarachnoidal space. Complete unilateral deafness and lasting facial palsy have been reported, even damage to the optic nerve with ensuing blindness has been described following attempts to inject the second division, when the needle has been pushed too far through the inferior orbital fissure.

*Recurrent nerve paresis* is seen after tractotomy if the incision is carried too deep into the medulla. The motor tenth nucleus—the nucleus ambiguus—is situated 4–4·5 mm. underneath the surface.

**4. Herpes.** Herpes of the face is seen following all types of interference with the trigeminal nerve or its pathways, usually on the lips or ala of the nose. The eruption usually starts on the second or third postoperative day. The origin of this complication is not yet fully explained. It may be seen after all types of fifth nerve operations, also after tractotomy—in one case even in spite of the fact that the nerve root had been cut in an earlier operation—but as pointed out by Epstein it is more frequent when the root has been interfered with close to the ganglion. Traumatism to the ganglion is in itself sufficient to give herpes, and the cause is presumably some sort of trophic lesion. Clinically it is insignificant, disappearing without special measures within a week's time. Fatty ointments should be avoided and the blisters allowed to dry and the crusts to fall off. Herpes is, however, always unwelcome. The author has the impression that numbness and paresthesia are more likely to occur among patients who develop herpes in the postoperative period.

**5. Keratitis.** Keratitis neuroparalytica is rightly feared as the most unfortunate complication. If not early recognized and energetically treated it may lead to complete blindness of one eye. This type of keratitis is apparently some sort of trophic lesion of the cornea comparable to herpes. It is only seen after operations which have rendered the first trigeminal division insensitive to all modalities of sensation. It is never seen after tractotomy although the corneal reflex always is missing after this operation and is never seen after root section close to the pons. In the days of the Krause operation when the ganglion was removed it was a common occurrence and it is also frequent after electrocoagulation of the ganglion. Should the cornea have been rendered anesthetic and a facial nerve palsy be added in the postoperative course, the danger of keratitis is imminent and ophthalmologic consultation should be sought at once. Should the corneal reflex be found absent after operation for tic doulouteux—except after tractotomy where no special measures are necessary—the eye should be kept moist and covered.

**6. Ataxia and hemianalgesia** are occasionally seen after trigeminal tractotomy. Ataxia may be brought about by lesion to the dorsal spino-cerebellar tract within the superior cerebellar peduncle (the restiform body) if the incision is placed too far cranially. But also if the incision is placed underneath the obex, ataxia may develop, if the incision is made too far medially injuring the nuclei of the dorsal column. The ataxia is usually most pronounced in the homolateral arm and noticeable in the finger-nose test. It rarely lasts more than a few weeks. Lasting ataxia—still of a mild degree—is very rare. This was seen only once by the present writer. Hemianalgesia finally will mean that the incision has been carried too far ventrally. It will affect the contralateral side and is usually incomplete and more marked in the upper part of the body. It may be lasting but of no clinical significance since it as a rule is not even observed by the patient himself.

### c) Postoperative Paresthesias. Anaesthesia dolorosa.

Disagreeable numbness of the face is not uncommonly felt by patients who have undergone trigeminotomy. The feeling of numbness is often combined with a tickling sensation. Occasionally there is also a feeling of soreness most frequently seen in the tongue, the mouth or in the eye, or there may be a feeling of heat or cold. In a few cases the disagreeable sensation is intensified into a severe aching or burning pain which is felt day and night, independent of sensory stimulation. This distressing clinical picture which will sometimes spoil a good operative result has been termed *painful anesthesia* or *anaesthesia dolorosa* (Olivecrona). It is most likely to occur after operations followed by heavy sensory loss and is rarely seen in young individuals. Old age and arterial hypertension seem to be predisposing factors. In this respect painful anesthesia bears a close resemblance to herpetic neuralgia. The pain is constant, is not brought about by tactile stimulation and there are no free intervals. All grades of severness are seen, from a slight feeling of numbness or tickling to the fullblown picture of intense burning pain. Very little is known of the etiology. Possibly it is of nuclear origin (SJÖQVIST): The lack of afferent impulses after section of the nerve fibers may cause secondary changes in the nuclei causing them to fire impulses in central direction. With the SPILLER-FRAZIER operation major trigeminal neuralgia lost much of its terror but on the other hand the accumulation of patients complaining of painful anesthesia became a problem to be faced by neurological surgeons. Unfortunately very little or nothing can be done for them in the way of therapy. All kinds of sympathectomy have been tried with no avail. Narcotic drugs should be refrained from since these patients easily become addicts. A small dose of luminal and atropine sometimes seem to be helpful. In desperate cases where the patient is a burden to himself and to his surroundings *frontal lobotomy* may be considered. This is the only therapeutic measure which can give at least partial relief to these poor sufferess. Further considerations of this problem will be found in capter 41.

## 6. Mortality. Final Results. Choice of Operation.

In the choice between the surgical procedures now available in major trigeminal neuralgia the degree of relief and the number of recurrences must be considered as well as the operative mortality and the rate of early and late complications. Large statistics concerning results in the various methods are since long at hand, and results in larger clinics seem uniform. Still, operative mortality in *temporal root section* varies from 2,3% (SACHS 1935: 182 patients) down to 0·77 (OLIVECRONA's series reported by GUIDETTI 1950: 515 patients), while the percentage of *recurrence* lies between 13·6 (BAKAY: 250 patients) and 3% (CRAIG 1941: 434 patients).

As to *complications* keratitis or iritis seem to vary widely: 15·1% (PEET and SCHNEIDER 1952: 544 patients), 1·1% (CRAIG 1941: 434 patients), while transitory facial paralysis seems to lie between 3 to 9%, undoubtedly diminishing in the latter years.

*Root section in the posterior fossa* (DANDY's procedure) is by most neurosurgeons used only on special indications (see above). WALKER has, however, reported 350 patients with only one (irrelevant) death and very few complications. Recurrence is definitely more frequent than by the temporal route when fractional root section is attempted—17·9% in OLIVECRONA's series of 145 patients, while the mortality rate was 3·4% (GUIDETTI 1950).

*Trigeminal tractotomy* (SJÖQVIST) in different series seems to carry an average mortality of 1–3% (SJÖQVIST's and OLIVECRONA's series together [160 patients]: 1%), but recurrence is definitely more usual following tractotomy than root section (25–30%) and seems dependant on the degree of sensory loss.

*Addendum.* The TAARNHØJ decompression was first introduced 1951 and adequate follow-up studies are consequently not yet available. The last control (1956) of the Copenhagen clinic showed a percentage of recurrence of 27%, including, however, the first tentative cases and counting every type of pain, even so slight that no treatment was necessary. Re-operation has been indicated in 10%. Most of the recurrences occurred during the first half-year following operation and seem at any rate not to be more frequent in the extradural operations. Even with this considerable percentage of recurrence the TAARNHØJ procedure seems a definite advantage and is the routine procedure in Copenhagen. In recurrences indicating surgery we usually perform a temporal trigeminotomy and have had no difficulty even in cases of previous intradural decompression.

It should once more be stressed that surgery should never be suggested to a patient until the diagnosis of major trigeminal neuralgia is certain. In so-called atypical neuralgia any surgical procedure which induces anesthesia to the face will invariably render the condition worse and the surgeon will have to bear the repeated reproach of having blocked the way to recovery for ever. If a case seems the least doubtful in this respect a novocaine-alcohol injection of the peripheral branches or the main divisions should be done. The clinical picture of major trigeminal neuralgia is, however, so typical and easily recognizable that one rarely is in doubt concerning the diagnosis.

In most neurosurgical centers the world over *extradural root section by the temporal approach* is still the method of choice. It is a safe and precise procedure with a very low mortality which is of primary importance in elderly patients and in a disease with no intrinsic mortality. Recurrencies are rare. The two main drawbacks of the temporal method is the risk of corneal complications and, especially, the high incidence of postoperative paresthesias and anaesthesia dolorosa.

The main indication for *the cerebellar approach* is a suspected cholesteatoma of the cerebellopontine angle. If a young individual presents the typical picture of tic douloureux the possibility of a cholesteatoma should always be kept in mind, especially, if he has had one or more periods of longstanding headache and fever of obscure etiology (intracranial cholesteatomas, especially in the neighbourhood of the large cisterns, may cause periodical aseptic meningitis). If exploration is negative the root can be sectioned according to DANDY's technique.

*Trigeminal tractotomy* has its principal advantage in the maintance of tactile sensation. It should be preferred in younger or middle aged patients—under 55 or 60 years of age—in which a lifelong anesthesia is especially undesirable. The difficulty of rendering the third division analgesic will exclude primary third division neuralgia from this operation. In larger statistics recurrencies after trigeminal tractotomy are practically only seen in primary third division neuralgia (SJÖQVIST, TÖNNIS and KREISSEL). Another group of cases in which tractotomy is advisable are *the bilateral neuralgias*, i.e. when the second side is operated on. A partial root section *can* be done on both sides but these patients have always great difficulties in taking food since the lips and tongue are insensitive. In major *neuralgia combined with disseminated sclerosis* pain is more likely to become bilateral than in ordinary cases and tractotomy may be preferred in this group. The small group of primary first division neuralgia is also best treated by tractotomy because of the risk of keratitis. On the other hand tractotomy is contraindicated in very fat and short-necked individuals and in poor surgical risks.

If the TAARNHØJ *procedure* should carry a low percentage of recurrence it will no doubt become the method of the future. It seems most unlikely that painful paresthesia and anaesthesia dolorosa—those nightmares in fifth nerve surgery—will occur after this operation. Technical difficulties in the operation still have to be overcome—mainly the risk of injury to the fourth nerve and to the trigeminal root itself.

*Alcohol injection into the* GASSER*ian ganglion or electrocoagulation of the ganglion* is never performed by the present writer. These procedures have precisely the same drawbacks as temporal root section and the incidence of complications from the cornea or other cranial nerves is higher.

## C. Atypical Facial Pain. Atypical Trigeminal Neuralgia so-called. Neuralgia Trigemini Minor.

This type of pain gives no clear-cut clinical picture and may appear in many variations which, however, have one thing in common, namely, that pain is *not* relieved by interruption of sensory conduction. The patient complains of a dull, aching pain somewhere in the teeth and jaws. He is convinced that there must be some local disorder in the jaw and usually wanders from one dental surgeon to another. Dental examination including X-ray will not reveal anything wrong, but finally some local treatment is tried and carried on until all teeth have been removed. The patient's condition is, however, not improved; on the contrary, usually it becomes worse. Finally the patient is told, that he—or she—these patients mostly belong to the female sex—is suffering from "neuralgia" and is referred to a neurologist. The neurological specialist refers the patient to a surgeon for operation on the trigeminal nerve. But woe the surgeon, who endeavours to perform a root section! The patient is not improved and a sensory loss is added of which the patient will complain even more than of the original pain.

Another type of atypical pain is the feeling of numbness of the lips and nose. There is no real pain, the patient explains, but the lips may feel swollen or "strange". This disagreeable sensation is bilateral and more or less symmetric. This is sometimes a serious symptom seen as a forerunner to a depressive psychosis and should never be treated by surgical measures.

A third type belonging to the same group corresponds to what has been described under the name *supraorbital neuralgia*. Pain is localized over one eye with irradiation toward the hair line. It may also be bilateral and is described as intense and aching. In these cases a frontal sinusitis should first be excluded, especially if the supraorbital region is tender to pressure.

All these types of facial pain fail to respond favourably to any type of surgery. Blocking of the peripheral branches or the main divisions, root section, tractotomy, and various types of operations on the cervical sympathetic ganglions have no effect. The picture has very adequately been termed "the syndrome of the many useless operations" (GLASER).

Concerning the origin of this syndrome it should in the first place be remembered: that, if pain is bilateral, it cannot be ascribed to one nerve only and consequently is no *neuralgia*, possibly a "polyneuralgia" but in the vast majority of cases a "psychalgia". Special attention should be given to the psychic background. There may be an economic claim directed against the dentist who first treated the case, a "Renten-neurose", or there may be some mental conflict related to marital or sexual matters. These patients sometimes respond favourably to medical treatment but should never the less as a rule be subjected to psychiatric examination. If the mental conflict is discovered and exposed, the patient may be cured.

Some of these patients ambulate from one neurologist or neurosurgeon to another for long periods of time. Again and again they are interrogated whether pain is flashlike or sudden and eventually they consent in their despair. That is the point of danger to the surgeons who may be tempted to suggest an operation which the patient herself always is extremely willing to undergo. A word of warning is here in place: If there is the *slightest* doubt concerning the diagnosis of major trigeminal neuralgia, an operation inducing permanent loss of sensation should *never* be undertaken as the first step. Here novocain and alcohol injections have their main indications. If the patient is not relieved he may be reassured that sensory loss is transient.

## D. Herpetic Neuralgia.

Herpes zoster of the face is most frequently seen in the first trigeminal division. As showed by HIS the GASSERian ganglion consist of two portions which are built up separately during embryonic life from two clusters of cells, one corresponding to the first division, the other corresponding to the second and third division. The reason why the first division much more often becomes the seat of herpes than the second and third is not known.

*Herpes zoster opthalmicus* (opthalmic zoster) is a disease belonging to the later decades of life. A clinical description of the acute stages will be found in textbooks of ophthalmology. The herpes blisters are scattered over the area innervated by the first trigeminal division, including the cornea, where scars can be left which may impair vision. Good results have been reported with aureomycin treatment in the acute stages of herpes zoster. The blisters heal leaving a number of white scars in the skin of the forehead. Sensory examination will reveal a more or less heavy hypoesthesia for all qualities of sensation. A more prolonged or more intense stimulation will, however, give a painful response. The condition thus correspond to what FOERSTER termed *hyperpathy*.

The etiology of herpes zoster and, especially, of herpetic neuralgia are not known in detail, at least not from a patho-physiological point of view. BÄRENSPRUNG discovered the inflammatory changes in the corresponding spinal ganglia, but meningomyelitic changes are also seen. In two autopsy specimens from patients having succumbed from ophthalmic zoster—the disease has a certain, though low mortality of its own—MAGNUSSON and WOHLFART found definite changes within the trigeminal nuclei. Whether these were primary or secondary remained undecided.

The characteristic features of herpetic neuralgia is local hyperpathy, i.e. painful response to tactile stimulation. Touching the skin of the forehead or combing of the hair will bring about pain of a burning character and a certain after-discharge. But in addition to this there is also a constant dull aching pain and soreness in the forehead and in the eye. This type of pain is felt day and night, never leaving its victim for a second, and described by the majority of patients as far worse than the local hypersensitivity. It seems likely that hyperpathy in herpetic neuralgia is accounted for by changes in the ganglion or in the peripheral part of the nerve or the nerve root, whereas the dull aching pain is produced by changes in the nuclei.

Herpetic neuralgia is rarely seen in individuals under 50 years of age. In younger patients the infection heals out entirely, without leaving any other sequels than the scars. The older the patients when the infection is aquired, the more predisposed will he be to become a sufferer from herpetic neuralgia. In this respect this painful condition has a considerable likeness to the painful anesthesia seen after a fifth nerve root section.

The *treatment* of herpetic neuralgia is difficult. Antalgic drugs may give some relief but the patient will run a very real risk of becoming addicts. Aureomycin seems to be ineffective as to the neuralgia, also vitamine B. It was early recognized that root section did not relieve the pain (FOERSTER in spinal zoster, PEET in ophthalmic zoster). Root section will relieve the local hyperpathy but not the dull, aching pain, which is the main complaint of the patient. The same result can be achieved by trigeminal tractotomy but even this operation does not give better results in the long run than root section. BUSCH has reportet favourable results by a sort of "circumcision" of the hyperpathic area leaving only a narrow bridge of skin and soft tissue (laterally in spinal herpes, upwards in ophthalmic herpes) and resuturing the flap. Tsu rationale of the operation would be that both cerebrospinal and autonomic innervation of the affected skin area is completely interrupted. Usually thn pain subsides, but may recur after 5–6 months. Since the pathologic-anatomic substratum of dull, aching pain in herpetic neuralgia may be situated within the nuclei, transection of the secondary neurone (mesencephalic spinothalamic tractotomy) has also been tried (WALKER, SJÖQVIST). Convincingly good results have not been gained with this operation. This is in conformity with the experience gained in spinal herpetic neuralgia, where spinal spinothalamic tractotomy (anterolateral chordotomy) fails to relieve pain (SJÖQVIST 1949). In these desparate cases finally nothing is left except psychosurgery. Frontal lobotomy doubtless gives a considerable relief to these poor sufferers, the more so if senile depression has been added to the picture, which is quite common.

## E. Facial Pain from Spread of Carcinoma.

Carcinoma of the lower jaw or of the maxilla and the paranasal sinuses occasionally may give rise to facial pain by infiltration of larger nerve trunks, usually in late stages of the disease, when the tumor is beyond surgery and even radiation. Facial pain in malignant disease is not always restricted to the trigeminal area since glandular metastases in the neck may affect also the nerves of the cervical plexus. Pain from nerve infiltration by malignant tumors is severe and constant with or without paroxysmal exacerbations. The skin area may be anesthetic, when nerve compression or infiltration has extinguished nerve conduction. Pain surgery can offer many of these patients relief, provided drug addiction has not already ensued. If so frontal lobotomy is of more use than nerve operations. Surgeons and radiologists dealing with the treatment of cancer should be familiar with the resources of neurosurgery in giving relief of pain and these methods should be resorted to *before* the patients are gived large doses of morphia. The drug addict is always a deeply unhappy individual, often aware of his own condition, constantly at conflict with his surroundings and with his own self. With the resources of modern neurosurgery no victim of generalized spread of malignant disease should need to suffer physical pain provided his life expectancy is long enough to warrant surgery.

In the relief of pain from carcinoma of the jaws trigeminal tractotomy combined with section of the glossopharyngeal nerve (cfr. p. 40) and of the upper cervical sensory roots is the method of choice (Fig. 20). Root section by the temporal approach is often difficult to perform if ulcerations are present or if the tumor has invaded the base of the skull, and insufficient, if the nerves of the cervical plexus are involved. If the third trigeminal division is the seat of pain complete section of the root at the pons could be considered as analgesia of this division is difficult to obtain by tractotomy. The operation—be it a root section or a tractotomy—is preferably done under intratracheal anesthesia. The tube should have an inflatable cuff in order to tighten off the trachea and bronchi from infectious material from the tumor.

## F. The Facial and Intermediate Nerves.

*Nervus facialis. Nervus intermedius. Seventh Cranial Nerve.*

### I. Surgical Anatomy and Physiology.

The facial nerve leaves the lateral part of the lower border of the pons about 3 mm. above and anterior to the acoustic nerve. The acoustic and facial nerves converge towards the internal auditory meatus. Between the two nerves, closely attached but separate from the latter, lies the tiny intermediate nerve (the nerve of Wrisberg) which is the sensory root of the seventh cranial nerve. The larger facial nerve is the motor root. The seventh nerve is thus really a mixed nerve (Ramsay Hunt), though predominantly motor. The facial and intermediate nerves enter the internal auditory meatus in its inferior anterior quadrant and run on through the temporal bone within the facial canal. Within this canal the sensory ganglion of the intermediate nerve—the geniculate ganglion—is situated and here—i.e. in the canal—the sensory end branches are given off. These are of three different kinds: 1. the *chorda tympani* fibers transmitting taste from the anterior two-thirds of the tongue, 2. *cutaneous* sensory branches for the skin of the external auditory meatus and its surroundings (cfr. page 5), 3. the *proprioceptive* fibers from the facial muscles which accompany the motor facial nerve. From the region of the geniculate ganglion the superior and inferior petrosal nerves are given off. These are autonomic nerves containing unmyelinated fibers and innervate the lacrimal gland and the mucuous glands in the upper part of the nose. Section of the superior petrosal nerve as done e.g. in Gardner's operation for migraine is followed by diminished tear secretion and a feeling of dryness in the nose. After having left the temporal bone by way of the stylomastoid foramen the nerve runs in an arch underneath the external auditory meatus to enter the parotid capsule, sometimes it is more deeply embedded in the glandular tissue, which should be remembered when the nerve is exposed surgically. 10 or 15 mm. from the stylomastoid foramen the nerve divides into two branches innervating the upper and lower mimic muscles. The bifurcation of the nerve is often situated within the parotid gland.

Fiber analysis of the facial nerve reveals the nerve to be composed of mainly large fibers of two classes. The larger fibers are obviously motor fibers innervating the facial muscles. The other class of fibers is believed to be involved with the maintainance of tonus of the muscles. The taste fibers of the chorda tympani have an average diameter of 4–5 microns.

The motor facial nucleus is situated in the upper and lateral part of the medulla oblongata. The taste fibers join the tractus solitarius together with the taste fibers of the glossopharyngeal nerve whereas finally the cutaneous sensory fibers of the intermediate nerve join the spinal fifth tract (BRODAL). Also the pain and temperature fibers of the glossopharyngeal nerve enter the same tract (BRODAL) which opens up an opportunity to relieve pain transmitted by the intermediate and glossopharyngeal nerves by trigeminal tractotomy.

Surgery of the seventh cranial nerve deals with 1. loss of motor function (facial nerve paralysis), 2. hyperfunction (facial tic, clonic facial spasm), 3. painful conditions related to the intermediate nerve. From a mere anatomic but also from a practical surgical point of view the facial nerve consists of three different portions: 1. the nerve root, situated in the cerebellopontine angle, 2. the petrous portion of the nerve situated within the facial canal, 3. the peripheral part of the nerve beyond the stylomastoid foramen.

Only the first and the third portions of the nerve belong to the neurological surgeon. Surgery of the second, i.e. petrous portion of the nerve falls within the domaine of the ear-, nose and throat surgeon. The close topographic relations of this portion to the inner ear will require special qualifications that the neurosurgeon does not possess. Dexterity in operations with hammer and chisel can only be aquired by perennial daily routine work. Repair of injuries to the nerve within the facial canal should therefore confidently be handed over to the otologic surgeon.

## II. Facial Paralysis. BELL'S Palsy.

The clinical picture was described by CHARLES BELL in the second decade of the nineteenth century. It is characterized by a complete paralysis of the facial muscles with inability to shut the eye, to point the lips and to show the teeth. The difference between facial paralysis of central or supranuclear and of peripheral type is so well known that it need not be entered upon here. If facial paralysis is allowed to persist for a long period of time atrophy of the facial muscles will take place, causing a secondary disfiguration of the face. The corner of the mouth will droop and the lower lip become everted, the lower eye lid will also become everted (ectropium). Depending on the site of the nerve lesion —whether central or peripheral to the exit of the chorda tympani fibers— the sense of taste of the anterior two-thirds of the tongue is lost or preserved. The normal rotation upwards of the bulbus oculi when the eyes are shut, which is normally not seen under the closed lid, is easily observed (BELL'S *phenomenon*). In examining a patient suffering from facial paralysis *electromyography* should not be omitted. It has replaced the oldfashioned electrical examination of the nerve, since it gives more reliable information concerning the function of the nerve and the degree of regeneration. The functional restoration after facial nerve palsy may be complete. More often regeneration is incomplete. A characteristic feature of this incomplete recovery is contracture of the facial muscles and mass function. The reason for this is an internal derangement in the nerve, the individual nerve fibers not finding their way to their original end stations. Contracture and mass function are always seen after nerve anastomosis. But frequently they will follow an ordinary "rheumatic" facial palsy which has healed spontaneously. All sorts of temporary facial nerve paralysis may heal with contracture and whether this will happen is unpredictable in the early stages of regeneration.

The chances of restoring function in facial paralysis depend on the site of and the type of the lesion. If the lesion is situated in the nucleus—as seen in tumors of the medulla oblongata—or in the cerebellopontine angle, e.g. brought about by the radical exstirpation of an acoustic tumor the damage is irreparable by direct methods. In such cases nerve anastomosis or plastic operations must be resorted to. In the facial canal the damaged nerve can be directly repaired by approximation of the cut ends or by the use of nerve grafts (BALLANCE and DUEL). If an edematous nerve has been incarcerated in the canal, which is probably the common cause of so-called rheumatic palsy and regeneration does not take place within reasonable time, a simple decompression of the nerve in the canal may facilitate recovery. Peripherally to the stylomastoid foramen direct repair is possible but often very difficult. If paralysis has followed the exstirpation of a parotid gland tumor, direct repair as a rule is not possible.

# III. Operations on the Nerve within the Facial Canal.

*(Decompression, Nerve Grafting, Nerve Suture.)*

By

Karsten Kettel.

Facial paralysis is serious, not because it endangers the patient directly, but because the person afflicted loses the language of facial expression. Therefore the aim of therapy is to restore the normal appearance with the face at rest, and to give back to the patient the power of expressing emotion. While the first task can be carried out in many different ways, it is only possible to restore the facial movements of emotion if the facial nerve can be made to function again. The symmetry and synchronism of the emotional movements of the face are dependent on close cooperation of the cortical facial centres of both hemispheres. Such cooperation can never be established between the facial centre of one cerebral hemisphere and some different centres of the other, as in anastomosis operations.

Consequently direct repair of the nerve at the site of the lesion is superior to any other procedure, but there are two necessary conditions for success. These are that the site of lesion is surgically accessible, and that the muscles have not degenerated but still respond strongly to the galvanic current.

Alt (1908) was the first to advocate direct exposure of the nerve trunk at the site of lesion, Ney in 1922 published a method of repairing the facial nerve intratemporally as worked out on the cadaver, but Bunnell was the first to perform a successful intratemporal nerve grafting as well as a nerve suture. He was followed by Martin and Smith (1931). Chief credit for the enormous advances which these operations have brought to the therapy of facial paralysis is howerer due to Sir Charles Ballance and Dr. Arthur B. Duel (1932) who established experimentally and clinically the foundation on which treatment rests.

## 1. Surgical Anatomy.

In its tortuous course through the temporal bone the nerve is enclosed in the narrow bony Fallopian canal and may be divided into four segments: the petrous, intratympanic, pyramidal and vertical portions. It bears an undeviating relationship to the horizontal semicircular canal and other structures which can readily be recognized and used as landmarks for its exact anatomical position (Fig. 29).

*The petrous or labyrinthine segment* begins where the nerve enters the internal auditory meatus and runs laterally in the horizontal plane between cochlea and vestibule to the geniculate ganglion. The facial nerve is a mixed nerve formed from a larger motor root and a smaller sensory root, the nerve of Wrisberg. The parts of the nerve coming from its two roots are intimately bound together in this segment. From this part of the nerve the sensory end branches are given off as described in a previous chapter.

*The intratympanic segment* is the only part of the nerve which is not buried deeply in the temporal bone. It begins at the geniculate ganglion and may be recognized as a rounded elevation running horizontally directly backwards across the upper limit of the tympanic cavity, above the promontory, immediately inferior and slightly medial to the anterior edge of the horizontal semicircular canal in the surgical dome of the vestibule. It is covered by extremely thin and brittle bone in which dehiscences may be present. The anterior limit of this segment is approximately represented by the point at which the tendon of the tensor tympani muscle is given off, the posterior limit by the ampullary end of the horizontal semicircular canal.

*The pyramidal segment* lies between the intratympanic and vertical portions in intimate relation to the inferior surface of the horizontal semicircular canal, on the superoposterior wall of the middle ear.

*The vertical segment* begins below the posterior end of the horizontal semicircular canal lying slightly medial to the eminence of the canal. It ends at the stylomastoid foramen, where the nerve emerges from the Fallopian canal. This point is located where the digastric ridge joins the posterior bony wall of the external auditory canal.

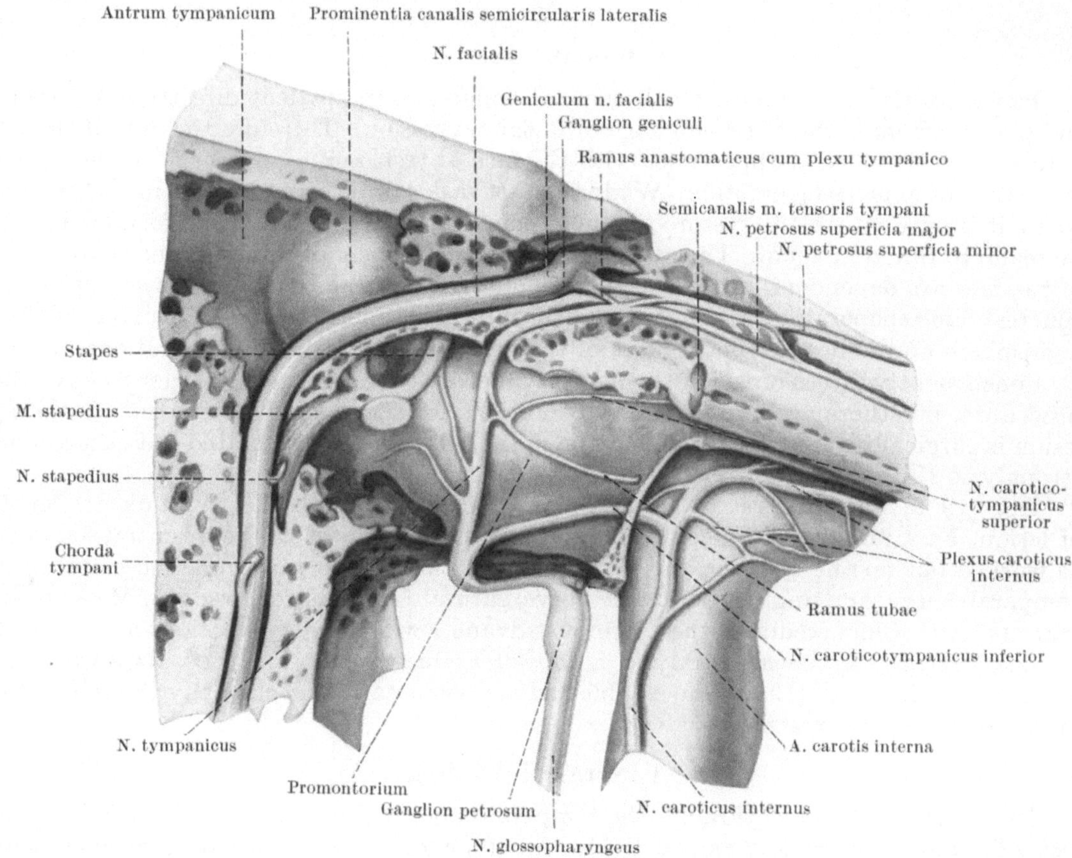


Fig. 29. Intratemporal course of the facial nerve. Reprinted from Spalteholtz.

In the lower part of the Fallopian canal the chorda tympani is given off from the postero-lateral aspect of the nerve. It contains the fibres transmitting taste from the anterior $^2/_3$ of the tongue.

The landmarks for exposure of the nerve within the temporal bone are the stylomastoid foramen, the horizontal semicircular canal and the processus cochleariformis. After location by means of these, the nerve may be exposed at any point within the temporal bone.

## 2. Technique.

Intratemporal operations on the facial nerve may be divided into three main groups: 1. decompression, 2. nerve grafting and 3. nerve suture.

*Decompression of the facial nerve.* To effect decompression the Fallopian canal is opened, the nerve exposed to view, and in some cases the nerve sheath is split. The facial nerve can be exposed to include all or any part of its vertical, pyramidal, intratympanic and petrous segments.

If the vertical portion is to be laid bare a retroauricular incision is preferable. If however the site of lesion is known to be in the pyramidal, intratympanic or petrous segments the endaural approach gives an easier and more direct access to the field.

*The vertical segment* is most easily isolated as the nerve emerges from the stylomastoid foramen. The foramen and the posterior end of the horizontal semicircular canal are the two landmarks which must be clearly defined in order to ensure a safe exposure of this portion.

To perform the finer details of these operations a dissecting microscope giving a magnification of ten diameters is necessary. The cells in the tip of the mastoid process and those covering the plate of the sigmoid sinus, as well as the posterior wall of the external auditory canal, are completely removed. By means of a burr and curettes the latter is skeletonized and thus the posterior end of the horizontal semicircular canal is brought into view at the floor of the aditus ad antrum. At the point where the digastric ridge joins the skeletonized posterior wall of the external auditory canal the inferior end of the FALLOPian canal and the stylomastoid foramen are found. Many surgeons remove the tip of the mastoid proces before starting to open the FALLOPian canal. This, however, may cause the patients discomfort and the nerve may instead be exposed from within the mastoid cavity. This is accomplished by means of a burr and curettes working parallel to the vertical portion of the nerve.

Having exposed the nerve at its exit, the posterior wall is shaved down until only a very thin layer of bone covers the nerve. By inserting a fine curette underneath the edge of this, the plate is removed. This procedure is repeated millimeter by millimeter until the horizontal semicircular canal is reached. It should be stressed that the nerve must be exposed in its full width, and due consideration paid to anomalies of its course.

In some cases e.g. ischaemic facial palsy, the nerve sheath is split. If however, infection is present, this should not be done, as intraneural infection with ensuing formation of scar tissue must be avoided.

*The pyramidal segment* of the nerve, situated in the superoposterior part of the wall of the middle ear, may be exposed using the posterior end of the horizontal semicircular canal as a landmark. Careful removal of bone lying immediately anterior and inferior to the horizontal canal will expose the nerve in this area.

To get access to the *intratympanic segment* a radical mastoidectomy is in most cases necessary. This part of the nerve is situated in the medial wall of the tympanic cavity, where it runs horizontally above the promontory, immediately below and slightly medial to the anterior end of the horizontal semicircular canal, covered only by a very thin layer of bone, which in some cases may even be lacking. This thin cover of bone is easily removed by small curettes and a suitable dental excavator.

In cases of facial paralysis resulting from fractures of the temporal bone involving the cochlea as well as the vestibular portion of the labyrinth, the *petrous segment* of the nerve may finally be reached by removing the superior semicircular canal, using the canal for the tensor tympani muscle as a landmark (SULLIVAN).

*Nerve grafting.* The value of nerve grafting to bridge a gap in an injured nerve has long been established. This is most often necessary with injuries due to operative traumata, but other conditions such as tumors of the nerve, fractures of the petrous or tympanic portions of the temporal bone and casualties of various art may be responsible for a lesion which needs such grafting.

The vertical portion of the nerve is most commonly injured in performing a simple mastoidectomy by creating an artificial antrum distal to the horizontal semicircular canal, and curetting outwards from this, thus tearing the nerve; or by removing infected retrofacial cells.

The pyramidal portion may be injured in planing down of the hypotympanon on the posterior wall of the tympanic cavity in a radical mastoidectomy, and the intratympanic segment in removing the contents of a middle ear destroyed by infection.

To secure a good result the proximal and distal ends of the facial nerve stumps must be refreshed, thus removing scar tissue or neuromas. A graft of equal calibre to the recipient nerve must be used (n. cutaneus femoris lateralis or better n. ilio-inguinalis). The approximation must be accurate and fixation as perfect as possible.

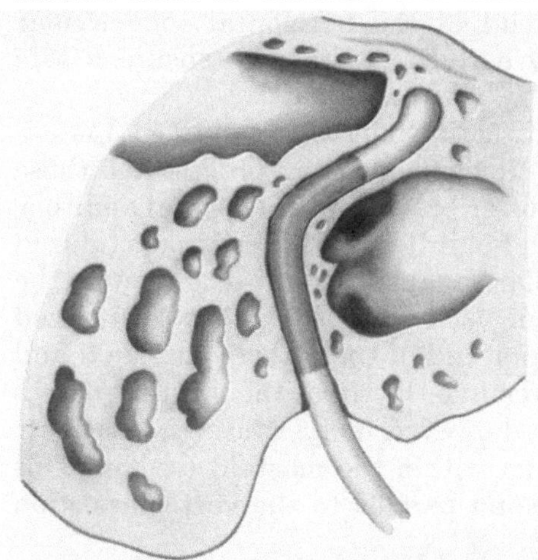

Fig. 30. Intratemporal nerve grafting according to Ballance & Duel.

In the temporal bone the graft can generally be placed in the Fallopian canal, or if this is destroyed, in an artificial groove made in the underlying bone by means of the burr. The oozing of tissue fluids will to some degree fix the graft but it is better to glue the nerve ends together with plasma whenever possible (Sullivan). Sutures should be avoided, as they produce endoneural scar tissue which is a hindrance to the downgrowth of neurofibrils through the graft (Fig. 30).

The site and nature of the lesion is important. Even though a single report is available (Tickle) in which the proximal end of the graft was fixed to the facial nerve where it pierces the dura, most surgeons agree that attempts to repair the nerve proximal to the geniculate ganglion are useless. If however the nerve is divided distal to the ganglion the prospects of success are good.

In many cases the grafting is performed strictly intratemporally, in others the distal end of the graft must be fixed to the distal stump of the facial nerve in the soft tissues both proximal and distal to the devision of the stem at the pes anserinus. In cases where the pes anserinus has been destroyed good results have been obtained by using a "cable graft" consisting of a bundle of smaller nerves instead of a single bigger nerve and suturing the ends of these strands to the peripheral ends of the facial nerve in the face (Lathrop, Maxwell). In partiel injuries of the nerve, where some strands have been left, good results have been obtained by leaving these intact and inserting a lateral graft (Cawthorne).

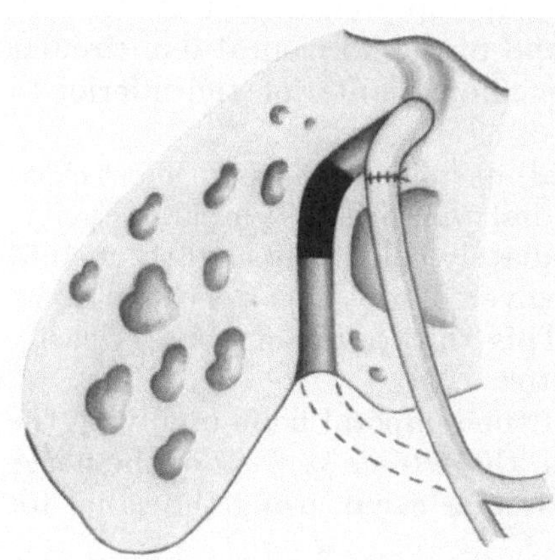

Fig. 31. Nerve suture after "re-routing" of the nerve according to Bunnell.

*Nerve suture.* If the facial nerve has been divided in the temporal bone by a clean cut, and if the distance between the ends is only 1–2 mm. it may be possible to mobilize the stumps and unite the nerve. This is however very rare. The gap is generally larger, and in these cases it has been suggested that the course of the nerve should be shortened by lifting it out of the Fallopian canal, suturing it across the promontory, the "re-routing method" [Bunnell (Fig. 31)]. Thus it may be possible to overcome a gap of up to 23 mm., and good results have been reported. Most surgeons however do not favour the re-routing procedure but prefer a nerve graft as by the latter, the nerve is left in its bed with blood supply intact. If the nerve graft is going to be fixed to the facial nerve outside the stylomastoid foramen (stem or branches) it should if possible be done by the plasma glue method, and if this cannot be accomplished sutures should only be placed in the nerve sheath to avoid intraneural formation of scar tissue.

## 3. Indications and Results.

Those facial paralyses for which an intratemporal operation may be considered can be divided into 2 main groups: atraumatic and traumatic palsies.

## a) Atraumatic Palsies.

**1. Ischaemic facial palsy.** The majority of the atraumatic facial palsies belong to this group. The term "Bell's palsy" or "rheumatic facial palsy" which generally is used is misleading, being a "collective diagnosis" covering all cases where it has been impossible to demonstrate a definite cause. Most of the socalled Bell's palsies are due to ischaemia near the stylomastoid foramen (AUDIBERT et al., SULLIVAN, KETTEL) probably caused by arteriolospasm (HILGER). Ischaemia is then the primary cause of the palsy and resulting from it various structural alterations take place in the facial nerve, between the lateral semicircular canal and the stylomastoid foramen where it leaves the FALLOPian canal, and in some cases also in the surrounding bone. The nerve becomes unduly constricted at the stylomastoid foramen and oedematous proximal to this point, while tiny haemorrhagic streaks are seen in the nerve sheath running longitudinally (CAWTHORNE). As a further result of the ischaemia there may be exudation in the mastoid cells and especially around the stylomastoid foramen together with bony necrosis in the walls of the cells and in the FALLOPian canal (KETTEL).

The swelling of the nerve within the lower part of the bony inelastic FALLOPian canal results in compression of the adjacent blood and lymph vessels, and consequently a vicious circle arises. This process is reversible, therefore the prognosis is on the whole good, but in severe cases the ischaemia is followed first by necrosis later by fibrosis. It seems that the course of the palsy and the pathological alterations are both connected with the environment, occuring more often and more severely in the northern countries (MARTIN).

Whereas the pathogenesis seems to be clear, our knowledge of the etiology is limited. The impetus to arteriolar constriction is derived from autonomous nervous impulsion (HILGER). The etiologic cause consequently should be searched for among factors, which may upset the ballance of innervation. Ischaemic facial palsy may occur after the patient has been exposed to draught, or it may arise in connection with sudden fright or anger, with extraction of a tooth or a tonsillectomy. In these cases the palsy is probably reflex-released.

Approximately 75–85% of the ischaemic facial palsies recover under conservative treatment. Prognosis of recovery must be based upon a careful history, physical findings and special tests. Sudden onset of the palsy accompanied by pain is considered a bad prognostic sign and of importance in deciding on operation (FINDLAY, SULLIVAN). Loss of Faradic response is by some authors considered most important and the principal indication for decompression (SULLIVAN, CAWTHORNE) while others do not find it a very reliable sign (MARTIN, KETTEL, MAXWELL). In exactly the same way opinions differ regarding the value of electromyography (SULLIVAN, COLLIER, MARTIN).

At present it is questioned whether better results can be obtained by surgical intervention performed on the present indications than by conservative therapy. It must be remembered that only 15% of the patients on whom a decompression has been performed after 6–8 weeks of observation recover completely and that some of them undoubtly would have recovered to some extent without operation. But that decompression may be effective is illustrated by the cases a) in which movements started in direct conjunction with the operation after weeks of unsuccesful conservative treatment and b) in the conservatively treated cases where the improvement had come to a standstill but where a further improvement was obtained by decompression.

The idea of decompression is unquestionably right, the present indications however insufficient.

Surgery does not correct the vascular disturbance that is the underlying cause of ischaemic palsy only the sequels, oedema and subsequent compression of the nerve in the FALLOPian canal (MARTIN). Therefore the only time for prophylaxis or prevention of a lasting ischaemic palsy is during the first few hours. Prompt decompression will keep the nerve alive. If decompression is not done then, ischaemia will result in a degree of damage to the nerve ranging from temporary palsy to permanent paralysis (BUNNELL).

Prompt surgical decompression will however be unneccessary in about 80 % of cases. We should decompress in the other 20 % at once, not days or weeks later for by then the irreversible damage has been done (BUNNELL). The problem is how to recognize the 20 % of serious cases. Electrodiagnosis and electromyography are useless as emergency guides as 3–21 days elapse before anything can be deducted from the reactions, and meanwhile the prophylactive value of immediate decompression has been lost.

Meanwhile we have to act on the present indications which certainly have given results, but which are not good enough. As stated above SULLIVAN and CAWTHORNE advise decompression in cases with loss of response to the Faradic current while KETTEL advocates operations in a) cases which from the start are accompanied by severe pains in or behind the homolateral ear, b) cases where after 2 months observation no signs of recovery have been noticed and c) cases where the improvement has come to a standstill without satisfactory recovery.

**2. Hemifacial spasm.** The surgical treatment of hemifacial spasm has been described in a previous chapter by SJÖQVIST.

It should however be mentioned, that decompression of the facial nerve in its vertical segment has been tried by WILLIAMS et al., SULLIVAN and KETTEL. From the clinical standpoint however the operation has been somewhat disappointing, as there is a tendency for the spasm to recur after a time, one year on the average. In spite of this many patients report considerable relief from the procedure.

**3. Tumors of the facial nerve.** The majority of intratemporal tumors of the nerve belong to the group termed neurinomas. These are benign tumors originating from the cells of SCHWANN in the nerve sheath and growing by expansion (ANTONI). Only 2 malign tumors have been reported (KETTEL, GUTTMAN & SIMON). The clinical picture has been described by ALTMANN and KETTEL.

The tumors generally develop in youngish people, and the first sympthom is facial paralysis, which may develop gradually or suddenly. This may often remain the only symptom for a long period. Generally the paralysis remains permanent but temporary improvement has sometimes been observed. The hearing remains intact for a while but later symptoms of a chronic otitis media develop resulting from ingrowth in the middle ear and subsequent secondary infection. When the condition advances further, labyrinthine and intracranial complications may ensue.

These tumors generally arise from the vertical segment of the nerve but have also been observed in the pyramidal as well as in the intratympanic portion. In the first case it is hardly possible to diagnose them before intervention, and most of such tumors have been detected at operation, a decompression having been made on the erroneous diagnosis of ischaemic facial palsy (CAWTHORNE, KETTEL). If, however, the tumor is situated in the pyramidal or the intratympanic segment of the nerve, it may sometimes be possible to diagnose it before operation. It may be visible as a swelling of the posterior wall of the external acoustic meatus feeling soft to the touch of a probe; it may appear as polyps bearing a disconcerting resemblance to the polyps seen in chronic otitis, or finally as an obturating tumor which in advanced cases grows in clusters like a bunch of grapes occupying all available space in the cavum conchae (WILLIAMS & PASTORE). If it arises from the intratympanic segment of the nerve the drum may be seen to bulge.

The lesion found at operation has ranged from a minor well defined focus around the vertical segment of the nerve, to extensive destructions of the mastoid process including the posterior and even the anterior wall of the acoustic meatus, the middle ear, the labyrinth and pyramid. In one case the tumor had penetrated the internal ear and had set up an abscess of the brain.

On the whole prognosis is favorable quoad vitam, although some reservation would be appropriate, as the site of the tumor near the middle ear and the labyrinth implies the risk of complications from the latter when the tumor grows into them. The prognosis as regards the future function of the nerve, on the other hand, is bad. Therapy is exclusively surgical, irradiation has been tried but without success. Not only the question of whether the tumor may be removed radically but also the possibility of sparing the middle ear depends on the time at which the patient applies for treatment. If the tumor is successfully removed a nerve graft should be inserted.

**4. Facial palsy of otogeneous origin.** Preoperative facial palsy may arise in conjunction with an acute as well as a chronic otitis media. In an acute otitis media the palsy is probably due to a toxic neuritis and the prognosis is good assuming an adaequate conservative treatment of the otitis. Decompression should only be considered in the extremely rare cases where the palsy does not disappear in spite of the treatment after at least 2 months of observation.

A facial palsy in conjunction with a chronic otitis media always indicates a radical mastoidectomy. At operation it may be impossible to demonstrate the cause of the palsy and the patient should only simply be observed, as in the group of palsies in acute otitis media. If on the other hand a fistula on the facial canal is found which in most cases will be due to a cholesteatoma which has erroded the FALLOPian canal, or an osteitis in its wall, the fistula should be widened until every sign of an osteitis in the canal and the surrounding bone is removed, and the nerve looks normal. In very rare cases the continuity of the nerve may be interrupted, and here a graft should be inserted.

a

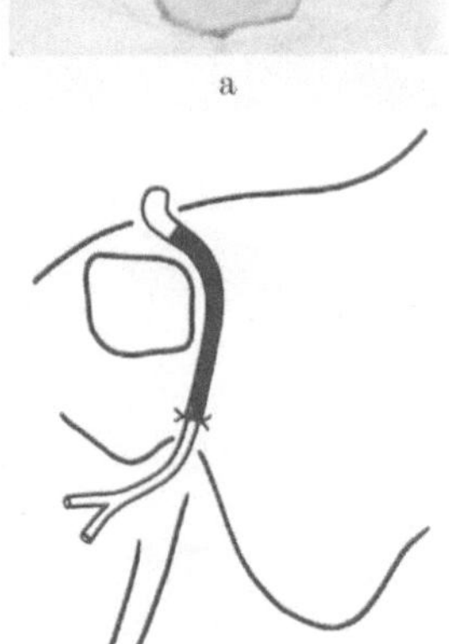

b

Fig. 32a and b. a Nerve grafting 14 mm left side. Patient before repair; b 14 mm graft intratemporally situated.

### b) Traumatic Palsies.

The nerve may be injured through various accidents among which should be mentioned surgical injuries, skull fractures, and lesions of the face.

#### α) *Intratemporal Injuries.*

**1. Surgical injuries.** The nerve may be damaged in the porus acusticus internus during removal of an acoustic neurinoma. If the nerve has been divided proximal to the geniculate ganglion direct repair is extremely difficult, only in one case has it been done successfully (DOTT). In most cases an anastomosis operation should be performed, provided that the muscles have not degenerated. If however the muscles have degenerated plastic operations may be indicated. If however the nerve has only been contused decompression has proved satisfactory in a few cases (SULLIVAN).

The majority of surgical injuries to the nerve are due to a simple or radical mastoidectomy. If the palsy arises in *direct conjunction* with the operation it nearly always means that the nerve has been divided or severely damaged. The only way to decide this is to uncover and inspect the nerve without delay. The palsy may be due to stretching of the nerve, to a haematoma, or to a bone spicule pushed into the sheath, and here a limited decompression and eventually removal of bone splitters is sufficient. In most cases however the nerve is severed, and a nerve graft should then be inserted. The prognosis after nerve grafting and nerve suture is good. A clinically satisfactory result meaning that the patient looked normal with the face at rest and was able to smile and close the eye, was obtained by CAWTHORNE, in 25 of 30 cases (83%), by BOTMAN & JONGKEES in 21 of 28 cases (78%) and by KETTEL in 52 of 58 cases (90%). It should be stressed that recovery after nerve grafting and nerve suture is never functionally perfect although often amazingly satisfactory when compared to the preceding paralysis (Fig. 32—35 incl.).

On the average the first signs of returning function may be expected after 10 months, but the delay may last longer. During these months every effort must be made to prevent overstretching and degeneration of the muscles, by the use of electrical stimulation, massage and a supporting hook, which can be fixed in various ways.

If, however, palsy arises only *after an interval* of freedom continuity is not interrupted, and the palsy is probably due to slight tearing of the sheath, a haematoma, or collateral oedema. In the majority of these cases the prognosis is good with conservative treatment, and decompression should only be considered if there is no sign of returning function after a reasonable time of observation.

**2. Fractures of the temporal bone.** The treatment of facial paralysis in fractures of the temporal bone has been purely conservative until recently; first, because prognosis with conservative therapy has been considered favourable and, second, because before the introduction of surgery of the facial nerve by Ballance & Duel the proper treatment could not be instituted.

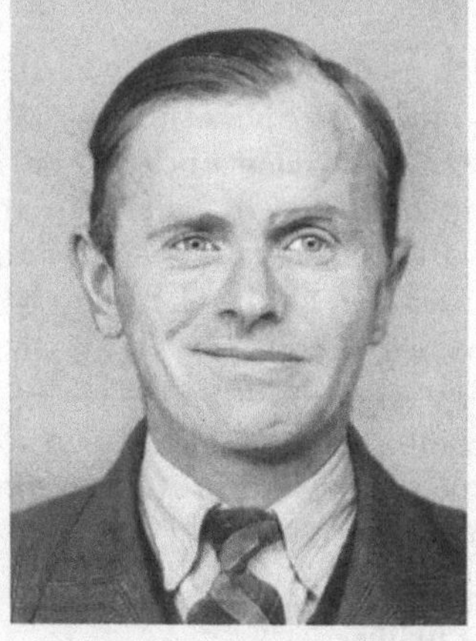

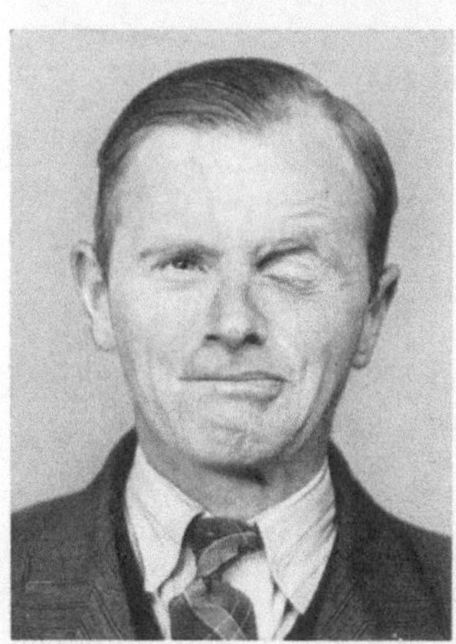

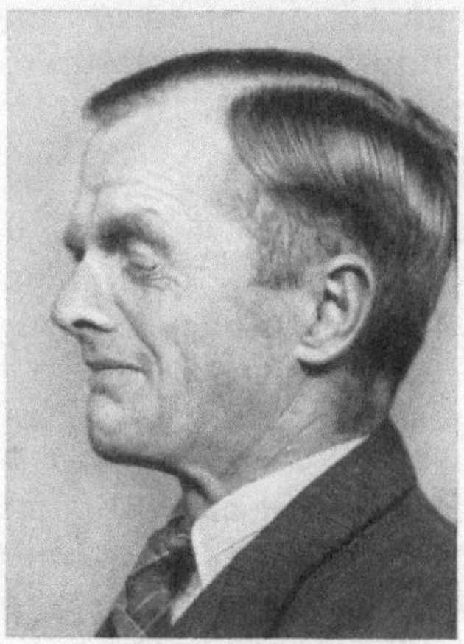

Fig. 33. Same patient as in fig. 32. 21 months after nerve grafting (Kettel). Note function of all major branches of the facial nerve.

Recent investigations, however, have shown that even if prognosis is good in most cases, there is, nevertheless, a limited number of cases in which the nerve ought to be repaired, and reports are available indicating that this has been done with success.

Fractures of the temporal bone involving the ear and the facial canal may be divided into two main groups, longitudinal, by far the commonest, and transverse.

In the *longitudinal* fractures the middle ear is always damaged. The drum is torn, and bleeding occurs. The incus may be dislocated and the ossicular ligaments torn. The labyrinth capsule remains undamaged, although marked perilymphatic haemorrhage in the scala tympani may take place, particularly near the round window.

Of the *transverse* fractures, there are two types; the internal, which transverses the internal auditory meatus, shattering the cochlea; and the external, which passes through the entire internal ear (cochlea and vestibule) and through the Fallopian canal. The middle ear may be entirely spared, although a haematotympanum may occur; the drum, is never torn and there is no bleeding from the external canal. The fracture is accompanied by a complete and permanent loss of function, both cochlear and vestibular.

Apart from these main types, longitudinal and transverse fractures, there is one to which Ramadier & Caussé drew attention: an uncommon fracture restricted to the mastoid process itself, which can open into the external auditory canal and the middle ear and also reach the facial nerve in its descending segment.

The *facial palsies* may be divided in two groups: immediate, occurring in direct conjunction with the accident and delayed, arising after a free interval. *Immediate paralyses* are usually due to an actual lesion of the nerve by the line of fracture, either in the Fallopian canal or at the internal auditory meatus. They are usually complete, caused by traction, tearing, compression (blood, oedema) or actual section of the nerve. According to the nature of the lesion, function may never return or the paralysis may disappear completely. *The delayed paralyses* appear during the first two weeks following the accident; they may be complete or incomplete, but cure results as the general rule. They are probably due to haemorrhage or oedema in the facial canal or in the nerve.

According to statistics longitudinal fracturs caused facial paralysis in from 10 to 18% of cases, and transverse fractures in about 50%.

Generally the prognosis of facial paralysis in conjunction with closed head injuries is good. TURNER reexamined 70 consecutive cases; in 36 the paralysis occurred immediately, but in 27 of these it disappeared completely (75%). In 6 it only disappeared partially, in 3 it remained massive. Of the 34 delayed palsies a complete recovery occurred in 32 cases, a partial in 2.

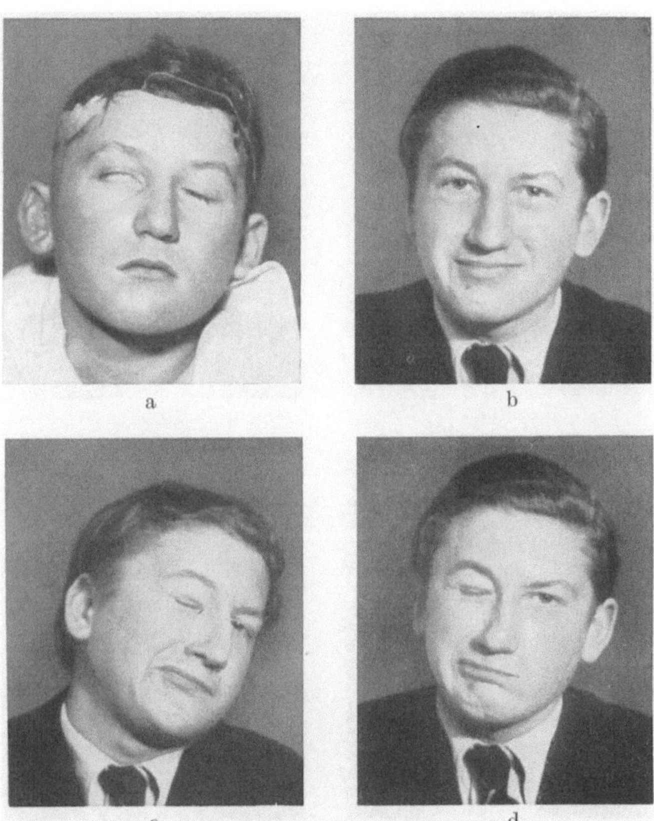

Fig. 34 a—d. Nerve grafting (35 mm) before (a) and 27 months after the operation (b, c, d). The proximal end of the graft has been placed just distal to the geniculate ganglion, the peripheral sutured to the distal stump of the faceal nerve just before the division at the pes anserinus (KETTEL).

Even if the prognosis of the palsy is relative good, there is consequently a limited but definite field for surgical intervention.

For determining the site of injury one must resort to such information as can be gained from roentgenographic studies and from noticing the extent to which the functions served by the facial nerve (sense of taste, salivation, lacrimation) are interrupted. CAWTHORNE points out that skull fractures in which facial paralysis is accompanied by signs of damage to the ear, particularly if the middle ear is affected, should be considered as possible instances of fracture involving the middle ear cleft and the facial nerve as it runs along its inner wall.

The patients should be examined electromyographically, and if the site of lesion is surgically accessible the nerve should be repaired as soon as definite proofs are at hand, indicating that complete denervation has taken place.

Even if the patient appears late with a paralysis, surgical intervention should be considered, if the site of lesion is surgically accessible and the muscles have not atrophied.

Following these lines good results have been obtained by intratemporal repair of the nerve either by nerve grafting or sealing the nerve stumps together (CAWTHORNE, BEHRMAN, MAXWELL) or by decompressing a nerve in which a haematoma was present, and removing bone splitters from the nerve sheath (FARRIOR and CALDWELL, KETTEL).

### β) *Extratemporal Injuries.*

The facial nerve may be injured outside the stylomastoid foramen by surgical procedures e.g. removal of a tumor in the parotid gland and by various accidents, including war injuries. Lathrop has an especially wide experience in dealing with the latter.

The possibility of repairing the nerve depends upon the extent of the damage; it is often impossible, always difficult to accomplish.

Strictly extratemporally, a nerve graft has been succesfully used to bridge a traumatic gap in the zygomatic branch of the facial nerve (Lathrop, Seeley); three strand cable graft have been sutured proximally to the stem of the facial nerve just before the division at the pes anserinus and distally to the three main branches (Maxwell).

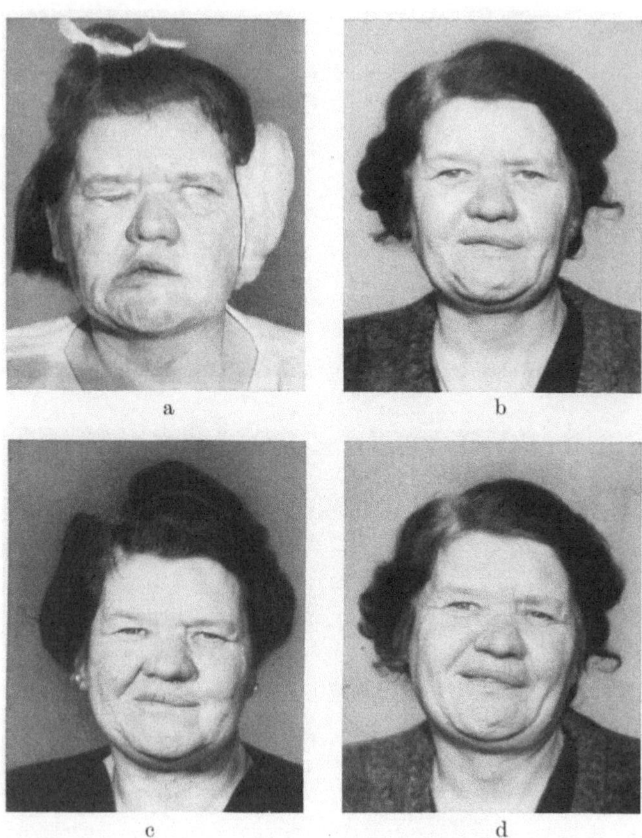

Fig. 35 a—d. Nerve suture after "re-routing" of the nerve according to Bunnell; before (a) and 27 months after the operation (b, c, d) (Kettel).

A combined intra- and extratemporal procedure has been employed in cases in which the facial nerve was injured proximally within the temporal bone, distally in the soft tissues. The gap has been bridged either by means of a graft or by nerve suture; a graft has been fixed proximally to the intratemporal stump of the facial nerve, distally to the peripheral stump of the facial nerve, either before the division at the pes anserinus or after, in the latter case after splitting of the peripheral end of the graft into three strands to be fixed to the three main branches of the facial nerve (Maxwell). To accomplish a direct suture of the facial nerve in these cases, the proximal end of the facial nerve must be "re-routed" (Bunnell, Maxwell), as earlier described.

## IV. Operations on the Nerve outside the Facial Canal.

### 1. Nerve Anastomosis.

In this operation the function of another nerve is sacrificed to restore the tonus of the facial muscles. After a successful anastomosis the face is entirely symmetric and not distorted when at rest. The patient need not feel constantly and watchfully observed in the streets or by fellow passengers in the train or street-car. The eye can be completely closed and a certain degree of mimic movement are possible. The facial movements are, however, always *mass movements*, and a certain degree of disfiguration will always be apparent when the patient laughs or smiles. The two nerves commonly used for the anastomosis are the spinal accessory nerve and the hypoglossal nerve. Spinofacial anastomosis was first performed by Drobnik in 1879. The technique was further elaborated by Cushing. Hypoglosso-facial anastomosis was first tried by Körte (1903). Coleman has published an extensive series of this operation (1940). Other nerves tried (trapezius branch of the spinal accessory nerve, ramus descendens of the hypoglossal nerve) have not given satisfactory results.

In the choice between the spinal accessory and the hypoglossal nerve the latter is to be preferred. It is of the same diameter as the facial nerve and the nerve sheath is firm which will ensure a better approximation of the nerve ends. The disability resulting from paralysis of the trapezius muscle is also more disabling than the hemiatrophy of the tongue which follows the transection of the hypoglossal nerve. No significant disturbance of speech and deglutition is seen after this operation but the patient should of course be informed in advance of the sequels.

### Operative Technique.

Although the operation is somewhat time-consuming—it lasts about an hour—it can well be performed under local anesthesia. The patient is placed in a recumbent position with his head turned to the opposite side and tilted a little backwards. Skin and muscles are infiltrated with 1 % novocain under ordinary precautions to avoid intravenous injection. The incision is made from the mastoid process obliquely downwards and slightly curved preferably in a skin fold to ensure an invisible scar. The external jugular vein is held aside or doubly ligated and the greater auricular nerve is identified and held aside. If the spinal accessory nerve is chosen for the anastomosis this nerve is exposed in front of the sterno-mastoid muscle, where it runs obliquely immediately underneath the fascia colli media, and freed upwards and downwards for about 4 cm. The hypoglossal nerve is best looked for at the point where it crosses the external carotid artery and freed peripherally to the corner of the hyoid bone. The exposure of the facial nerve is often difficult. The paralysed nerve is always more or less degenerated, of greyish colour and of a smaller diameter than normally. Electric stimulation can not be used for identification since the nerve is rather inexcitable. The nerve runs from inwards in an outward direction and is found rather close to the external auditory meatus within the parotid capsule or embedded in the glandular tissue where it divides into its two main branches. The posterior auricular artery may be in the way and sometimes has to be ligated. By pulling the digastric muscle downwards the tiny muscular branch from the facial nerve can occasionally be identified and followed upwards to the facial nerve. When the nerve has been identified with certainty it is cut as far centrally as possible with a sharp knife. The spinal accessory or hypoglossal nerve, depending on which nerve was chosen, is then divided peripherally and the central stump reflected and sutured to the peripheral stump of the facial nerve with 4 or 5 stitches in the nerve sheath of finest possible silk with smallest possible needles. All tension on the line of suture should, of course, be avoided. After careful control of all oozing—hematomas in the loose connective tissue in the neck can reach considerable dimensions and endanger the result—the wound is closed in layers.

The first signs of regeneration cannot be expected until after 8 or 10 weeks. Sometimes up to 3 months will pass until signs of regeneration are seen and the final result still be completely satisfactory. Early signs of regeneration may be seen by electromyography. Facial muscle tonus is first improved, later come voluntary movements. After hypoglosso-facial anastomosis the act of swallowing is always accompanied by a grimace, after spino-facial anastomosis elevation of the arm or shoulder will cause twitching of the face. Intelligent patients can utilize this for maintaining a certain symmetry of the face when laughing or smiling.

## 2. Facial Tic. Clonic Facial Spasm.

The French term "tic facial" refers to a condition characterized by involuntary twitching movements of the facial muscles. The twitchings appear in volleys of clonic contractions usually first seen around the eye in the orbicularis oculi muscle, but often spreading to the triangularis and risorius. They are more marked when the patient feels himself observed or in moments of mental strain. In one of my patients, a business man, twitchings appeared when he was about to sign important documents, a fact which often caused him embarrassment. Facial spasm is not painful, but may nevertheless bring about discomfort and suffering, especially since it has a drawn-out course over years and has a tendency to involve more and more of the mimic muscles and since medical treatment can offer little or no relief. Such cases often are referred to the neurosurgeon. Several surgical procedures have been suggested in clonic facial spasm (alcohol injection [PEET],

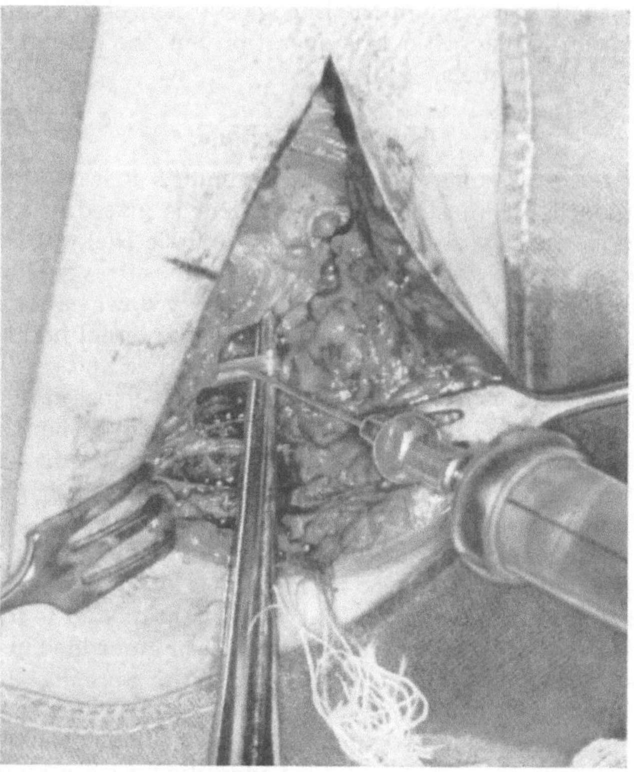

Fig. 36. Facial tic. Operation.

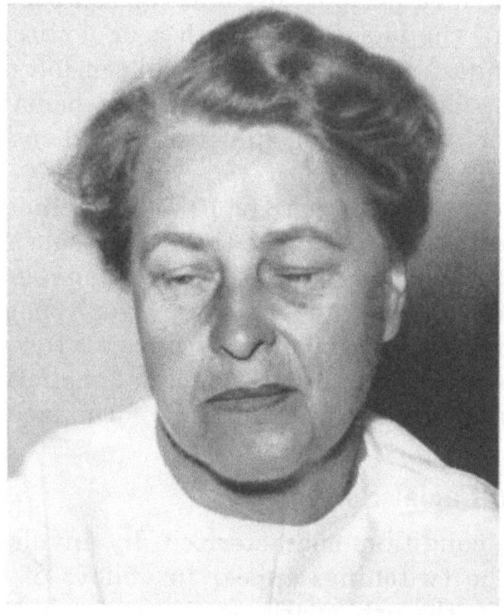

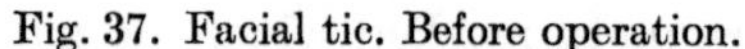

Fig. 37. Facial tic. Before operation.

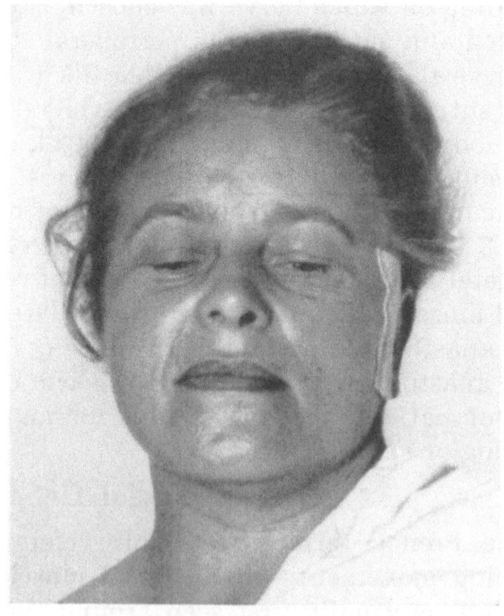

Fig. 38. Facial tic. After operation.

crushing of the peripheral seventh nerve branches [COLEMAN], partial section of the main branches [GERMAN] and even complete nerve section followed by primary hypoglosso-facial anastomosis). Facial tic should not be confused with *tonic facial spasm* which is symmetric and usually seen in the upper facial muscles (blepharospasmus).

In the comparatively rare cases of clonic facial spasm where surgical measures are called for the present writer perfers crushing the upper facial branches. Under local anesthesia a small curved incision is made in front of the tragus and the facial end branches are exposed at the anterior margin of the parotid gland. Starting from upwards the nerve branches are crushed by an artery forceps one by one under control of facial muscle function. When the twitchings around the eye have ceased a silk thread is tied very loosely around each of the crushed branches. The resulting partial facial paralysis will last from 3 to 6 months and the patient can compare this discomfort to the inconvenience of the spasm. If he is satisfied, the nerves that have been crushed can readily be identified by the loose ligatures and sectioned with lasting effect. In the most severe cases nerve section and anastomosis may be considered. In only one case in the author's series was this deemed advisable.

### 3. Geniculate Neuralgia.

It is the merit of RAMSAY HUNT to have completed our knowledge of the sensory function of the seventh nerve and to have identified herpes oticus and postherpetic otalgia as related to the geniculate ganglion. In this form of herpes zoster the eruptions appear in the external auditory meatus and its surroundings. It is, however, a very rare disease and, therefore, of small practical importance. In spite of some experience with painful conditions of the face and head the present writer has so far never seen a case of herpes oticus or postherpetic geniculate neuralgia. The existence of a non-herpetic neuralgia related to the nervus intermedius of WRISBERG is doubtful. The one case published over 40 years ago (by CLARKE and TAYLOR 1909) seems "reasonable authentic" (PEET), but no more reports have followed.

In the light of the poor results of neurosurgery in post-herpetic neuralgia in general it seems unlikely that much can be gained by surgical measures in geniculate neuralgia following after herpes oticus. Trigeminal tractotomy may be worth trying since the cutaneous sensory fibers of the intermediate nerve enter the spinal fifth tract (BRODAL). In non-herpetic geniculate neuralgia—if this disease exists—tractotomy should be the method of choice and safer than section of the intermediate nerve itself which must be a difficult procedure to perform without damage to the acoustic or motor facial nerve.

## G. The Acoustic Nerve.

### 1. Eight Cranial Nerve. Nervus acusticus.

Even if isolated attempts were made by KRAUSE, FRAZIER a. o. to section the acoustic nerve for invalidating tinnitus, it is the merit of DANDY to have brought the eight nerve within the domain of neurosurgery by his pioneer work in the middle if the 1920'ies on the operative treatment of aural vertigo. Since the establishment of otology as a speciality the surgery of the organ of hearing and equilibrium has been taken care of by this group of specialists. Operations on the auditory nerve root situated, as it is, within the cerebellopontine angle, requires neurosurgical technique and is, consequently, a neurosurgical task.

#### Surgical Anatomy.

The root of the eight cranial nerve runs transversely across the cerebellopontine angle from its origin at the lateral part of the lower border of the pons to its entrance into the internal auditory meatus. It is entirely situated within the cerebello-pontine cistern, but as soon as the posterior cistern is opened the cistern collapses and the nerve is seen covered by a thin layer of arachnoid which has to be torn to approach the nerve. A loop of the inferior anterior cerebellar artery crosses the nerve more or less at right angles on its dorsal aspect, but can easily be pushed medially. The inferior anterior cerebellar artery usually gives off the internal auditory artery; it runs parallel to the nerve and enters the internal auditory meatus. Sometimes the artery runs within the nerve between the vestibular and the cochlear portions. In such cases the artery may be torn when the nerve is divided and can give a troublesome hemorrhage.

The eight nerve posesses a glial cone of considerable length, about 6–8 mm. The vestibular and cochlear portions run more or less parallel, the vestibular portion occupying the anterior-superior, the cochlear portion the posterior-inferior part. The vestibular portion is the larger of the two, but may be atrophic in Ménière's disease. The two portions may be difficult to separate close to the porus. More medially it is usually easy to separate the two by gentle pressure from above with a blunt instrument. The internal architecture of nerve fibers within the eight nerve is still insufficiently known.

## 2. Ménière's Disease. Aural Vertigo.

This clinical entity was described in 1861 by Prosper Ménière. It consists of the following trias of clinical symptoms: 1. unilateral *tinnitus,* 2. increasing *deafness* of one ear and 3. sudden *attacks of intense vertigo* associated with nystagmus, nausea and vomiting.

The most disabling symptom to the patient is the attacks of vertigo. They usually set on with sudden violence, often forcing him to lay down immediately, or even to fall over. The surroundings seem to rotate, usually from one side to another, sometimes obliquely or even vertically. The patient feels extremely nauseated and soon starts vomiting. The attack lasts for one or two hours, sometimes more. The intervals between the attacks can vary within wide limits—from one or two attacks a year to several attacks a week, when the patient is completely incapacitated. The disease usually starts in the third or fourth decade of life and befalls men and women in about equal degree. The course is usually progressive. Tinnitus is present between the attacks, but is reinforced during the attack. The loss of hearing is also progressive and finally leads to deafness of one ear. It was early noticed that when deafness was complete, the attacks of vertigo would cease.

From the nature of symptoms and also from the relief gived by section of the vestibular nerve it was early concluded, that the causative factors were situated within the labyrinth. From Hallpike's and Cairns' and Mygind's studies it seemed likely that the acute attack would be produced by acute hydrops of the labyrinth. The cause of this acute hydrops is not known with certainty. Allergic factors have been considered. In the majority of cases only one ear is involved. Bilateral involvement is said to occur in 10% (Peet).

The diagnosis is not difficult in typical cases: A history with unilateral tinnitus, loss of hearing on one ear and the description of the attacks. Neurogenic loss of hearing is the only objective sign. There is, however, a considerable confusion concerning terminology from the time Ménière himself believed the syndrome described by him to depend on an intralabyrinthine hemorrhage. Attacks of vertigo without accompanying deafness and tinnitus have been called Ménière's *disease* in contradistinction to Ménière's *syndrome,* by Dandy "*pseudo*-Ménière's *disease*". According to the writers opinion Ménière's name should be attached only to the clinical entity described by him—aural vertigo or Ménière's disease (syndrome). It is this clinical entity that is amenable to surgical interference with the eighth nerve.

Medical treatment has been tried with considerable success. Setting out from the assumption that the changes in the salt and water balance of the body would influence hydrops of the labyrinth, Fürstenberg inaugurated the treatment with ammonium chloride and restriction of the fluid intake. According to the writer's experience a daily dose of 6 grams of ammonium chloride, with or without restricted fluid intake has a marked effect on the frequency of the attacks of vertigo. The cases which react favourably to this treatment are also favourable cases for operation. Good results have been reported from the use of nicotinic acid and thiamine chloride.

The surgical treament consists of complete or partial section of the eighth nerve. The operation introduced by Frenckner (1952) should also be mentioned. It consists of opening the labyrinth and plugging one of the semicircular canals with a small piece of cartilage combined with excision of the tympanic plexus. FRENCKNER's operation can by no means claim the same consistently good results as seen after section of the eighth nerve.

The cases in which surgical treatment should be considered are the severe ones with frequent attacks rendering the patient more or less incapacitated. A strictly unilateral localization is desirable. Even such cases in which the attacks are kept reasonably well under control by ammonium chloride treatment often ask for an operation since their digestion in the long run suffers from the large doses of ammonium chloride and the patient becomes weary of the treatment.

## Section of the Eighth Nerve in MÉNIÈRE's Syndrome.

Partial section of the eighth nerve, saving the cochlear portion and transecting only the vestibular fibers was introduced by McKENZIE in 1932. Independently of him also DANDY performed this operation in 1933. It has since then become the method of choice, as hearing is preserved and even improved after the operation. Large series of cases in which this technique has been applied were published by DANDY, OLIVECRONA a. o. If the ear is already deaf the whole nerve can be transsected.

The operation is preferably performed under general (intratracheal) anesthesia. Section of the vestibular nerve is not painful but the patient is seized by a sudden most violent giddiness, feeling himself "hurdled through space", and may have difficulties in keeping his head still. Nausea and vomiting is also often seen when air enters the subarachnoidal space. The author prefers a recumbent position with the head supported in a head rest. A unilateral cerebellar exposure is made of the same type as has already been described in cerebellar section of the fifth nerve (Fig. 14). The opening in the bone can be made a trifle smaller, since the auditory nerve lies more superficial and is more accessible than the fifth, but should pass well out laterally and upwards to the edge of the sigmoid sinus. The dura is opened in a T-shaped fashion and the edges held apart by sutures. Sometimes it may be expedient first to empty the posterior cistern but, if the anesthesia is smooth and the pressure in the posterior fossa not unduly high, the cerebello-pontine angle can be approached directly by gently elevating the cerebellar hemisphere until the cistern is encountered and opened. The acoustic nerve is easily identified. It runs laterally and a little upwards. The glossopharyngeal and vagus filaments are situated more caudally. The arachnoid is carefully stripped from the eighth nerve together with a loop of the inferior anterior cerebellar artery, which usually crosses the nerve. The nerve is freed as far medially as possible. As pointed out by OLIVECRONA it is easier to avoid damage to the seventh nerve, and also easier to separate the two portions of the nerve, medially than close to the internal auditory meatus. If gentle pressure is exerted on the nerve from above with a blunt narrow dissector it is usually easy to separate the vestibular portion, which is situated upwards and anteriorly. This portion is then gently elevated on a blunt hook and divided by means of a long, narrow, buttoned, sickle-shaped knife. It is most important to treat the nerve gently and not pull on it. This may damage the facial nerve which is as a rule entirely hidden under the auditory nerve. The only complication of importance that can occur, except injury to the facial nerve, is hemorrhage from the internal auditory artery, which may be inadvertently sectioned together with the nerve.

The artery is small, but the bleeding may still be sufficiently brisk to obscure the field entirely. It can be controlled by application of muscle, fibrine foam or oxycel, but there is a real risk of contusion of the facial nerve. The only case of facial palsy following this operation seen by the author took place because of lesion of the internal auditory artery. After the vestibular nerve has been sectioned, the field is irrigated and the dura closed by interrupted silk sutures. The wound is closed in layers and the patient put under ordinary postoperative control for at least 48 hours.

The postoperative course is usually smooth and the patient may leave his bed on the sixth or seventh day. For the first two or three days he usually complains of double vision.

The mechanism of this symptom is not clear. It may be caused by the lack of normal vestibular impulses from the nuclei to the dorsal longitudinal tract. Nystagmus is also usual in the first postoperative period. Before discharge the caloric reactions should be tested and should, following a successful operation be completely absent on the affected side.

The exclusion of one vestibular apparatus is compensated for gradually. For the first weeks the patient has some giddiness and for one to two months some difficulty in walking in the dark, but equilibrium is gradually restored. As mentioned above hearing may improve somewhat after section of the vestibular nerve. Recurrence is never seen, but *tinnitus* will remain unchanged—and this whether the whole eight nerve has been cut or only the vestibular portion. As mentioned above section of the eight nerve has been performed in serious tinnitus and good results have been reported (Frazier). In the author's experience tinnitus in a deaf ear is inaccessible to surgery. This condition is seen in elderly individuals, almost always combined with marked mental depression. It seems to resemble the syndrome of painful anesthesia following section of the fifth nerve and it is believed that the mechanism is the same in both instances, viz. nuclear changes from lack of the normal influx of impulses. In the two cases in which transection of the eight nerve for intractable tinnitus was tried by the author the results were entirely negative.

## H. The Glossopharyngeal Nerve.

### 1. Surgical Anatomy and Physiology.

The glossopharyngeal nerve emerges from the lateral aspect of the medulla oblongata immediately cranial to the uppermost vagus filaments at the level of the upper pole of the olivary eminence and runs laterally and somewhat cranially to the foramen jugulare. The diameter of the intracranial portion of the nerve is a little more than one mm. Towards the jugular foramen converge also the root filaments of the vagus and the spinal accessory nerves. These filaments are smaller in diameter than the ninth nerve root, which is easy to distinguish from the other two nerves, even if they run closely together. The glossopharyngeal nerve is mainly, perhaps entirely, a sensory nerve (Dandy), which is contrary to previous concepts, according to which the nerve is mixed. After transsection of the glossopharyngeal nerve there is no lateral shift of the posterior wall of the pharynx ("signe de rideau") and no impairment of the act of deglutition. The area innervated by the glossopharyngeal nerve covers the tonsillar region and extends upwards including the ostium of the Eustachian tube. Most of the pyriform recess and the base of the tongue is also innervated by this nerve. The taste fibres from the posterior third of the tongue also run in this nerve. The sensory ganglia of the nerve are the ganglion superius and the ganglion petrosum. It receives an important branch of partly unmyelinated fibres from the carotid sinus (the nerve of Hering). If the acidity, i.e. the carbon dioxide content of the blood, is increased, respiration will be accelerated by way of a reflex mechanism in which the glossopharyngeal nerve forns the afferent part, as has been conclusively proved in animal experiments. It is therefore remarkable that transsection of the nerve in man does not affect respiration.

### 2. Glossopharyngeal Neuralgia and its Treatment.

A paroxysmal type of pain localized to the tonsillar region was described in 1920 by Sicard and Robineau. Harris was the first to associate this type of neuralgia with the glossopharyngeal nerve. Already in 1910 Weisenburg had described a case of aching pain in the throat from tumor involvement, which he supposed to be mediated by the glossopharyngeal nerve. Extracranial section of the ninth nerve was performed by Adson 1924. Intracranial section of the nerve was introduced by Temple Fay (1926) and Dandy (1927).

Glossopharyngeal neuralgia is a rare disease. Only two cases were seen by the author in the last 13 years. The largest series of glossopharyngeal tic which has been published was presented by PEET in 1935, comprising 14 cases of which two were bilateral.

There is a close clinical resemblance between glossopharyngeal neuralgia and major trigeminal neuralgia. In both instances pain is paroxysmal and brought about by external stimulation, and in both instances periods of pain alternate with completely free intervals. The localization of pain is, however, different: In glossopharyngeal neuralgia pain is felt in the throat, in the tonsillar region with irradiation towards the ear, and is elicited by the act of swallowing. Pain is said to be even worse than in trigeminal neuralgia, and the condition still more unbearable because of the patient's inability to avoid the involuntary swallowing movements. An important diagnostic criterion is the cocainization of the tonsillar region, which will arrest the paroxysms immediately.

Intracranial section of the glossopharyngeal nerve is the best and safest way to relieve this condition. In accordance with the investigations of BRODAL tractotomy also should relieve glossopharyngeal pain, but, due to the ease and safety of glossopharyngeal nerve section, this must remain the method of choice. The nerve is accessible either from a small unilateral exposure or from a midline incision with removal of some of the bone around the foramen magnum. After the dura has been opened and the posterior cistern evacuated by suction, the glossopharyngeal nerve, which is unaccompanied by vessels is picked up by a blunt hook and divided. According to DANDY the uppermost vagus filaments may be transected also. In the two cases seen by the author section of the ninth nerve alone was sufficiently completely to stop the pain.

In dull aching pain from malignant tumor invasion of the glossopharyngeal nerve trunk—seen especially in carcinoma of the base of the tongue and of the hypopharynx—the nerve should be sectioned intracranially and the operation combined with tractotomy and section of the upper cervical roots (Fig. 20). In these cases a midline incision is preferable with removal of the two upper cervical laminae.

As to other cranial nerves the *spinal accessory nerve* and its role in the treatment of spastic torticollis is reported in vol. IV. The *vagus* nerve has not been the subject of surgery with exception of peripheral section in gastric and duodenal ulcer, which procedures fall outside the scope of neurosurgery. It should be mentioned, however, that damage to the vagus rootlets, e.g. in the removal of tumors of the cerebello-pontine angle will result in recurrent nerve paresis with hoarseness, disturbances in swallowing and also in the motor function of the oesophagus with reflux of gastric contents. This is an extremely dangerous condition carrying imminent risk of aspiration and pneumonia.

The *hypoglossal* nerve, finally, is used in nerve anastomosis with the facial nerve, as described above.

## References.


ADSON, A. W.: Surgical treatment of glossopharyngeal neuralgia. Arch. of Neur. **12**, 487 (1924).

— Diagnosis and surgical treatment of trigeminal neuralgia. Ann. of Otol. **35**, 601 (1926).

ALTMANN, F.: Mschr. Ohrenheilk. **69**, 1032 (1935); **71**, 1287 (1937).

ANTONI. N. R. E.: Über Rückenmarkstumoren und Neurofibrome. München: J. F. Bergmann 1920.

AUDIBERT, V., D. MATTEI et A. PAGANELLI: La paralysie faciale périphérique dite "à frigore" est fonction d'une atteinte artérielle des vasa nervorum. Presse méd. **1936**, 1049.

BÄRENSPRUNG, A. v.: Beitrag zur Kenntnis des zoster. Annat. Charite-Krankh. **11**, 96 (1863).

BAKAY, L.: Zit. Pain, Its Mechanisms and Neurosurgical Control by J. C. WHITE and W. H. SWEET. Springfield: Ch. C. Thomas 1955.

BALLANCE, C. A.: Operative treatment of chronic facial palsy of peripheral origin. Brit. Med. J. **1903**, 1288

—, and A. B. DUEL: Operative treatment of facial palsy. Arch. of Otolaryng. **15**, 1 (1932).

BEHRMAN, W.: Surgical treatment of peripheral facial paralysis in fractures of the cranial base. Acta oto-laryng. (Stockh.) **37**, 189 (1949).

BELL, CHARLES: The nervous system. 3. edit. London 1844.

BRODAL, A.: Central course of afferent fibres for pain in facial, glossopharyngeal and vagus nerves. Arch. of Neur. **57**, 292 (1947).
BUNNELL, S.: Surgical repair of the facial nerve. Arch. of Otolaryng. **25**, 235 (1937).
— Summation of papers on management of facial paralysis. Arch. of Otolaryng. **55**, 417 (1952).
BUSCH, E.: Personal communication.
CASTELLANO, F.: Ménière's disease and its surgical treatment. Report of 300 cases. J. of Neurosurg. 8, 173 (1951).
CAWTHORNE, T.: Nerve grafting in facial paralysis. Trans. Med. Soc. Lond. 171 (1938).
— Peripheral facial paralysis. Some aspects of its pathology. Laryngoscope **56**, 653 (1946).
— Proc. Roy. Soc. Med. **44**, 565 (1951).
— The rôle of surgery in the investigation and treatment of peripheral facial palsy. Lancet **1952** 1219.
CLARKE, L. P., and A. S. TAYLOR: Tic douleureux of the sensory filaments of the geniculate ganglion: Operation, recovery. J. Nerv. Dis. **37**, 242 (1910).
COLEMAN, C. C.: Results of facio-hypoglossal anastomosis in treatment of facial paralysis. Ann. Surg. **111**, 958 (1940).
— Surgical treatment of facial spasm. Ann. Surg. **105**, 647 (1937).
COLLIER, J.: The present position of facial nerve surgery. Ann. of Otol. **58**, 686 (1949).
— The treatment of facial paralysis. Proc. Roy. Soc. Med. **43**, 746 (1950).
CRAIG, W. McK.: Diagnosis and treatment of trigeminal neuralgia. South. Surg. **10**, 17 (1941).
CUNNINGHAM, J.: Textbook of anatomy, 2. edit. Edinburgh and London 1906.
CUSHING, H.: A method for total exstirpation of the GASSERian ganglion for trigeminal neuralgia. J. Amer. Med. Assoc. **34**, 1035 (1900).
— Surgical treatment of facial paralysis by nerve anastomosis. Ann Surg. **37**, 641 (1903).
DANDY, W. E.: Section of the sensory root of the trigeminal nerve at the pons. Bull. Johns Hopkins Hosp. **36**, 105 (1925).
— An operation for the cure of tic douleureux. Arch. Surg. **18**, 687 (1929).
— Operative relief from pain in the mouth, tongue and throat. Arch. Surg. **19**, 143 (1929).
— Certain functions of the roots and ganglia of the cranial sensory nerves. Arch. of Neur. **27**, 22 (1932).
— The brain. Dean Lewis's Practice of Surgery. Hagerstown 1932.
— Ménière's disease. Diagnosis and treatment. Amer. J. Surg. **20**, 693 (1933).
— Ménière's disease. Arch. Surg. **16**, 1127 (1928).
— Treatment of Ménière's disease by section of only the vestibular portion of the acoustic nerve. Bull. Johns Hopkins Hosp. **53**, 52 (1933).
DAVIS, L. E.: The deep sensibility of the face . Arch. of Neur. **9**, 283 (1923).
— Neurological surgery. London 1936.
—, and H. A. HAVEN: Surgical anatomy of the sensory root of the trigeminal nerve. Arch of Neur. **29**, 1 (1933).
DODGE, H. W., and J. G. LOVE: Surgical treatment of trigeminal neuralgia in the older age groups. J. Amer. Geriatrics Soc. **2**, 467 (1954).
DOGLIOTTI, M.: First surgical section in man of the lemniscus lateralis (pain-temperature path) at the brain stem for the treatment of diffuse rebellious pain. Anesth. a. Analg. **17**, 143 (1938).
— Chirurgia del n. trigemino e del n. faciale. Arch. ital. Chir. **44**, 667 (1936).
EPSTEIN, L.: Herpes zoster following operations for facial pain. Acta psychiatr. (Københ.) **23**, 13 (1948).
FALCONER, M. A.: Intramedullary trigeminal tractotomy and its place in the treatment of facial pain. J. Neurol., Neurosurg. a. Psychiatry **12**, 297 (1949).
FALLOPPIO, G.: Observationes anatomicae. Venice 1561.
FARRIOR, J. B., and P. C. CALDWELL: Facial nerve paralysis resulting from fracture of the temporal bone: report of a case. New Orleans Med. a. Surg. J. **100**, 23 (1947).
FAY, TEMPLE: Intracranial division of glossopharyngeal nerve combined with cervical rhizotomy for pain in inoperable carcinoma of the throat. Ann. Surg. **84**, 456 (1926).
FINDEISEN, L., u. W. TÖNNIS: Über intrakranielle Epidermoide. Zbl. Neurochir. **2**, 301 (1938).
FINDLAY, J.: Facial paralysis. Published by the author, Sydney 1950.
FOERSTER, O.: Die Leitungsbahnen des Schmerzgefühls und die chirurgischen Behandlung der Schmerzzustände. Berlin u. Wien 1927.
FOTHERGILL, J.: A painful affection of the face. London 1776. Zit. L. DAVIS.
FRAZIER, C. H.: A surgeon's impression of trigeminal neuralgia. J. Amer. Med. Assoc. **70**, 1345 (1918).
— Pain phenomena of the face, their origin and treatment. Amer. J. Med. Sci. **169**, 469 (1925).
— Subtotal resection of sensory root for relief of major trigeminal neuralgia. Arch. of Neur. **13**, 378 (1925).
— Operation for the radical cure of trigeminal neuralgia. Ann. Surg. **88**, 534 (1928).
— Atypical neuralgia. Arch. of Neur. **19**, 650 (1928).
— Bilateral trigeminal neuralgia. Ann. Surg. **100**, 770 (1934).
—, and F. H. LEWY, and S. N. ROWE: Origin and mechanism of paroxysmal neurologic pain and the surgical treatment of central pain. Brain **60**, 44 (1937).
—, and E. C. RUSSELL: Neuralgia of the face: Analysis of 754 cases. Arch. of Neur. **11**, 563 (1924).

FRAZIER, C. H., and E. WHITEHEAD: The morphology of the GASSERian ganglion. Brain **48**, 458 (1926).
FRENCKNER, P.: Some view-points in the treatment of Ménière's disease. Arch. of Otolaryng. **55**, 420 (1952).
FÜRSTENBERG, A. C., F. H. LASHMET and F. LATHROP: Ménière's symptom complex. Medical treatment. Ann. of Otol. **43**, 1015 (1934).
— G. RICHARDSON and F. LATHROP: Ménière's disease. Addenda to medical treatment. Arch. of Otolaryng. **34**, 1083 (1941).
GALEN: Galeni opera omnia, edit. C. G. KÜHN. Leipzig 1821—1833.
GARDNER, W. J., and J. A. BABBITT: Occurrence of tympanic hemorrhage follow. radical operation for relief of trigeminal neuralgia. Ann. of Otol. **38**, 1040 (1929).
— A. STOWELL and R. DUTLINGER: Resection of greater superficial petrosal nerve in treatment of unilateral headache. J. of Neurosurg. **4**, 105 (1947).
GERMAN, W. J.: Surgical treatment of spasmodic facial tic. Surgery **11**, 912 (1942).
GLASER, M. A.: Atypical neuralgia, so-called. A critical analysis of 143 cases. Arch. of Neur. **20**, 537 (1928).
— Atypical facial neuralgia: Diagnosis, cause and treatment. Arch. Int. Med. **65**, 340 (1940).
GRANIT, R., L. LEKSELL and C. R. SKOGLUND: Fibre interaction in injured and compressed region of nerve. Brain **67**, 125 (1944).
GRANT, F. C.: Major trigeminal neuralgia. Amer. J. Surg., N. S. **27**, 430 (1935).
— Results in operative treatment of major trigeminal neuralgia. Ann. Surg. **107**, 14 (1938).
GUIDETTI, B.: Tractotomy for the relief of trigeminal neuralgia: Observations in 124 cases. J. of Neurosurg. **7**, 499 (1950).
GUTTMAN, M. REESE, and U. MARSHALL SIMON: Neurofibrosarcoma of the facial nerve involving the tympanomastoid. Arch. of Otolaryng. **54**, 162 1951.
HÄRTEL, F.: Behandlung der Trigeminusneuralgie mit intrakraniellen Alkoholeinspritzungen. Dtsch. Z. Chir. **126**, 429 (1914).
HALLPIKE, C. S., and H. CAIRNS: Observations on the pathology of Ménière's syndrome. J. of Laryng. **53**, 625 (1938).
HARRIS, W.: Alcohol injection of the GASSERian ganglion for trigeminal neuralgia. Lancet **1912, I**, 218.
— Neuritis and neuralgia. London: Oxford Univ. Press 1926.
— The Facial Neuralgias. London: Oxford Univ. Press 1937.
HARTLEY, F.: Intracranial neurectomy of the second and third divisions of the fifth nerve. A new method. N. Y. Med. J. **55**, 317 (1892).
HILGER, J. A.: The nature of Bell's palsy. Laryngoscope **59**, 228 (1949).
HORRAX, G., and J. L. POPPEN: Trigeminal neuralgia: Experiences with and treatment employed in 468 patients during the past ten years. Surg., Gynec. Obst. **61**, 394 (1935).
HORSLEY, V., and O. MAY: The mesencephalic root of the fifth nerve. Brain **33**, 175 (1910).
HOVELAQUE, A.: Anatomie des nerfs craniens et rachidiens et du systeme grand sympathique chez l'homme. Paris 1927.
HULLES, E.: Beitrag zur Kenntnis der sensiblen Wurzel der Medulla oblongata. Arb. neur. Inst. Wien. **13**, 392 (1906).
JIMENEZ GONZALES, L.: Topografia del tractus spinalis nervi trigemini en relacion con la operacion de la tractotomia. Arch. españ. Morf. **4**, 23 (1944).
KETTEL, K.: Bell's palsy. Arch. of Otolaryng. **46**, 427 (1947).
— The prognosis of nerve grafting and nerve suture in pheripheral facial palsies. Acta otolaryng. (Stockh.) Suppl. **74**, 180 (1948).
— Peripheral facial paralysis in fractures of the temporal bone. Arch. of Otolaryng. **51**, 25 (1950).
— Neurinoma of the facial nerve. Arch. of Otolaryng. **44**, 253 (1946).
KIRSCHNER, M.: Zur Elektrochirurgie. Arch. klin. Chir. **167**, 761 (1931).
— Punktionstechnik und Elektrokoagulation des Ganglion Gasseri. Arch. klin. Chir. **176**, 581(1933).
— Zur Behandlung der Trigeminusneuralgie. Arch. klin. Chir. **186**, 325 (1936).
KÖLLIKER, A.: Mikroskopische Anatomie und Gewebslehre des Menschen. Leipzig 1850.
KÖRTE, N., u. M. BERNHARDT: Fall von Nervenpropfung des n. facialis auf den n. hypoglossus. Dtsch. med. Wschr. **1903**, 293.
KRAUSE, F.: Die Neuralgie des Trigeminus nebst der Anatomie und Physiologie des Nerven. Leipzig 1896.
LATHROP, F. D.: The repair of traumatic lesions of the facial nerve secondary to war wounds. The Surgical Clinics of North America, June 1946, Lahey Clinic number.
— Facial nerve surgery in the European theater of operations. Laryngoscope **56**, 665 (1946).
— Management of traumatic lesions of the facial nerve. Arch. of Otolaryng. **55**, 410 (1952).
— The practical anatomical and surgical considerations for exposure of the facial nerve. Laryngoscope 58, 743 (1948).
LOVE, J. G.: Decompression of the GASSERian ganglion and its posterior root for trigeminal neuralgia. Post-Graduate J. Med. **15**, 1 (1954).

Love, J. G., and H. J. Svien: Results of decompression operation for trigeminal neuralgia. J. of Neurosurg. **11**, 499 (1954).
Magnusson, J. H., u. G. Wohlfart: Beitrag zur Klinik und Pathologie der Zostererkrankung mit besonderer Rücksicht des Vorkommens meningo-encephalitischer Veränderungen. Dtsch. Z. Nervenheilk. **153**, 225 (1941).
Martin, R. C.: Bell's palsy. Arch. of Otolaryng. **55**, 405 (1952).
— Intratemporal suture of the facial nerve. Arch. of Otolaryng. **13**, 259 (1931).
McKenzie, K. G.: Intracranial division of the vestibular portion of the auditory nerve for intractable vertigo. Trans. Acad. Med. Toronto **14** (1932/33).
Ménière, P.: Sur une forme de surdite grave dependant d'une lesion de l'oreille interne. Bull. Acad. imp. med. **26**, 241 (1861).
Meynert, Th.: Vom Gehirn der Säugethiere. In Strickers Lehrbuch von den Geweben, Bd. 2, S. 694. 1872.
Ney, K. W.: Facial paralysis and the surgical repair of the facial nerve. Laryngoscope **32**, 327 (1922).
Norlén, G.: Personal communication.
Olivecrona, H.: Tractotomy for relief of trigeminal neuralgia. Arch. of Neur. **47**, 544 (1942).
— The surgery of pain. Acta psychiatr. (Københ.) **46**, 268 (1948).
— On section of the trigeminus at the pons. Acta chir. scand. (Stockh.) **61**, 366 (1927).
— Über doppeltseitige Trigeminusneuralgie. Arch. klin. Chir. **164**, 196 (1931).
— Die chirurgische Behandlung der Ménièreschen Krankheit. Münch. med. Wschr. **1943**, 466. Siehe Castellano.
Peet, M. M.: Post-herpetic trigeminal neuralgia: Persistence of pain after section of sensory root of Gasserian ganglion. J. Amer. Med. Assoc. **92**, 1503 (1929).
— Glossopharyngeal neuralgia. Ann. Surg. **101**, 256 (1935).
—, and D. H. Echols: Surgery of disorders of cranial nerves. In surgical treatment of the nervous system (edit. Bancroft and Pilcher), p. 249. Philadelphia 1946.
—, and R. C. Schneider: Trigeminal neuralgia: 689 cases with follow-up study of 65 pct. of the group. J. of Neurosurg. **9**, 367 (1952).
Pitres, J. A., et T. P. H. Verger: Nevralgie faciale traitée par les injections modificatrices d'alcool. Soc. de Med. et de Chir. de Bourdeaux 1902.
Portugal, J. Ribe: O tratamento cirurgico da trigeminalgia, neurotomia retrogasseriana por via temporal, intradural. O Hospital **1946**, 501.
Ramsay Hunt, J.: The sensory system of the facial nerve and its symptomatology. J. Nerv. Dis. **36**, 321 (1909).
— Geniculate neuralgia (neuralgia of the nervus facialis). A further contribution to the sensory system of the facial nerve and its neuralgic conditions. Arch. of Neur. **37**, 253 (1937).
Retzius, G.: Untersuchungen über die Nervenzellen der cerebrospinalen Ganglien und der übrigen peripherischen Kopfganglien mit besonderer Rücksicht auf die Zellausläufer. Arch. f. Anat. **4**, 369 (1880).
Sachs, E.: Diagnosis and treatment of trigeminal neuralgia. Tri-State Med. J. **7**, 1416 (1935).
Schloesser, C.: Erfahrungen in der Neuralgiebehandlung mit Alkoholeinspritzungen. Verh. Kongr. inn. Med. **24**, 49 (1907).
Shelden, C. Hunter, Robert H. Pudenz, Donald B. Freshwater and Benjamin L. Crue: Compression wather than decompression for trigeminal neuralgia. J. of Neurosurg. 12, 123 (1955).
Sicard, J. A., et Robinaeu: Communications et presentations. I. Algie velopharyngée essentielle. Traitement chirurgical. Revue neur. **34**, 256 (1920).
Sjöqvist, O.: Neue Operationsmethode bei Trigeminusneuralgie: Durchschneidung d. tractus spinalis trigemini. Zbl. Neurochir. **2**, 274 (1938).
— Studies on pain conduction in the trigeminal nerve. A contribution to the surgical treatment of facial pain. Acta psychiatr. (Københ.) Suppl. **17** (1938).
— Trigeminal neuralgia. A review of its surgical treatment and some aspects of its etiology. Acta chir. scand. (Stockh.) **82**, 201 (1939).
— Ten years experience with trigeminal tractotomy. Brasil Med.-Cir. **10**, 259 (1948).
— Surgical section of pain tracts and pathways in the spinal cord and brain stem. IV. Congr. Neurol. Internat. Paris 1949, p. 119.
—, and E. Weinstein: Effect of section of the medial lemniscus on proprioceptive functions in chimpanzees and monkeys. J. of Neurophysiol. **5**, 69 (1942).
Spiller, W. G., and C. H. Frazier: Tic douloureux. Anatomic and clinical basis for subtotal section of sensory root of trigeminal nerve. Arch. of Neur. **29**, 50 (1933).
Stender, A.: "Gangliolysis" for the surgical treatment of trigeminal neuralgia. J. of Neurosurg. **11**, 333 (1954).
Sullivan, J. A.: The practical anatomical and surgical considerations for exposure of the facial nerve. The American Laryngo-rhinootological Soc., Inc. Atlantic City, New Jersey, april 7, 1948.
— A modification of the Ballance-Duel technique in the treatment of facial paralysis. Trans. Amer. Acad. Ophthalm. a. Otolaryng. **1936**.

SULLIVAN, J. A.: The surgical treatment of facial palsy by an autoplastic nerve graft. Canad. Med. Assoc. J. **34**, 474 (1934).
— The otological concept of Bell's palsy and its treatment. Ann. of Otol. **59**, 1148 (1950).
— Recent advances in the surgical treatment of facial paralysis and Bell's palsy. Laryngoscope **62**, 449 (1952).
TAARNHØJ, P.: Ny operation ved trigeminusneuralgi. Dekompression af trigeminusroden og gangliets bageste del. Nord. Med. **47**, 360 (1952).
— Decompression of the trigeminal root and the posterior part of the ganglion as treatment in trigeminal neuralgia. Preliminary communication. J. of Neurosurg. **9**, 288 (1952).
TICKLE, T. G.: The surgical treatment of facial paralysis. In S. KOPETZKY, Surgery of the ear. New York: Thomas Nelson & Sons 1939.
— Surgery of the facial nerve in 300 operated cases. Laryngoscope **1945**.
TÖNNIS, W., u. H. KREISSEL: Die Traktotomie nach SJÖQVIST in der Behandlung der Trigeminusneuralgie. Zbl. Chir. **75**, 873 (1950).
TURNER, J. W. A.: Facial palsy in closed head injuries: prognosis. Lancet **1944**, 756.
VESALIUS, GABRIEL: De humani corporis fabrica libri septem. Basle 1543.
WALKER, E. A.: Anatomy, physiology and surgical considerations if the spinal tract of the trigeminal nerve. J. of Neurophysiol. **2**, 234 (1939).
— Origin, course and terminations of the secondary pathways of the trigeminal nerve in primates. J. Comp. Neur. 71, 59 (1939).
— Mesencephalic tractotomy. A method for the relief of unilateral intractable pain. Arch. Surg. **44**, 953 (1942).
— Relief of pain by mesencephalic tractotomy. Arch. of Neur. **48**, 865 (1942).
— The neurosurgical treatment of intractable pain. Lancet **1950** I, 279.
— Section of the sensory root in the posterior fossa. New York Acad. Med. **1953**.
WEINBERGER, L. M., and F. C. GRANT: Experiences with. intramedullary tractotomy. Arch. of Neur. **49**, 665 (1943).
WEISSENBURG, T. H.: Cerebello-pontine tumor diagnosed for six years as tic doulereux. The symptoms of irritation of the ninth and twelth cranial nerves. J. Amer. Med. Assoc. **54**, 1600 (1910).
WILLIAMS, H. L. et al.: The problem of synkinesis and contracture in cases of hemifacial spasm and Bell's palsy. Ann. of Otol. **61**, 850 (1952).
—, and P. N. PASTORE: Neurofibroma of facial nerve in facial canal: destruction of labyrinth and mastoid process. Arch. of Otolaryng. **29**, 977 (1939).
WOHLFART, G.: Über den inneren Bau der peripheren Nervenstämme. Z. mikrosk.-anat. Forsch. **1938**.

# Die Chirurgie der extrapyramidalen Hyperkinesen.

Von

K. Schürmann.

Mit 52 Abbildungen.

Es gibt zur Zeit noch keine Standardoperation in der chirurgischen Behandlung der unkontrollierten Bewegungen.

Bei einem geschichtlichen Rückblick ist man verblüfft über die Vielzahl und die Unterschiedlichkeit der Auffassungen, auf welche Weise man das Problem der unwillkürlichen Bewegungen chirurgisch zu lösen versuchte. Insbesondere haben die vergangenen 2 Jahrzehnte eine Fülle von Beiträgen zur operativen Behandlung bestimmter Formen von Hyperkinesen gebracht. Dennoch sind die bisherigen Ergebnisse auch heute noch weit davon entfernt, sowohl den Kranken als auch den Operateur restlos zufriedenzustellen, obgleich eine Reihe beachtenswerter Resultate erzielt werden konnte. Nun sind es die jüngsten Erfahrungen, welche vor allem mit der weiteren Entwicklung der gezielten Ausschaltungen günstigere Zukunftsaussichten für die chirurgische Beeinflußbarkeit derartiger Krankheitszustände erhoffen lassen.

## Historisches.

Als Parkinson im Jahre 1817 bei einem seiner Tremorkranken mit Eintreten eines apoplektischen Insultes auf der Seite der Hemiplegie den Tremor vollständig verschwinden und dann parallel mit der nachfolgenden Rückbildung der Lähmung auch die Tremorsymptome wiederkehren sah, waren noch keine chirurgisch-therapeutischen Konsequenzen daraus zu ziehen. Ebensowenig waren solche nach der viel später gemachten Beobachtung von Jacob (1923) erfolgt, welcher in gleicher Weise eine halbseitige athetoseähnliche Hyperkinese infolge einer auf der gleichen Körperseite eingetretenen apoplektischen Hemiplegie verschwinden sah. Die abnormen Bewegungen sind aber in diesem Falle, im Gegensatz zum Tremorpatienten von Parkinson, auch nach weitgehender Rückbildung der Halbseitenlähmung *nicht* wiedergekehrt. Diese frühen Beobachtungen, deren weittragende Bedeutung nicht sofort erkannt worden ist, hätten bereits zu einer interessanten und richtungweisenden Schlußfolgerung führen können: *die dauerhafte Unterdrückung der Tremorsymptome scheint weitgehend an eine möglichst vollständige Unterbrechung der langen Pyramidenbahnen gebunden zu sein, während athetotische Bewegungen anscheinend schon durch eine unvollständige Schädigung dieser (und benachbarter Systeme) gedrosselt werden können.* Umgekehrt ist viel später von Kinnear Wilson (1940), unabhängig von den klinischen Ergebnissen, vermutet worden, daß *der Tremor in der Hauptsache von der Integrität der Pyramidenbahnen abhängig sei, während die Choreoathetose in hohem Grade mit der Aktivität des extrapyramidalen Systems in Beziehung stehe.* Diese Mutmaßungen werden jedenfalls durch die bisherigen experimentellen und chirurgischen Erfahrungen weitgehend bestätigt.

Nachdem man sich lange Zeit praktisch vergeblich bemüht hatte, den Kranken mit mehr oder weniger grotesken unwillkürlichen Bewegungen zu helfen, war es dem Pionier der Chirurgie des Zentralnervensystems VICTOR HORSLEY als erstem vergönnt, diesen hilflosen Kranken neue und konkrete Hoffnungen zu machen. Im Jahre 1909 erscheint HORSLEYs erster Bericht über die Rindenexcision bei unwillkürlichen Bewegungen. Entsprechend seiner bescheidenen Art ist diese Mitteilung von HORSLEY nicht etwa in der Form eines enthusiastischen chirurgischen Erfolges aufgemacht worden, sondern im Rahmen einer „Untersuchung über die Funktionen der motorischen Rinde" gegeben worden. Seine klinischen Forschungen zu einer chirurgischen Behandlungsmöglichkeit unwillkürlicher Bewegungen hatten zudem in ausgedehnten tierexperimentellen Untersuchungen eine gut fundierte Grundlage. Man hat ihm unter anderem nachgesagt, daß das Gehirn wohl jedes für ihn irgendwie erreichbaren Tieres durch elektrische Reizversuche untersucht worden sei. In der erwähnten Arbeit von 1909 beschreibt nun HORSLEY auch die Operation eines Knaben, welcher an einer Athetose des linken Armes litt. Er

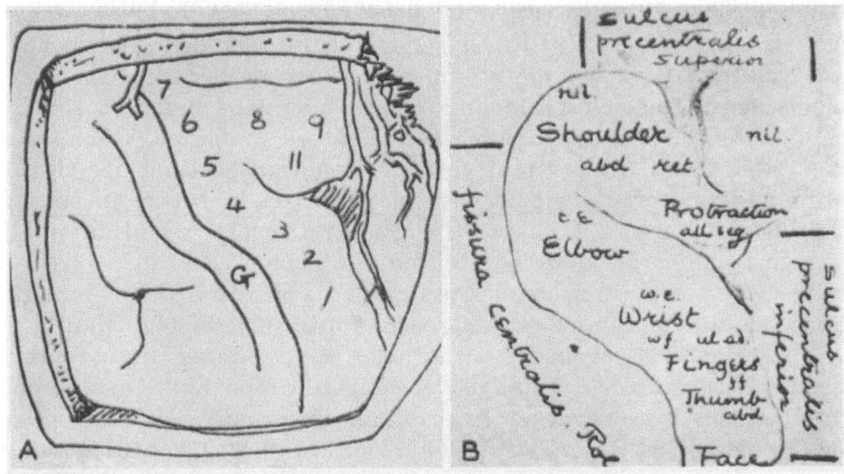


Abb. 1A u. B. HORSLEYs Originalskizze vom Operationsfeld (A) und der Ausdehnung der Rindenresektion (B) in seinem Fall von Athetose. (Aus WALKER.) A Die elektrische Reizung der Punkte *1—11* in A ergab: *1* Bewegung der linken Gesichtsseite; *2* Abduktion des linken Daumens, und bei Wiederholung der Reizung dazu noch eine Beugung aller Finger; *3* Beugung der Finger, Beugung des Handgelenks mit Ulnarabduktion und verzögerter Beugung des Ellenbogengelenks; *4* Streckung der Finger, Ulnarabduktion des Handgelenks, fragliche Beugung des Ellenbogengelenks; *5* Streckung des Handgelenks, Ellenbogengelenk in einem rechten Winkel gehalten; *6* dieselbe Bewegung wie *5* und darüber hinaus eine Abduktion der Schulter; *7* keine Bewegung der oberen Extremität; *8* Ellenbogengelenk in einem rechten Winkel gehalten, kraftvolles Zurückziehen der Schulter; *9* Ellenbogen in einem rechten Winkel, Streckung des Armes und Streckung des Handgelenks; *10* keine Reaktion; *11* Streckung des Armes, Ellenbogen zu einem stumpfen Winkel, Streckung des Handgelenks und fragliche Streckung der Finger. B Die Abkürzungen in B bedeuten: *abd.* Abduktion; *ret.* Retraktion, Zurückziehen; *e. e.* Streckung des Ellenbogens; *w. f.* Beugung des Handgelenks; *ul. ad.* Ulnarabduktion; *f. f.* Fingerbeugung.

schildert darin, wie er zuerst durch eine elektrische Reizung das gesuchte Rindenfeld, welches als Reizantwort eine Bewegung des kontralateralen Armes entstehen läßt, bestimmt, und wie er dann dieses Feld durch eine subpiale Resektion entfernte. Dieser Patient war 13 Monate nach der Operation noch frei von unwillkürlichen Bewegungen, obgleich eine gewisse motorische Funktion des linkenArmes, wie HORSLEY ausdrücklich betont, wiedergekehrt war. Obschon mit diesem Eingriff bereits der Grundstein zu einer Chirurgie der unwillkürlichen unkontrollierten Bewegungen gelegt worden war, wurden damals jedoch die sich aus dieser Pioniertat ergebenden therapeutischen Möglichkeiten noch nicht in ihrer ganzen Bedeutung erfaßt (Abb. 1). In den folgenden Jahren ist dieser Eingriff nur sporadisch ausgeführt worden. Die deutschen Chirurgen ANSCHÜTZ (1910) und PAYR (1921) haben in entsprechender Weise in je einem Falle von Athetose das corticale Armfeld mit angeblich gutem Erfolg abgetragen bzw. unterschnitten. NASAROFF (1927) berichtete an Hand einiger Fälle über die Erfahrungen russischer Chirurgen mit HORSLEYs

Technik. Er selbst unternahm in 2 Fällen von Athetose den originellen Versuch, Alkohol in das motorische Armfeld zu injizieren. In beiden Fällen seien die abnormen Bewegungen gebessert worden, aber leider wurden die Kranken nur wenige Monate weiter verfolgt. Die 1937 von NAFFZIGER nochmals aufgegriffene intracorticale Alkoholinjektion hat jedoch unter 4 Fällen nur in einem Falle zu einer gewissen Besserung geführt.

Der Bericht HORSLEYs war, von den genannten Ausnahmen abgesehen, schon fast in Vergessenheit geraten. Erst einige Jahrzehnte später, nachdem das Interesse für die Funktionen der Hirnrinde dank der neurophysiologischen Untersuchungen FULTONs und seiner Schule (1932—1936) wiederbelebt wurde, hat man sich jener Mitteilung erinnert und wurde die Neurochirurgie erneut angeregt, sich dem Problem der Bewegungsstörungen zu widmen.

## Anatomische, physiologische und pathophysiologische Vorbemerkungen.

In der Hirnanatomie und Hirnphysiologie sind seit den klassischen Forschungsergebnissen Ende des 19. Jahrhunderts mit Verbesserung der klinischen, experimentellen und histologischen Untersuchungstechnik beachtliche neue Erkenntnisse hinzugewonnen worden. Es überschreitet aber die Aufgabe des Autors, in diesem Abschnitt einen genauen Plan vom anatomischen Aufbau und von der Funktionsleistung der Großhirnrinde und des extrapyramidalmotorischen Systems zu geben, da hierüber im ersten Band dieses Handbuches berichtet wird. An dieser Stelle seien aber einige einführende Bemerkungen zu diesen noch recht wechselhaft beurteilten Problemen erlaubt.

Den frühen *Anatomen* war schon bekannt, daß die Hirnrinde kein einheitlicher, sondern in Durchmesser und Zusammensetzung sehr unterschiedlicher Mantel ist. Die von CAMPBELL im Jahre 1905 gegebene ausführliche Beschreibung der cytoarchitektonischen Gliederung der Hirnrindenfelder hat in der Folgezeit eine Flut von beispiellosen Untersuchungen über den histologischen Aufbau der Hirnrinde ausgelöst. Doch waren die Forschungsergebnisse von BRODMANN (1909), von C. und O. VOGT (1919) und von ECONOMO und KOSKINAS (1925) trotz ihrer Exaktheit so verschieden, daß die Grenzen der cytoarchitektonischen Felder bei jedem Untersucher woanders lagen. Die ursprüngliche Unterteilung ist von jedem neuen Bearbeiter abermals unterteilt worden und nur die Anzahl der Rindenneurone schien für eine exakte Begrenzung der Felder konstant zu sein. LASHLEY und CLARKE (1946) fanden schließlich, daß beim Affen nur einige Rindengebiete cytoarchitektonisch übereinstimmten und nur wenige Grenzen mit einem gewissen Grad an Wahrscheinlichkeit zu bestimmen waren. Kurz darauf haben dann v. BONIN und BAILEY (1947) darauf hingewiesen, daß diese Abgrenzungsschwierigkeiten auch aus den älteren Karten vom Menschen hervorgingen. Die jüngste Karte von der Hirnrinde, welche auf v. BONIN (1949) zurückgeht, zeigt die folgenden Felder in der Präzentralregion (s. Abb. 2).

Die Anschauungen über *die Funktion der motorischen Rinde* waren gleichfalls manchem Wechsel unterworfen. Das Hauptschema der frühen Autoren, wie das von FERRIER (1876), ist in seinen Kernpunkten später bestätigt worden. Gewisse neue Erkenntnisse ließen sich diesem ohne Zwang hinzufügen.

Im Jahre 1937 wurde dann von M. HINES entdeckt, daß die Reizung eines Rindenstreifens, welcher im vorderen Teil der reizbaren motorischen Rinde gelegen war, eine „Unterdrückung“ (Suppression) der Muskelkontraktion der Gegenseite hervorruft. Die Entfernung dieses „Unterdrücker“-Streifens (Suppressorband) verhindere, wie er behauptet, das Auftreten von Spastizität an der kontralateralen Gliedmaßenmuskulatur. DUSSER DE BARENNE (1941) hat den von dieser Beobachtung abgeleiteten Gedanken mit Hilfe der Strychninneuronographie weiter verfolgt und ausgearbeitet. Er kam zu der Auffassung, daß noch andere „Suppressor“-Streifen in den Stirn- und Scheitellappen bestehen. Die Hypothese von der Existenz eines ganzen „Unterdrücker“-Systems führte zur Aufstellung sorgfältig ausgearbeiteter Schemata über die Wechselbeziehungen zwischen Hirnrinde und Stammganglien. Schließlich wurden aber berechtigte Zweifel an der wirklichen Existenz dieser „Suppressor"-Streifen beim Affen, zumindest in ihrer ursprünglich angenommenen Form, geäußert. Beim Menschen konnte von vornherein kein schlüssiger Beweis für das Vorhandensein eines derartigen „Unterdrücker"-Systems erbracht werden, obzwar bei Reizung bestimmter Rindengebiete eine „Unterdrückung", „Hemmung" bzw. „Bremsung" in dem genannten Sinne erzeugt werden konnte. Dagegen scheint die Aufdeckung der zweiten motorischen und sensorischen Rindenfelder durch ADRIAN (1950) von größerer Bedeutung zu sein. Seine Befunde konnten im Tierexperiment von WOOLSEY (1947) und beim Menschen von PENFIELD u. a. (1950) erweitert werden. Die gegenwärtige Auffassung von der Organisation der motorischen Rinde wird in der Karte von PENFIELD und RASMUSSEN wiedergegeben.

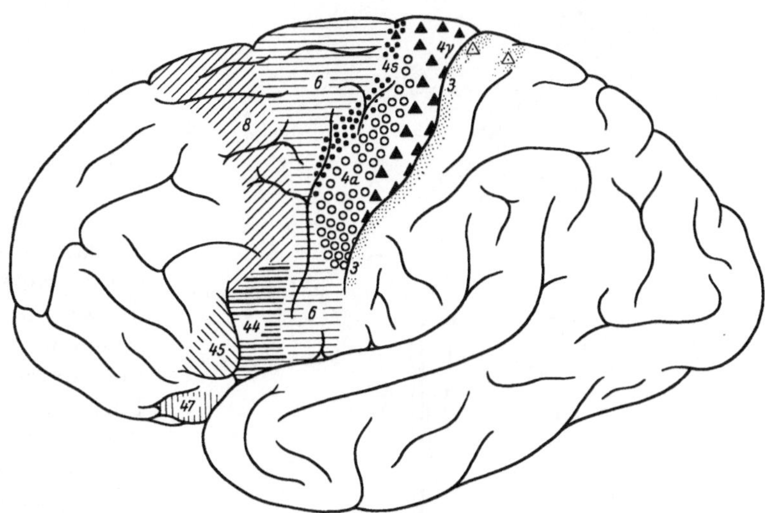


Abb. 2. Von BONINS Karte der cytoarchitektonischen Felder der Hirnrinde in der Präzentralregion.

*Area 4γ* Area gigantopyramidalis (BETZsche Riesenzellen), von welcher die langen Fasern ausgehen, welche mehr als 10% der Pyramidenbahnen ausmachen; *Area 4a* ähnlich der Area 4, enthält aber keine BETZschen Zellen; *Area 4s* ist gekennzeichnet durch das Vorhandensein von großen Pyramidenzellen in der 4. Schicht; *Area 6* ist ein Feld ohne Körnerschicht, welche ein Säulenmuster besitzt.

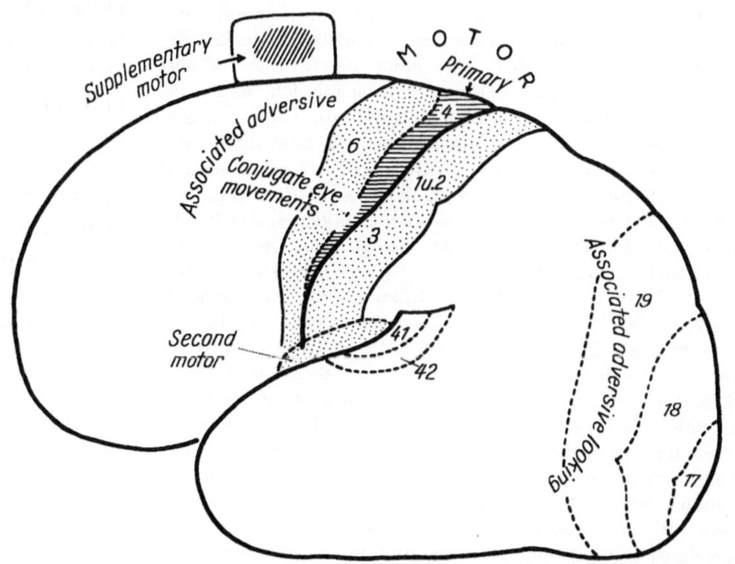


Abb. 3. PENFIELD und RASMUSSENS Karte von der Organisation der motorischen Rinde beim Menschen.

Von WALKER (1952) wird schließlich mit Nachdruck hervorgehoben, daß die prä- und postzentralen Windungen — reizphysiologisch gesehen — equipotentiale motorische Felder sind, da auf elektrische Reize gleichartige Reaktionen erfolgen. Nach seinen Angaben ist allerdings der vordere Rand des Sulcus centralis vom motorischen Hauptfeld durch seine niedrigere Reizschwelle zu unterscheiden.

Die klinischen, pathologisch-anatomischen und experimentellen Untersuchungen über die *Funktion der Stammganglien* machten wahrscheinlich, daß die subcorticalen Ganglien auf ein „Bewegungsmuster" regulierend einwirken.

Schon JACOB (1923) vertrat die Auffassung, daß das extrapyramidale Hauptsystem die Impulse des Mittelhirns und Hirnstamms mit ihren cerebellaren Verstärkungen

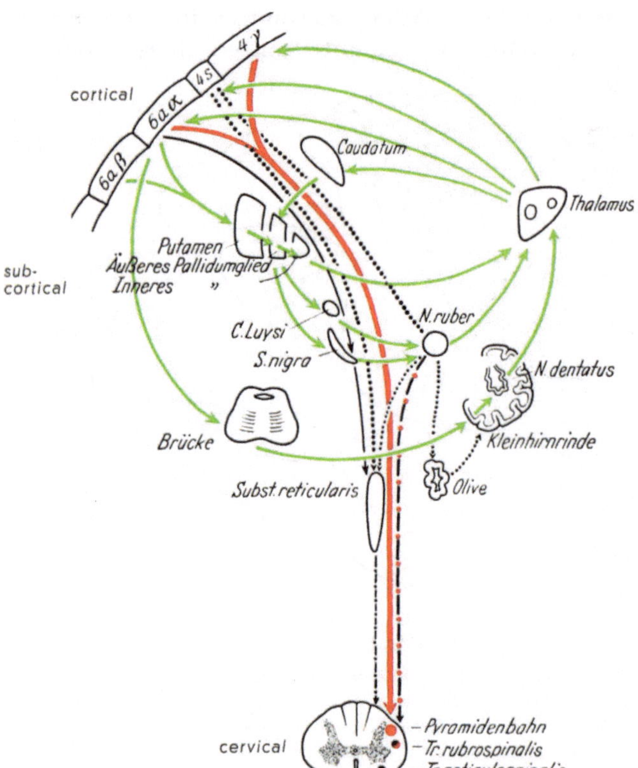


Abb. 4. Schematische Darstellung des sog. „Rücksteuerungssystems" zur Eigenkontrolle des motorischen Impulses, welches im wesentlichen aus drei neben- und nacheinandergeschalteten cortico-subcortico-corticalen Erregungskreisen besteht. Die *erste* ringförmige Rücksteuerung zur Rinde verläuft wahrscheinlich über das Striopallidum und den Thalamus direkt zur Rinde zurück. Die *zweite* führt über die Substantia nigra bzw. auch über das Corpus subthalamicum Luysi, den Nucleus ruber und den Thalamus zur Rinde zurück. Die *dritte* schließlich erreicht wahrscheinlich über die Brückenkerne, das Kleinhirn und den Thalamus wieder die Rinde. Das sind im wesentlichen die der *Eigenkontrolle* des motorischen Impulses dienenden Apparate. Hinzu kommt die *Fremdkontrolle* der Körperhaltung, -lage usw. und der bereits ablaufenden Bewegungen. Die dieser Fremdkontrolle dienenden afferenten Impulse (von den Muskeln, Sehnen, Gelenken usw.) werden über die Hinterwurzeln und den sensiblen Apparat der spinalen Reflexe und über die spinocerebellären Bahnen und Hinterstrangsysteme geleitet. Die Ableitung der so eingesteuerten Bewegungsimpulse zu den spinalen Segmenten geschieht einmal über die *Pyramidenbahn* und des weiteren über eine *mehrgliedrige Bahn*, welche von den Stammganglien zu den spinalen Segmenten führt. Der orale Teil der letzteren ist die „zentrale Haubenbahn" und als weiter nach caudal ableitende Bahnen kommen in erster Linie der *Vorderstrang* und wohl auch der Vorderseitenstrang in Betracht (ZÜLCH).

koordiniere und damit ein hochentwickeltes, insbesondere „der Motilität dienendes Koordinationssystem" darstelle, daß es gewissermaßen als ein „efferentes Organ des Thalamus" anzusehen sei. Hierdurch befähige das extrapyramidale Hauptsystem mit seinen Zentren neben dem fronto-ponto-cerebellaren System zu höher differenzierten motorischen Eigenleistungen. Der Thalamus erfülle dabei die Aufgabe eines großen, mit dem Gesamtcortex in zu- und ableitender Verbindung stehenden Sammelbeckens von proprio- und exteroceptiven Reizen und von Kleinhirnimpulsen, wodurch er das Individuum nicht nur über die jeweiligen Zustandsänderungen des eigenen Körpers unterrichte, sondern auch mit der Außenwelt in einer innigen Beziehung halte.

Das Striatum ist dem Pallidum übergeordnet, beide sind somatotopisch gegliedert und stehen, wie auch das Corpus Luysi und wohl auch die Substantia nigra, beiden Körperhälften vor, jedoch mit besonderer Betonung der Gegenseite. Die Reizung des Striatum ergibt nach WALKER — bei Fehlen einer Körperstellung oder -bewegung — keine sichtbare Reaktion. Bei aktiver Muskelinnervation dagegen ruft nach den Untersuchungen von TOWER (1936) die Reizung des Striopallidums eine sehr wirksame „Unterdrückung" bzw. „Hemmung" einer Muskelkontraktion hervor. Dieser Effekt ist von METTLER u. a. (1939) für solche Bewegungen bestätigt worden, welche durch eine elektrische Rindenreizung erzeugt wurden. Die Studien von DUSSER DE BARENNE u. a. (1941) mit der Strychninneuronographie ließen ja die Vermutung aufkommen, daß bestimmte Rindenfelder (die „Suppressor"-Streifen) einen Einfluß auf das Striatum haben, welcher in der Bewegungs-„hemmung" eine Rolle spiele (sog. „Unterdrückungs"- oder „Brems"effekt). Nachdem die Verbindungen des Striatum zum Thalamus via Pallidum und Ansa lenticularis seit langem als erwiesen gelten können, war es die fast selbstverständliche Folgerung, einen cortico-strio-thalamo-corticalen Erregungskreis anzunehmen, welcher in den Rindenfeldern 4 und 6 endigt, und welcher motorische Leistungen aufeinander abzustimmen vermag (WALKER). In schlüssiger Form hat ZÜLCH (1954) eine sehr schöne Darstellung von der heute geltenden Auffassung über das Zustandekommen einer normalen, harmonisch ablaufenden Willkürbewegung gegeben. Danach kommt bei der Entstehung einer isolierten Willkürbewegung dem Impuls des Feldes 4 zur Vorderhornzelle auf direktem Wege oder über ein Schaltneuron die größte Bedeutung zu. Wie vermutet werden darf, würde dieser Impuls aber gleichzeitig noch einmal mit dem „motorischen Gesamt" (von Körperhaltung und -lage, Tonus und zu gleicher Zeit ablaufenden anderen Bewegungen usw.) koordiniert, womit er sich selbst „einsteuere". Dies geschieht wahrscheinlich durch seine Einwirkung auf den Stammganglienapparat. Bekannt sind ja einerseits einige direkt nach spinal verlaufende Bahnen und andererseits eine Reihe von Ringverbindungen („Rücksteuerungskreise"), welche über das extrapyramidal-motorische System und den Thalamus zur motorischen Rinde zurückführen. Neben dem ableitenden Weg für die Impulse der Pyramidenbahn („Willkürbahn 1. und 2. Ordnung") besteht also ein zweites System für die Impulse vom extrapyramidal-motorischen Apparat. Auf welchem Wege dieses seine Impulse dem Rückenmark vermittelt, sei allerdings nur in groben Zügen bekannt. Wahrscheinlich handelt es sich um eine mehrgliedrige Bahn („Willkürbahn 3. Ordnung"), welche von den Stammganglien zu den spinalen Segmenten führt. Ihr oraler Anteil sei die „zentrale Haubenbahn" und als weiter nach caudal ableitende Bahnen kämen der Vorderstrang bzw. der Vorderseitenstrang in Betracht. ZÜLCH sieht eine Stütze für diese Zusammenhänge darin, daß die Pyramidenbahn zunächst ventral, später nach ihrer Kreuzung aber vorwiegend dorsolateral gelegen ist, während umgekehrt die von den extrapyramidalen Kernen zu den spinalen Segmenten verlaufenden Bahnen („zentrale Haubenbahn" usw.) zunächst dorsal, nach ihrer vermutlichen Kreuzung aber ventral bzw. ventromedial zu liegen kommen. Die *erste* ringförmige Rücksteuerung zur Rinde aber verliefe wahrscheinlich über das Striopallidum und den Thalamus direkt zur Rinde zurück, die *zweite* über die Substantia nigra bzw. das Corpus subthalamicum Luysi, den Nucleus ruber und den Thalamus zur Rinde zurück, während die *dritte* wahrscheinlich über die Brückenkerne, das Kleinhirn und den Thalamus die Rinde wieder erreiche. Dies wären die zur Verfügung stehenden Apparate für die Selbststeuerung bzw. „*Eigenkontrolle*" des Impulses für eine intendierte Bewegung. Hinzu kommt aber noch die „*Fremdkontrolle*" der Körperhaltung, -lage usw. und der bereits ablaufenden Bewegungen, deren afferente Impulse von den Muskeln, Sehnen, Gelenken usw. über die Hinterwurzeln und den sensiblen Apparat der spinalen Reflexe und über die spinocerebellären und Hinterstrangsysteme laufen. Nach ZÜLCH dürfte die *Eigensteuerung* im wesentlichen dazu dienen, die isolierte Bewegung in die großen Muskelverbände für Bewegung und Haltung einzufügen, während die *Fremdkontrolle* den glatten Ablauf der Bewegung und die Koordination von Agonisten und Antagonisten garantiere.

Da sich der zu einer Hyperkinese führende pathologische Prozeß im Gebiet der zur *Selbststeuerung* bzw. *Eigenkontrolle* dienenden Reglerkreise abspielt, muß in der chirurgischen Behandlung derartiger Störungen zwischen solchen operativen Eingriffen unterschieden werden, welche *an den Steuerungskreisen selbst* (bzw. an den von diesem Apparat direkt ableitenden Wegen, wie z. B. dem Vorderstrang) ansetzen, oder welche *am Pyramidenbahnsystem* angreifen.

## Die operativen Methoden.

Durch operative Maßnahmen irgendwelcher Art wird es kaum jemals möglich sein, das Krankheitsbild, welches eine Hyperkinese hervorruft, d. h. das Grundleiden, zu heilen. Ebensowenig wird es auch zukünftig schwerlich einmal zu verwirklichen sein, die gestörte Motorik völlig zu normalisieren, sondern wird die willkürliche motorische Funktion — selbst nach gut gelungener und auch vollständiger chirurgischer Ausschaltung der Hyperkinese — stets auf einem niedrigeren Niveau stehen.

Der Beitrag der Chirurgie in der Behandlung der Hyperkinesen besteht vorerst lediglich darin, das eine oder andere Symptom der Erkrankung beseitigen oder wenigstens verringern zu können. Das ist aber eben bei fast allen im Augenblick üblichen Operationen nur um den Preis einer gewissen, wenn auch manchmal nur vorübergehenden Parese zu erreichen. Diese kann einmal so gering sein, daß der Kranke sie gar nicht bemerkt bzw. nicht beachtet, oder aber so erheblich, daß durch die Lähmung eine ernsthafte Behinderung entsteht. Obgleich auch gelegentlich ein ideales Ergebnis mit Aufhebung der unkontrollierten Bewegungen ohne merkliche Lähmung erzielt werden kann, so bildet derzeit ein solches Resultat noch eher eine Ausnahme als die Regel. Immerhin kann bei jüngeren Kranken mit einer guten Rückbildung der anfänglichen Parese gerechnet werden, nicht dagegen bei älteren Leuten. Weiterhin ist zu berücksichtigen, welches Symptom des Leidens im Vordergrund steht. So kann z. B. im Falle eines PARKINSON-Syndroms die Starre und Bewegungsarmut störender als der Tremor sein. Starre und Akinese sind aber, wenigstens zur Zeit noch, chirurgisch mit viel geringerer Aussicht auf Erfolg als die Tremorsymptome zu behandeln, wohingegen sie glücklicherweise auf die moderne konservative Therapie gut anzusprechen scheinen. Mit dem Tremor verhält es sich dagegen gerade umgekehrt; dieser ist gegenüber der medikamentösen Behandlung gewöhnlich außerordentlich resistent und einer chirurgischen Beeinflussung zugänglicher. Auf der anderen Seite kann im Falle einer Dystonie oder Athetose eine so erhebliche geistige Schwäche vorliegen, daß selbst nach einer geglückten operativen Beseitigung der Bewegungsstörung der Kranke sozial nicht einzugliedern sein wird. Darüber hinaus wird man auch zwischen stationär bleibenden Defektzuständen und progredienten Krankheitsbildern, gerade beim Parkinsonismus, zu unterscheiden haben.

Auf jede Besonderheit des Krankheitsbildes kann verständlicherweise erst im Einzelfalle eingegangen werden. Aus den vorhergehenden Andeutungen ist aber zu entnehmen, daß die Kranken für eine Operation streng ausgesucht werden müssen. Bestimmte Regeln lassen sich für die Anzeige zu einem Eingriff nicht aufstellen, sie hängen zudem weitgehend von der subjektiven Einstellung des Operateurs und der von ihm bevorzugten Methode ab. Dennoch dürften gewisse Richtlinien für die Indikation zur Operation inzwischen Allgemeingültigkeit gewonnen haben.

**Indikation.** 1. Das Lebensalter und der körperliche Zustand müssen den Eingriff am Zentralnervensystem erlauben, ohne daß ein zu großes Operationsrisiko eingegangen wird. Unterhalb des 6.—8. und oberhalb des 50. Lebensjahres sollte nicht operiert werden.

2. Die unwillkürlichen Bewegungen müssen unbedingt das hervorstechendste Symptom des Leidens sein, gegen das die Begleitsymptome zurücktreten.

Akinese und Starre beim Parkinsonismus bzw. Debilität bei Dystonie oder Athetose sind, ebenso wie eine erheblichere Hirnatrophie, Gegenanzeigen.

3. Zu bevorzugen sind einseitige Hyperkinesen, weil diese gegenüber den doppelseitigen Syndromen die besseren Chancen haben. Ein in diesen Fällen erlaubtes radikaleres Vorgehen ermöglicht die Beseitigung der Bewegungsstörung mit einer größeren Sicherheit und die Operationsmortalität ist geringer, selbst wenn die Operation bei bilateralen Störungen in 2 Sitzungen ausgeführt wird.

4. Nicht zuletzt sollte der Patient in vollem Umfang über die begrenzten Möglichkeiten einer operativen Behandlung und deren nicht sicher vorauszusehende Nebenfolgen aufgeklärt werden.

## I. Die Eingriffe an der Hirnrinde.

VICTOR HORSLEYs Priorität, als erster mit gutem Erfolg durch eine Rindenresektion im motorischen Feld eine Hyperkinese (Athetose) gebessert zu haben, ist unumstritten. Der Gedanke, daß die Entfernung des motorischen Rindenfeldes unwillkürliche Bewegungen ausschalten könne, war zwar anscheinend schon um die Wende des 20. Jahrhunderts aufgekommen. So berichtete FRAZIER (1906) von einer Craniotomie und Excision des corticalen motorischen Armfeldes bei einer Athetose, wodurch allerdings der

Zustand anscheinend nicht gebessert wurde. Bedauerlicherweise fehlen Angaben über Einzelheiten der von ihm gewählten Technik.

Das unzweifelhafte Verdienst HORSLEYs, mit seiner gelungenen Operation die Chirurgie der Hyperkinesen begründet zu haben, hat jedoch, wie eingangs erwähnt wurde, zunächst nur wenig Widerhall gefunden. Es bedurfte erst der experimentell gesicherten Ergebnisse der auf einer breiteren Basis ausgeführten neurophysiologischen Untersuchungen FULTONs und seiner Schule (1932—1936), um die Neurochirurgie wieder für die Probleme einer operativen Therapie der Hyperkinesen zu gewinnen.

FULTON, LIDDELL und RIOCH (1932) konnten zeigen, daß der Entfernung des Kleinhirns bei der Katze ein Tremor der Extremitäten folgt, welcher nur bei willkürlichen Bewegungen auftritt (Intentionstremor). Darüber hinaus stellten sie fest, daß dieser experimentell hervorgerufene Tremor in den kontralateralen Gliedmaßen zur Ruhe kommt, wenn die entsprechende Großhirnhemisphäre entfernt wird. Eine weitere grundlegende Beobachtung wurde dann von ARING und FULTON (1936) an Affen gemacht. Sie sahen, daß dieser Intentionstremor, welcher von einer experimentell erzeugten Kleinhirnläsion herrührt, durch eine Exstirpation des Feldes 4 vorübergehend verschwindet oder sogar permanent vermindert wird, daß er durch eine Exstirpation des Feldes 6 eher verstärkt wird und daß er schließlich nach einer Entfernung des Feldes 4 *und* 6 dauerhaft auszuschalten ist.

## 1. Cortectomie.

Die experimentell gewonnenen Erkenntnisse begann PAUL C. BUCY (1932, 1937, 1942, 1947, 1950) für die neurochirurgische Praxis nutzbar zu machen. Zusammen mit BUCHANAN (1932) hat BUCY die Operation eines 7jährigen Mädchens mitgeteilt, welches an einer Hemiparese und Athetose des linken Armes als auch an fokalen Krampfanfällen der gleichen Körperseite litt. Durch vorherige elektrische Reizung wurde die Begrenzung des abzutragenden Rindenfeldes exakt lokalisiert, d. h. die Ausdehnung der Exstirpation festgelegt. Nachdem auf diese Weise, durch faradische Reizung, der „Athetoseherd“ bestimmt worden war, wurde die Rinde der Area 6a α und der Area 4, der Ursprungsort der langen Pyramidenfasern, entfernt. Die choreoathetotische Bewegungsstörung war postoperativ verschwunden und das Ergebnis dauerhaft, wie eine Nachuntersuchung nach 9 Jahren gezeigt hat. — Im Falle eines posttraumatischen Hemiparkinsonismus mit rechtsseitiger Hemiparese bei einem 33jährigen Mann wurde von BUCY und CASE (1939) wie folgt vorgegangen: Da die Erscheinungen des grobschlägigen Tremors im Arm erheblich stärker als im Bein waren, haben sie durch faradische Rindenreizung die Repräsentationszone der rechten Schulter, des rechten Unterarmes, des rechten Handgelenkes und der Finger in den Areae 4 und 6 der linken präzentralen Windungen ausgetestet und anschließend dieses Segment exstirpiert. Es enthielt den vorderen Wall der Fissura Rolandi hinunter bis zum Fuß und dehnte sich nach vorn bis einschließlich der hinteren Teile der angrenzenden frontalen Windungen aus. Ausgespart blieb die „Gesichts“-Area. Es wurde die vollständige Höhe der Rinde und etwas von der unmittelbar darunter gelegenen weißen Substanz, bis zu einer Tiefe von etwa 1—1,5 cm, reseziert. Der nachträgliche Defekt an der Hirnoberfläche hat 2,3 × 3,5 cm betragen. Nach der Operation bestand zunächst eine komplette rechtsseitige Hemiplegie. Während die Lähmung des Gesichts und des Beines nach wenigen Wochen nahezu vollständig abgeklungen war, blieb die Rückkehr der motorischen Funktion am Arm fast ganz aus. Es waren nur langsame und ungeschickte Bewegungen im Sinne von Massenbewegungen, aber keine feineren Bewegungen der Hand und der Finger möglich. Der Tremor war permanent beseitigt.

Während BUCY in seinen frühen Fällen (1932, 1937) die reizbare Rinde entfernte, welche der betroffenen Gliedmaße entsprach, beschränkte er seine späteren Rindenexcisionen (1942) auf bestimmte ventral vom Sulcus centralis gelegene cytoarchitektonische Felder. Nachdem bekannt wurde, daß der Tremor von der Unversehrtheit des

Pyramidenbahnsystems abhängig war, vermutete BUCY (1947), daß eine auf die hintere Hälfte der präzentralen Windung (Area 4 γ) begrenzte Exstirpation zur Beseitigung des Tremors ausreichen müsse. Er schloß, daß die Impulse, welche den Tremor leiten, durch den hinteren Teil der Präzentralwindung — Area 4γ — ziehen, so daß die Areae 4a, 4s und 6 geschont werden könnten. Die klinische Erfahrung hat dagegen gezeigt, daß eine solch eng umschriebene Abtragung den Tremor lediglich zu verringern, aber nicht zu beseitigen vermochte. BUCY hat aber noch kürzlich die Ansicht vertreten (1950), daß die auf die präzentrale Windung — auf das Feld 4 — beschränkte Exstirpation genüge, um den Tremor zu beseitigen, daß es aber im Gegensatz dazu eine viel ausgedehntere Exstirpation der präzentralen motorischen Rinde erfordere, um die Bewegungen der Choreoathetose auszuschalten. Um die letzteren zu bessern, entfernte BUCY die präzentrale Windung einschließlich des vorderen Walls der Fissura Rolandi und eines Teiles der frontalen Windung, welche *vor* dieser gelegen ist. Er kam auch früh zu der Erkenntnis, daß die bis dahin häufig übliche, auf die Area 6 beschränkte Rindenexcision für eine dauerhafte Besserung der choreoathetotischen Bewegungen nicht ausreicht, sondern daß es in jedem Falle notwendig ist, Teile der Area 4 in die Abtragung mit einzubeziehen, wenn man nicht eine nur vorübergehende Besserung erhalten wolle!

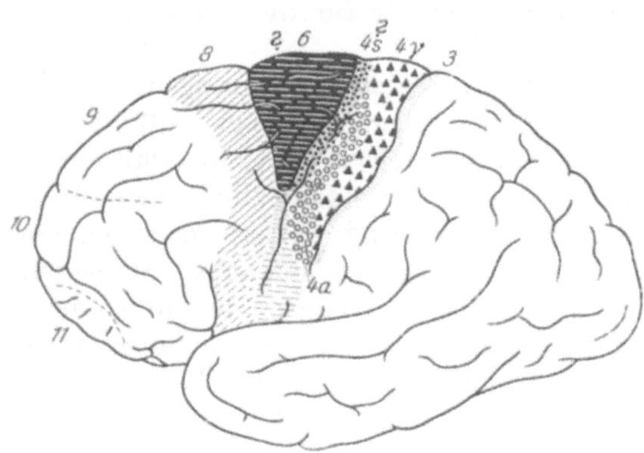


Abb. 5a—i. Verschiedene Modifikationen der Cortectomie. ■ totale Zerstörung der Rinde; ▨ Teilschädigung der Rinde. a KLEMMES mutmaßliche Rindenabtragung bei Athetose und PARKINSON-Tremor (1940).

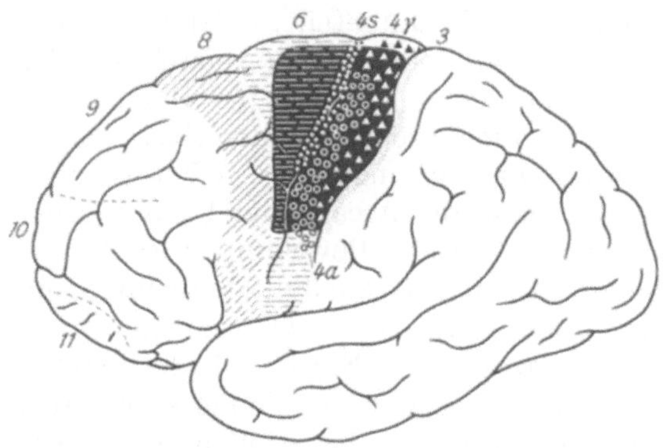


b BUCY und CASE bei einem Hemiparkinsonismus (1939), BUCY bei Choreoathetose.

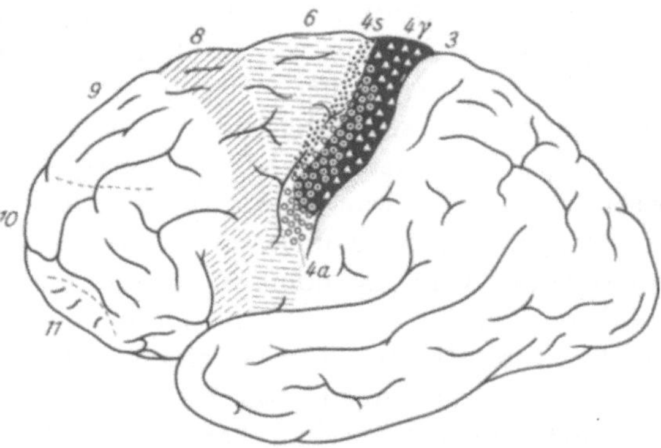


c BUCY beim Parkinsontremor (1950).

Im Gegensatz hierzu stehen die Angaben von KLEMME (1940), welche jedoch mit einer großen Zurückhaltung aufzunehmen sind, da er weder seine operative Technik noch die Lokalisation und Ausdehnung seiner corticalen Abtragungen jemals in konkreter Weise beschrieben hat. Im Jahre 1937 begann KLEMME mit einer Serie von „prämotorischen Rindenresektionen“, welche wohl, wie einem Brief an PUTNAM zu entnehmen ist, in der Frontalregion und unmittelbar vor der elektrisch reizbaren Rinde (Area 4) ausgeführt wurden, also offenbar auf die Area 6 beschränkt geblieben sind. Trotzdem gibt KLEMME in 100 Fällen von „Dystonie“, über deren Art — ob Athetose oder Tremor — ebenfalls nähere Angaben fehlen, in 36 Fällen Heilung und in 24 Fällen eine Besserung der Bewegungsstörung an.

In den folgenden Jahren (1942—1954) wurde eine ganze Reihe klinischer Erfahrungen mit der *Cortectomie* gewonnen (PUTNAM, SACHS, THIÉBAUT, WOLINETZ und GUIOT,

ALAJOUANINE, LE BEAU und HOUDART, PAILLAS, BOUDOURESQUE und PELLEGRIN, VERBIEST, PUECH, FISCHGOLD, GIBERT und DREYFUS-BRISAC, DAVID, HÉCAEN und TALAIRACH, DE LISI, PERRIA und SACCHI, MEYERS u. v. a.). Die Ergebnisse der verschiedenen Autoren können aber nicht im einzelnen besprochen werden. Selbst die exakteste

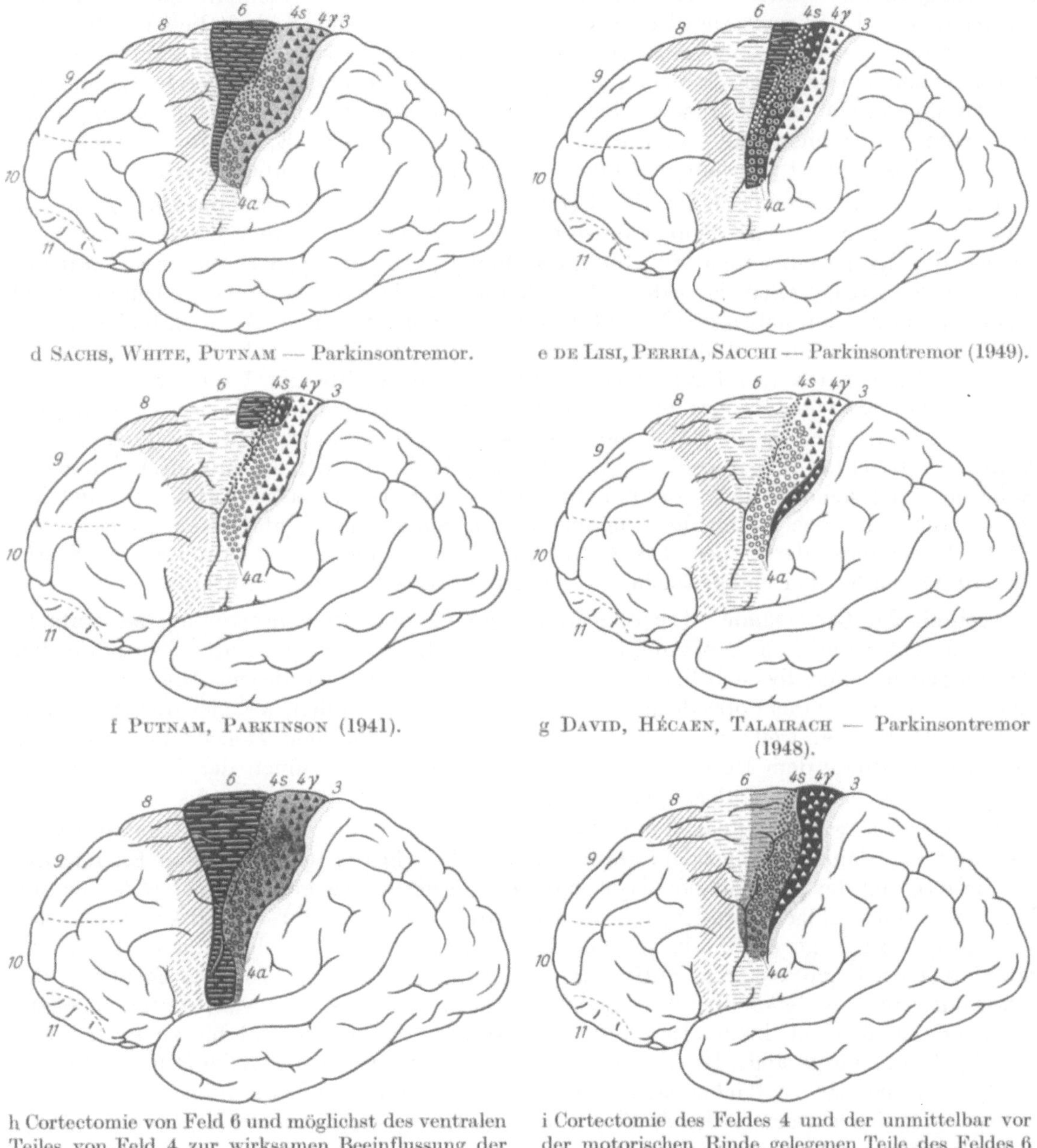

d SACHS, WHITE, PUTNAM — Parkinsontremor.

e DE LISI, PERRIA, SACCHI — Parkinsontremor (1949).

f PUTNAM, PARKINSON (1941).

g DAVID, HÉCAEN, TALAIRACH — Parkinsontremor (1948).

h Cortectomie von Feld 6 und möglichst des ventralen Teiles von Feld 4 zur wirksamen Beeinflussung der Choreoathetosen (s. Text).

i Cortectomie des Feldes 4 und der unmittelbar vor der motorischen Rinde gelegenen Teile des Feldes 6 zur wirksamen Beeinflussung der Tremorformen (s. Text).

Festlegung der Grenzen der entfernten Rindenareale ist bei verschiedenen Operateuren dennoch großen Schwankungen unterworfen und die Beurteilung des Operationsresultates hängt auch zu sehr von der subjektiven Einstellung des Operateurs ab, als daß sich ein wirklich objektives Urteil finden ließe.

Immerhin scheint nach kritischer Würdigung der Literatur heute soviel gesichert, daß bei den *Choreoathetosen* die Abtragung des Feldes 6 und des vorderen Randes von

Feld 4 am erfolgversprechendsten sind. Die Exstirpation der Area 6 für sich allein beeinträchtigt die willkürliche motorische Funktion zwar überhaupt nicht, ist aber offensichtlich in der Mehrzahl der Fälle auf die unkontrollierten Bewegungen nur vorübergehend von günstigem Einfluß. Man muß hiernach stets mit einem Wiederkehren der Bewegungsautomatismen — auch in ihrem vollen Umfang — rechnen. Nach Excision der Area 6 und des ventralen Teiles der Area 4 wurden durchschnittlich in 40—60% gute und dauerhafte Ergebnisse erzielt. Allerdings kommt es stets danach zum Auftreten vorübergehender oder auch permanenter Paresen. In der Regel klingen aber die Lähmungserscheinungen nach einigen Wochen bis auf geringe Residuen ab. Als Dauerstörung muß mit einem motorischen Funktionsausfall im Gebiet der distalen Extremitätenabschnitte, mit einer Insuffizienz für feinere Fingerbewegungen u. a. gerechnet werden.

Beim *Tremorsyndrom* scheint der Erfolg der Rindenabtragung um so sicherer und dauerhafter, je mehr vom Feld 4 entfernt wird, jedoch mit einem in gleichem Maße wachsenden Risiko einer nicht rückbildungsfähigen postoperativen Hemiparese. Mit der Excision der Area 6 allein ist jedenfalls in keinem Falle auszukommen! Dennoch wird allgemein empfohlen, neben der Resektion der motorischen Rinde (Area 4), insbesondere im Gebiet des vorderen Walles vom Sulcus centralis Rolandi, auch die ventral davon gelegene Rinde (Area 6) mitzuentfernen. In über der Hälfte der Fälle ist mit diesem Vorgehen ein fast vollständiges und auch dauerhaftes Verschwinden der Tremorsymptome zu erwarten. In der Regel bildet die postoperative Hemiparese bzw. Monoparese des Armes bei Beschränkung des Eingriffs auf das „Armfeld" sich in einigen Wochen bis Monaten weitgehend zurück. Permanent bleibt ein Verlust der motorischen Funktion an den distalen Abschnitten der Gliedmaßen im Sinne einer Unfähigkeit zu isolierten Willkürbewegungen der Finger. Die Symptome der Bewegungsarmut (Akinese) und Starre (Rigidität) werden bei einem solchen Vorgehen praktisch nicht beeinflußt!

**Technik der Cortectomie.** Die operative Technik der Rindenabtragung ist einfach. Nach einer der üblichen Lappenbildungen werden die präzentralen und frontodorsalen Windungen in einer übersichtlichen Ausdehnung freigelegt. In diesem Augenblick muß sich der Patient in einem oberflächlichen Dämmerschlaf befinden, welcher die unkontrollierten Bewegungen weitgehend unterdrückt, aber mit geringen Reizströmen von der motorischen Rinde dem Reizort entsprechende Einzelkontraktionen der Muskulatur an der Körpergegenseite auszulösen gestattet.

Die Grenze zwischen Feld 4 und Feld 6 wird durch die elektrische Rindenreizung bestimmt und danach die Ausdehnung des Rindenbezirkes festgelegt, dessen Entfernung zur Beseitigung der vorliegenden Hyperkinese erforderlich scheint[1]. Die Größe des zur Resektion notwendigen Rindengebietes ist durch die Art und die Lokalisation der Bewegungsstörung gegeben, wie aus den im vorhergehenden Abschnitt gemachten Angaben zu entnehmen ist. Zur Entfernung der Rinde wird, nach Versorgung der in die Rinde eintretenden Gefäße, heute allgemein der subpialen Resektion der Vorzug gegeben. Die Rinde wird durch kleine Incisionen der weichen Häute subpial bis zu einer Tiefe von 10—15 mm ausgesaugt. Hierdurch werden ausgedehntere Läsionen der Hirnoberfläche, welche postoperativ zu flächenhaften Verwachsungen mit der Dura führen, vermieden. Zu einer Rindenzerstörung durch Elektrokoagulation (Guillaume und Paillas 1948), welche auch subpial ausgeführt werden kann, wird man aber nur an den für eine Resektion unzugänglicheren Stellen, wie im Bereich des Mittelspaltes oder auch für sehr eng umschriebene Läsionen im Gebiet der motorischen Rinde (Area 4), raten können. In der Regel dürfte jedenfalls nach der allgemeinen Auffassung die Entfernung der Rinde ihrer Zerstörung durch Elektrokoagulation vorzuziehen sein.

[1] Von uns wird das Thyratron-Entladungsgerät (Nr. 24811) der Elektromedizinischen Werkstätten Hamburg benutzt. Die Reizung wird bipolar bei einem Elektrodenabstand von etwa 5 m/m mit einer Stromstärke von 4—6 Volt ausgeführt. Das Kaliber der Silberknopfelektroden beträgt 0,4 mm, der Durchmesser des Knopfes am distalen Ende der Elektrode 1,8—2,5 m/m.

Die Angabe von DE LISI, PERRIA und SACCHI (1949/50), daß die Hyperkinesen durch eine schichtweise Schädigung der Rinde, welche direkt von ihrer Gefäßarchitektonik abhänge, zu beseitigen seien, muß als sehr zweifelhaft erscheinen. Sie behaupten, daß nur die vier äußeren Schichten der Rinde durch Gefäße der Pia mater versorgt würden, während die 5. und 6. Schicht, welche die BETZschen Zellen enthalte, von Gefäßen aus der Tiefe ihre Versorgung erhielten. Nun kommen sie zu der Schlußfolgerung, daß eine Seidenligatur der oberflächlichen Rindengefäße ausreiche, um die Tätigkeit der äußeren 4 Rindenschichten außer Funktion zu setzen, aber die Blutversorgung der BETZschen Zellen in der 5. und 6. Schicht zu erhalten, wodurch einerseits die Hyperkinesen beseitigt und andererseits die Willkürmotorik nicht beeinträchtigt würde. Aber es läßt sich weder von anatomischer Seite diese einzig dastehende Auffassung von der Gefäßversorgung der Rinde, noch von pathophysiologischer Seite die Ansicht aufrechterhalten, daß das Verschwinden der abnormen Bewegungen an die Zerstörung der ersten 4 Rindenschichten gebunden ist. Eine praktische Bedeutung wird dieser Methode sicher versagt bleiben.

## 2. Die lineare Rindenincision.

Der Vollständigkeit halber und zur Vermeidung von zwecklosen Operationen muß dieser Eingriff mit den Bedingungen, denen er seine Anwendung verdankt, kurz skizziert werden.

Zu der Zeit, als die — heute in ihren wesentlichen Punkten wieder verlassene — Anschauung von dem Suppressorsystem in manchen Kreisen Anerkennung gewann, wurde die Rindenresektion auf das „Suppressor-Feld", d. h. den schmalen „Suppressor-Streifen" der Area 4 (Area 4s) zu beschränken versucht.

REID (1948) vermutete, daß der „Suppressor-Streifen" unter dem Einfluß von Feld 6 stehe und daß seine Entfernung eine wirksamere Hemmung der subcorticalen Strukturen zur Folge haben würde, wodurch eine bessere Verminderung der unwillkürlichen Bewegungen zu erreichen sein müsse. Deshalb bemühte er sich, das motorische Feld (Area 4) und den „Suppressor-Streifen" (Area 4s) mit Hilfe der elektrischen Rindenreizung, durch elektrocorticographische Aufzeichnungen und durch die Reaktionen des Tremors auf die Reizung genau festzulegen. Wenn die Reizung eines bestimmten Punktes in diesem Gebiet den Tremor und die spontane elektrische Aktivität der Rinde für länger als 90 sec beseitigen ließe, dann müsse dieser Punkt als zum „Unterdrücker-Streifen", zur Area 4s, gehörig angesehen werden. Die so ausgetestete Region wurde von REID als die hintere Grenze des Segmentes, welches entfernt werden muß, angesprochen. Die übrigen 3 Grenzen der zu entfernenden Region versuchte er durch eine anatomische Untersuchung herauszufinden. Dann wurde von ihm das auf diese Weise begrenzte Gebiet durch vorsichtige subpiale Resektion, unter sorgsamer Schonung der Präzentralwindung selbst (Area 4), entfernt.

Den Vorteil dieses gezielten Vorgehens bei der Cortectomie sah REID insbesondere in den geringeren postoperativen Lähmungserscheinungen bei angeblich ausreichender Verminderung der unkontrollierten Bewegungen. Doch hat dieser Eingriff nicht regelmäßig befriedigende Resultate gezeigt. In verschiedenen späteren Fällen hat REID die vordere Begrenzung der Resektion immer mehr nach ventral, bis in das Feld 8, verlegt und seine Ergebnisse sollen danach ermutigender geworden sein. Ohne Zweifel scheint mit REIDs Vorgehen die Willkürmotorik weniger in Mitleidenschaft gezogen zu werden, aber das Ergebnis ist gewiß hinsichtlich einer Beeinflussung des Tremors zweifelhaft, obgleich REID unter seinen 15 Fällen nur 5 Mißerfolge angegeben hat. Zwei Todesfälle dieser Serie wurden allerdings nicht mit eingerechnet.

Im April 1948 hat RUSSEL MEYERS, zusammen mit SWEENY und SCHWIDDE, auf dem Treffen der HARVEY-CUSHING-Society in San Francisco die erfolgreiche Besserung der Symptome eines *Hemiballismus* durch einen *Längsschnitt in die Rinde zwischen Area 4 und 4s*, in einer Ausdehnung von 6 cm Länge und einer Tiefe von 2,5 cm, mitgeteilt. Er führte diesen Eingriff in 2 Fällen aus, aber in keinem von beiden konnte der „Suppressor-Streifen" einwandfrei gezeigt werden. Ein Patient hat die Operation bedauerlicherweise nicht länger als 1 Monat überlebt, während der andere ganz gesund geworden sein soll.

Zwei Monate später, im Juni 1948, wurde von WYKE auf dem Kongreß der American Neurological Association dieses Verfahren, allerdings zur *Durchtrennung der U-Fasern* zwischen Area 6 und 4s, als eine um vieles einfachere Operationsmethode zur Behandlung von *Starre und Tremor* bei der Paralysis agitans empfohlen. WYKE, ein Assistent REIDs, nahm nach dessen auf den „Suppressor-Streifen" beschränkten Rindenabtragungen an, daß die Unterbrechung der U-Fasern zwischen den Feldern 4s und 6 die entscheidende Rolle für eine Verminderung des Tremors und der Rigidität spiele. Jedoch wurde diese Auffassung von anderen Autoren nicht geteilt. Im Gegenteil, es erwies sich, daß die lineare Rindenincision beim Tremor einen vollständigen Mißerfolg gibt.

Auf Grund dieses mündlichen Berichtes von WYKE, welcher vor der Veröffentlichung von REIDs Arbeit gegeben wurde, ist eine Gruppe amerikanischer Neurologen und Neurochirurgen veranlaßt worden, diese Technik in insgesamt 9 Fällen von Paralysis agitans zu erproben. Das Ergebnis wurde im Jahre 1950, nach einer etwa einjährigen postoperativen Beobachtungszeit, gemeinsam veröffentlicht (COBB, POOL, SCARFF, SCHWAB, WALKER, WHITE). Es handelte sich in diesen unabhängig voneinander, aber mit gleicher Technik operierten Fällen um 5 einseitige und 4 doppelseitige Syndrome. Bei der Operation wurde in jedem Falle versucht, durch elektrische Reizung den „Suppressor-Streifen" (Area 4s) zu bestimmen, aber nur in einem von diesen Beispielen soll es dem Operateur gelungen sein, einen „Suppressor-Punkt" zu erhalten. Bestätigt wurde, daß der Tremor durch die elektrische Reizung der *motorischen Rinde* (Area 4) vorübergehend zu beseitigen ist. Aber es soll nicht möglich gewesen sein, *vor* diesem Feld einen Streifen festzulegen, bei dessen Reizung die Tremorbewegungen zu beseitigen gewesen wären! Die Längsincision der Rinde wurde im Anschluß an die Reizung ventral von dem reizbaren Feld ausgeführt, um die von der Area 6 zur Area 4s ziehenden U-Fasern zu unterbrechen. Auf diese Weise operierte SCARFF 3 Fälle, WHITE 2 Fälle, POOL 3 Fälle und WALKER 1 Fall. Jedoch blieben die Symptome des Tremors und der Starre in allen 9 Fällen völlig unbeeinflußt (!). Auch die Nachuntersuchung nach Verlauf eines Jahres nach dem Eingriff ließ keine Aussicht auf eine noch später folgende Besserung erwarten. In 6 Fällen waren dagegen die Erscheinungen infolge eines Fortschreitens der Grundkrankheit inzwischen sogar verschlimmert.

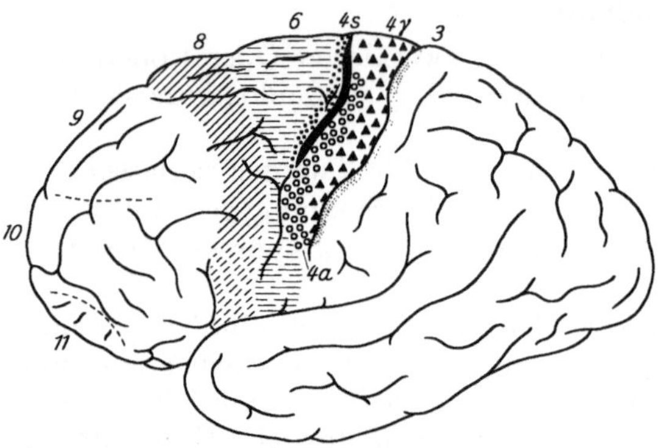

Abb. 6. Die lineare Rindenincision von MEYERS, SWEENY und SCHWIDDE beim Hemiballismus (1948).

## 3. Die Subcorticotomie.

Als jüngste in der Reihe der corticalen Operationen zur Behandlung der Hyperkinesen wurde die „Subcorticotomie" von dem Japaner TAKEBAYASHI (1951) in Vorschlag gebracht. Wegen der Eigenart der Schnittführung wurde dieser Eingriff von ihm auch mit „T-Tomy" benannt. Das Prinzip dieser Methode liegt darin, die von den Rindenfeldern 4, 6, 8, 9, 10 und eventuell sogar 46, 47 zu den Stammganglien ziehenden Faserverbindungen durch eine Rindenunterschneidung zu durchtrennen. Für diese Unterbrechung der Kommunikation der parapyramidalen Assoziationszentren mit den basalen Ganglien mittels einer Durchschneidung der in der weißen Substanz verlaufenden Verbindungsfasern hat der Autor ein sehr einfaches Verfahren gewählt, welches dem Vorgehen von FREEMAN und WATTS bei der präfrontalen Lobotomie gleicht.

**Technik der Subcorticotomie („T-Tomy").** Nach der Originalmethode TAKEBAYASHIs wird in Höhe der Kranznaht ein Bohrloch angelegt, und zwar an einem Punkt, welcher 2—2,5 cm dorsal vom äußeren Orbitalrand und 5—6 cm oberhalb des oberen Jochbogenrandes gelegen ist. Dann wird das Leukotom im Gebiet der Pars triangularis der unteren Frontalwindung eingestochen. Die Einstichstelle ist an der bezeichneten Stelle gewählt worden, um der Gefahr zu entgehen, den Seitenventrikel zu perforieren oder die zur Mediagruppe gehörigen Arterien und Venen zu verletzen, welche im ventralen Abschnitt der Insel verlaufen. Das Leukotom wird dann in Richtung auf die Markierung C, welche in der Mittellinie 11—12 cm von der Glabella entfernt durch eine cutane Seidennaht angebracht wurde, etwa 6,5 cm tief eingestochen (Abb. 8). Durch eine entsprechende Schwenkung des Leukotoms werden ventral vom Vorderhorn des Seitenventrikels die Markfasern in nahezu vertikaler Richtung und bei nach oben konvexer bogenförmiger Schnittführung schließlich oberhalb vom Vorderhorn in horizontaler Richtung durchschnitten, bis die Leukotomspitze auf die Markierung *D* zeigt, welche 3—4 cm dorsal von der Marke *C* liegt und die ungefähre hintere Begrenzung der Area 4 anzeigen soll.

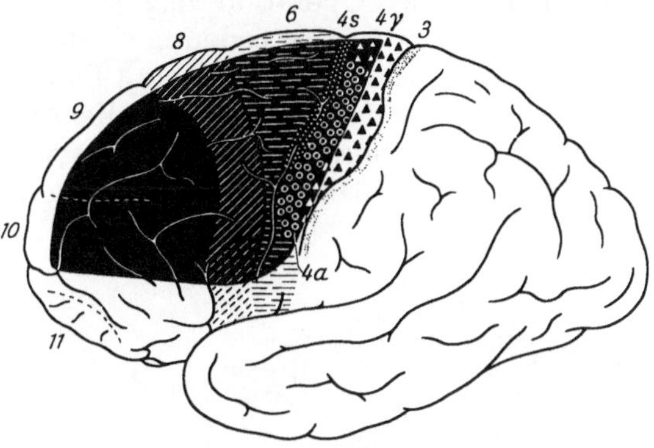


Abb. 7. TAKEBAYASHIS Subcorticotomie = Unterschneidung der Rindenfelder 4, 6, 8, 9 und 10.

Die dorsale horizontale Einschneidung bis zum Markierungspunkt *D* trennt die Rinde bis zum hinteren Teil des motorischen Feldes (Area 4) und eignet sich deshalb vornehmlich für die Tremorsyndrome. Bei Athetosen wird die Unterschneidung der Rinde nicht so weit nach dorsal ausgeführt, sondern nur bis knapp hinter Markierungspunkt *C*, womit die Einflüsse der Felder 6 und 8 und des vorderen Anteiles der Area 4 ausgeschaltet werden können. In jedem Falle wird die vordere, fast schon senkrechte Subcorticotomie ventral vom Vorderhorn unter den Feldern 8 bis einschließlich 10 vorgenommen, um hiermit eine weitgehende Ausschaltung auch der psychischen Einflüsse auf das subcorticale motorische System zu erreichen.

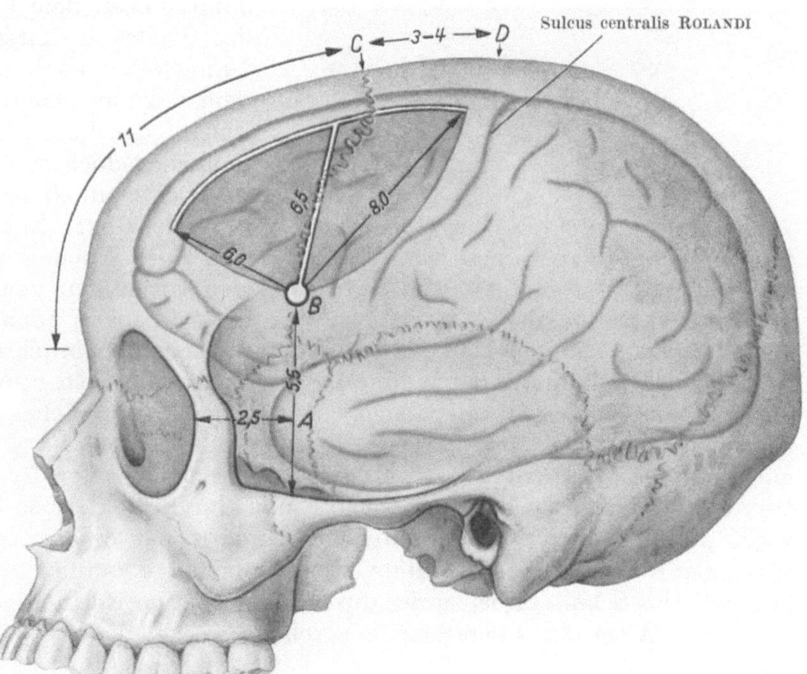


Abb. 8. Technik von TAKEBAYASHIS Operation. Markierungspunkte: *A* 2,5 cm dorsal vom lateralen Orbitalrand; *B* 5—6 cm oberhalb des oberen Jochbogenrandes; *C* 11—12 cm dorsal von der Glabella in der Mittellinie; *D* 3—4 cm dorsal von Punkt C in der Mittellinie. (Erklärung s. Text.)

In einer etwas abgewandelten Technik haben wir diese Methode doppelseitig in 3 Fällen einer Athétose double des Kindesalters angewandt. Hierzu wurde von einer osteoplastischen frontotemporalen Trepanation aus der hintere untere Frontallappen bis zur Präzentralregion übersichtlich freigelegt und dann die Rindenunterschneidung unter Sicht des Auges mit dem Sauger zwischen 2 Hirnspateln vorgenommen. Auf diese Weise scheint es uns sicherer, sowohl die Ausdehnung der Subcorticotomie besser begrenzen als auch unangenehme Gefäßverletzungen vermeiden zu können.

TAKEBAYASHI hat seine Subcorticotomie nicht allein bei unwillkürlichen Bewegungen, sondern auch bei Epilepsien und postapoplektischen spastischen Hemiplegien versucht. Insgesamt 300 Fälle wurden von ihm diesem Eingriff unterzogen und etwa die Hälfte von diesen konnte postoperativ 20 Monate und länger verfolgt werden. Leider wird in seiner Arbeit eine gute Kasuistik vermißt. Takebayashi gibt lediglich an, daß in 43 Fällen von Athetose „alle Fälle ein fast völliges Sistieren der Athetose mehrere Wochen nach der Operation zeigten“. Drei Fälle einer chronischen familiären Chorea zeigten postoperativ eine bedeutende Besserung, aber die Symptome seien in einer milden Form wiedergekehrt. Unter den 13 Fällen von Paralysis agitans zeigten „die Patienten, bei denen während der Operation die Area 4 genügend unterschnitten worden war, ein vollständiges Aufhören der Symptome wie Tremor, Schmerz, Schlaflosigkeit, Nervosität und Zuckungen“. Diese spärlichen Angaben, denen übrigens ein Hinweis über das Ausmaß einer Schädigung der Willkürmotorik fehlt, lassen kein Urteil über die wahre Wirksamkeit dieser Methode zu.

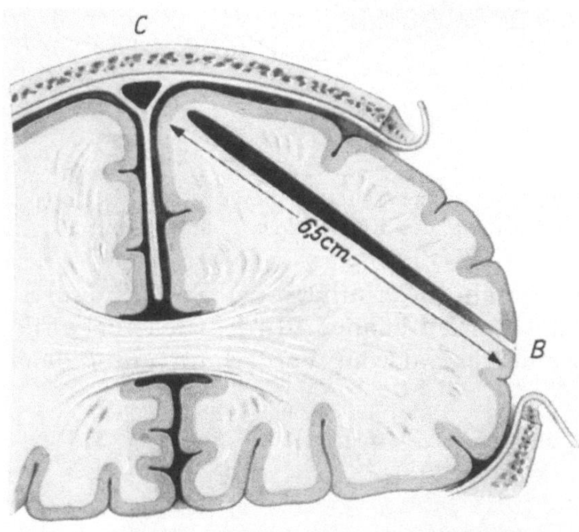

Abb. 9. Frontalansicht zu Takebayashis Subcorticotomie.

Bei drei von uns doppelseitig operierten Kindern mit einer Athétose double haben wir, wie oben erwähnt, die Subcorticotomie von einer übersichtlichen osteoplastischen Craniotomie aus durchgeführt. Die horizontale Unterschneidung haben wir nach dorsal bis zu einem Punkt, welcher in der Mitte zwischen den Marken C und D gelegen war, ausgeführt. Nach Takebayashis Angaben müßte damit neben dem Feld 6 die vordere Hälfte des Feldes 4 unterschnitten worden sein. Unmittelbar nach der Operation war in jedem Falle und nach jeder Sitzung die Hyperkinese deutlich vermindert, die Willkürmotorik jedoch nicht beeinflußt, so daß man vielleicht annehmen darf, daß die Unterschneidung gar nicht bis zur Höhe der Area 4 gereicht hat. Nach einer vorübergehenden Besserung der Hyperkinese für die Dauer von 6—8 Wochen sind die unkontrollierten Bewegungen etwa in der alten Stärke wieder vorhanden gewesen. Trotz des relativ geringen Operationsrisikos haben wir den Eingriff später nicht mehr ausgeführt. Vor allem schien uns die außen an der Kopfschwarte angebrachte Markierung C und D, welche zur Bestimmung der hinteren Begrenzung von Feld 6 und Feld 4 dienen soll, zu unsicher und ungenau, um danach einen Eingriff von solcher Bedeutung auszuführen. Vielleicht kann die Methode von Takebayashi dadurch an Boden gewinnen, wenn nach einer ausgedehnten osteoplastischen Freilegung der frontalen und präzentralen Windungen zunächst die motorische Rinde durch elektrische Reizung exakt bestimmt wird. Dann kann die Rindenunterschneidung in der beschriebenen Weise von der Pars triangularis der unteren Frontalwindung aus vorgenommen werden, da nun die Ausdehnung des Schnittes bis zu der durch die vorherige Reizung genau festgelegten Region durch das Auge des Operateurs kontrolliert werden kann.

## Epikrise zu den corticalen Operationsmethoden.

Die Rindenoperationen werden kontralateral zur Lokalisation der Hyperkinese ausgeführt.

1. Unter den Eingriffen an der Hirnrinde wird der *Cortectomie durch die subpiale Resektion* der Vorzug gegeben.

2. Die ausgedehnte *flächenhafte Rindenabtragung* und auch die *elektrochirurgische Rindenzerstörung* scheint mit häufigeren postoperativen Komplikationen belastet zu sein (Epilepsie).

3. Die *intracorticale bzw. subcorticale Alkoholinjektion* ist in ihrem Ergebnis zu unsicher.

4. Die auf den — beim Menschen heute nicht mehr anerkannten — *„Suppressor-Streifen“ (Area 4s) beschränkte Rindenexcision* hat sich nicht bewährt.

5. Die *lineare Rindenincision* zwischen Feld 6 und 4s beim PARKINSON-Tremor war ein vollständiger Mißerfolg in allen Fällen.

Allerdings scheint ein solcher Längsschnitt in die Rinde zwischen Area 4 und 4s beim Hemiballismus in einem Falle MEYERS zu einem vollen Erfolg geführt zu haben.

6. Die *Subcorticotomie* („T-Tomy“) nach der Originalmethode von TAKEBAYASHI ist zweifellos infolge einer unzureichenden Genauigkeit zu unsicher, da die Unterschneidung der Rindenfelder gewissermaßen „im Dunkeln“ ohne die Möglichkeit einer exakten Lokalisation der Präzentralwindung (Area 4) ausgeführt werden muß. Die Ergebnisse mit der Rindenunterschneidung lassen sich möglicherweise mit ausgedehnteren osteoplastischen Freilegungen und vorheriger genauer Bestimmung des Feldes 4 durch elektrische Reizung verbessern.

Zur Behandlung der Bewegungen der *Choreoathetosen* ist eine möglichst vollständige Entfernung bzw. Isolierung des Feldes 6 erforderlich, und es empfiehlt sich, immer darüber hinaus auch den vorderen Rand der elektrisch reizbaren Rinde, welche der Area 4 angehört, mitzuentfernen, um ein befriedigendes Resultat erreichen zu können. Die hiernach in Erscheinung tretenden kontralateralen Paresen sind gewöhnlich nur vorübergehend, bis auf gelegentlich permanent bleibende Störungen der willkürlichen motorischen Funktion an den distalen Abschnitten der Gliedmaßen.

Die Behandlung der verschiedenen Formen des *Tremors* erfordert stets eine möglichst weitgehende Entfernung bzw. Zerstörung oder Isolierung des Feldes 4, insbesondere im Gebiet des vorderen Walls des Sulcus centralis Rolandi. Die ventral davon gelegene Rinde (Area 6) sollte unter Umständen mit entfernt werden. Die nach diesen Eingriffen auftretenden kontralateralen Paresen sind im allgemeinen zunächst total und schlaff. Nach Wochen werden diese spastisch und noch später kehrt in der Regel eine gewisse Willkürmotorik zurück bis auf eine dauerhafte Unfähigkeit zu isolierten Willkürbewegungen an den körperfernen Gliedmaßenabschnitten, wie z. B. der Finger. Die Symptome der Bewegungsarmut (Akinese) und der Starre (Rigidität) werden bei einem solchen Vorgehen wenig bzw. gar nicht beeinflußt.

*Vorteile der Cortectomie.* Wenn eine Hyperkinese lediglich eine einzelne Extremität betrifft, so kann der Eingriff auf den der isolierten Hyperkinese entsprechenden Teil des kontralateralen Rindenfeldes beschränkt werden. Damit bleibt die Gefahr einer postoperativen Parese ebenso nur auf die Extremität beschränkt, welche von der Hyperkinese betroffen ist. Man geht also lediglich das Risiko einer Monoparese ein.

*Nachteile der Cortectomie:*

1. Gefahr des Auftretens aphasischer Störungen bei Operation an der führenden Hemisphäre.

2. Möglichkeit der Entstehung eines postoperativen Anfallsleidens (BUCY sah unter seinen ersten 8 Fällen 2 postoperative Epilepsien!).

3. Erschwerte Nachoperation nach unzureichendem Ergebnis infolge der Hirndura-vernarbungen.

4. Wachsendes Operationsrisiko bei doppelseitigen Operationen.

Die *Mortalität* der corticalen Eingriffe hat bei BUCY, bei MEYERS und beim Verfasser 0%, bei KLEMME unter 100 Fällen 17%, bei REID unter 15 Fällen 13,3% und bei DAVID, HECAÉN und TALAIRACH unter 13 Fällen 15,3% betragen.

## II. Die Eingriffe an den subcorticalen Strukturen.

Im Jahre 1940 wurde zum ersten Male von RUSSELL MEYERS versucht, zur Beeinflussung des Tremors und anderer Symptome der Paralysis agitans an den Stammganglien selbst zu operieren. MEYERS' verschiedene Operationsversuche waren auf eine Unterbrechung der Impulsleitung im Gebiet der subcorticalen Erregungskreise gerichtet.

Aber obgleich er seine Eingriffe immer weiter ausgedehnt hat, blieb ihnen ein wirklich durchschlagender Erfolg eigentlich versagt. Das Wesentlichste an MEYERS' Eingriffen, welche infolge des transventrikulären Vorgehens übrigens mit einem ungewöhnlich großen Risiko einhergehen, sind jedoch ohne Zweifel die auf diese Weise gewonnenen sehr interessanten physiologischen Erkenntnisse gewesen. Als MEYERS (1942) seine ersten Erfahrungen bekanntgab, hatte er bereits Eingriffe an verschiedenen subcorticalen Strukturen durchgeführt, ohne aber ein Standardverfahren gefunden zu haben. Mitunter hat er am gleichen Kranken in einer einzelnen Sitzung mehrere Eingriffe in der Tiefe hintereinander vorgenommen, bis schließlich der Tremor verschwand. In seinem ersten Fall, unter insgesamt 41 derartig operierten Patienten, hat er sich auf eine Zerstörung des Kopfes vom Nucleus caudatus beschränkt. Nachdem sich aber die Unzulänglichkeit dieses Vorgehens erwiesen hatte, wurden von ihm bei den darauffolgenden Operationen so lange bestimmte Strukturen in Angriff genommen, bis, noch auf dem Operationstisch, die Tremorsymptome ausgeschaltet waren. Auf diese Art hat MEYERS im Verlauf der gleichen Operation nacheinander die Radiatio subcallosa durchtrennt, den Kopf des Nucleus caudatus exstirpiert, dann die vordere Hälfte und schließlich auch noch den hinteren Teil des ventralen Schenkels der inneren Kapsel durchschnitten. Das Endergebnis hat jedoch nicht zufriedengestellt, da später der Tremor nur noch geringgradig vermindert und die Starre kaum beeinflußt war. In den nächsten beiden Fällen wurde nun von MEYERS auch das vordere Drittel des Putamen und in Verbindung damit der orale Teil des Globus pallidus zerstört und die Fasern in den vorderen $^3/_4$ des ventralen Schenkels der inneren Kapsel durchtrennt. Der Tremor soll in diesen beiden Fällen nahezu aufgehoben und auch die Starre vermindert worden sein. Dennoch hat das Ergebnis nicht voll befriedigt, und MEYERS hat, übrigens auch um der möglichen Verletzung eines zum Versorgungsgebiet des hinteren Schenkels der inneren Kapsel gehörigen Gefäßes aus dem Wege zu gehen, seinen Eingriff nochmals modifiziert. Nach Entfernung des Kopfes vom Schwanzkern durchtrennte er durch ein besonderes Vorgehen — am Fornix entlang — das pallidofugale Bündel. Diese in den letzten Fällen durchgeführte Unterbrechung der pallidofugalen Einflüsse mit einer Durchschneidung der Ansa lenticularis hatte offenbar zu den besten Resultaten geführt.

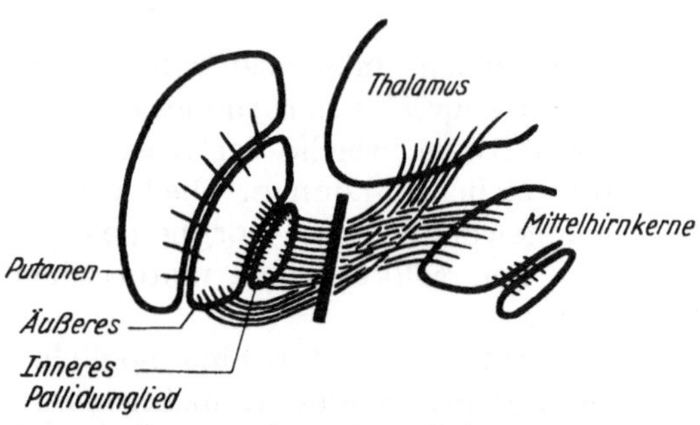

Abb. 10. Unterbrechung der pallidofugalen Faserverbindungen (schematisch, in Anlehnung an MEYERS).

Ein Urteil über den Wert der von MEYERS angewandten verschiedenen Techniken muß nach den von ihm mitgeteilten Operationsergebnissen zu finden versucht werden. MEYERS hat insgesamt 38 PARKINSON-Kranke, darunter 9 doppelseitige Syndrome, operiert. In 7 Fällen soll eine sehr gute Besserung, in 18 Fällen ein ausreichendes Resultat und in 7 Fällen ein Mißerfolg erzielt worden sein. Nicht einbezogen wurden 6 Todesfälle (etwa 16%). Bei 3 von den 7 *sehr gut gebesserten* Fällen hat MEYERS lediglich eine Durchschneidung der pallidofugalen Verbindungen im Gebiet der Ansa lenticularis durchgeführt und bei 2 anderen hat er zusätzlich den Kopf des Nucleus caudatus abgetragen und die Fasern des ventralen Schenkels der Capsula interna durchtrennt. Bei einem weiteren sehr gut gebesserten Fall wurde die prämotorische Rinde unterschnitten und eine Exstirpation des Kopfes vom Schwanzkern vorgenommen. Allerdings hat sich 4 Jahre später auf derselben Seite eine Hemichorea eingestellt. Bei dem siebenten, ebenfalls sehr gut gebesserten Kranken ist neben einer Entfernung des Kopfes vom Nucleus caudatus eine Durchtrennung der Fasern des oralen Schenkels der inneren Kapsel durchgeführt worden. — Unter den 18 *ausreichend gebesserten* Fällen wurden 7mal lediglich die pallidofugalen Fasern durchschnitten, davon einmal doppelseitig. In 2 Fällen dieser

Gruppe sind zusätzlich die Fasern des vorderen Schenkels der Capsula interna und eine Entfernung des Schwanzkernkopfes ausgeführt worden und in einem 3. Fall wurde darüber hinaus noch eine Zerstörung des oralen Teils vom Putamen hinzugefügt. In weiteren 4 Fällen derselben Gruppe bestand die Operation in einer Abtragung des Schwanzkernkopfes und einer Durchtrennung des ventralen Schenkels der inneren Kapsel. Dasselbe, doch zusätzlich mit einer Entfernung des vorderen Drittels vom Putamen, wurde in 2 anderen Fällen dieser Gruppe durchgeführt. Schließlich hat MEYERS in den letzten beiden Fällen dieser Gruppe mit einer ausreichenden Besserung der Bewegungsstörung zum letztgenannten Vorgehen noch eine Zerstörung auch des vorderen Drittels vom Globus pallidus hinzugefügt. — In den 13 *nicht beeinflußten* Zuständen wurde 5mal nur der Schwanzkernkopf abgetragen und gleichfalls 5mal nur eine vordere Capsulotomie und schließlich 3mal eine Durchtrennung des pallidofugalen Bündels allein oder in Verbindung mit Zerstörungen anderer Strukturen durchgeführt.

Ohne aus MEYERS' großen Erfahrungen endgültige Schlüsse ziehen zu wollen, läßt sich an ihrem Beispiel zeigen, welche Stellen der subcorticalen Steuerungskreise für eine Leitungsunterbrechung krankhafter motorischer Impulse geeignet erscheinen bzw. welche Strukturen sich bereits als ungeeignet hierfür erwiesen haben. MEYERS hat selbst von den verschiedenen Verfahren zuletzt nur noch die Unterbrechung pallidofugaler Erregungszuflüsse zum Thalamus und zu tiefer gelegenen Kernen mittels einer Durchschneidung des pallidofugalen Bündels, einschließlich Ansa lenticularis, zusammen mit einer Durchtrennung der im vorderen Schenkel der Capsula interna absteigenden Fasern, durchgeführt. Dieses Vorgehen, auch in Verbindung mit einer Entfernung des Kopfes vom Nucleus caudatus, schien ihm am verheißungsvollsten.

Das ohne Zweifel beinahe etwas heroische Vorgehen von MEYERS hat in den folgenden Jahren nur wenig Nachahmer gefunden. Anscheinend erfolgreich hat einmal PUTNAM durch die Resektion des Schwanzkernkopfes und einer damit verbundenen Durchschneidung der im vorderen Schenkel der inneren Kapsel verlaufenden Fasern die Symptome eines einseitigen Tremors zu bessern versucht. HAMBY, welcher 1947 über ein gutes Ergebnis nach einer einseitigen Durchschneidung der pallidofugalen Faserverbindungen berichtete, hatte aber nachfolgend mehrere Todesfälle nach der ein- und zweizeitig ausgeführten bilateralen Operation zu beklagen!

JEFFERSON BROWDER (1947) hat MEYERS' Fälle katamnestisch verfolgt. Er kam dadurch zu der Auffassung, daß der bedeutsamste Faktor an MEYERS verschiedenen Techniken die Unterbrechung der parapyramidalen Fasern im vorderen Schenkel der inneren Kapsel sei. Die Resultate nach diesem Eingriff sollen denen nach der Rindenexcision und selbst denen nach einer Durchschneidung der pallidofugalen Fasern überlegen sein. BROWDER hat 1948 das Ergebnis der transventrikulär durchgeführten *Capsulotomie* an einer Serie von 15 PARKINSON-Kranken mitgeteilt. Darunter bestanden in 9 Fällen die Erscheinungen eines vorwiegend einseitigen grobschlägigen Tremors. Sie sind durch den Eingriff in 6 Fällen vollständig beseitigt worden. In einem Falle wurde eine befriedigende Besserung des Tremors erreicht und in 2 Fällen war der Erfolg nur vorübergehend, da schon nach 2 Wochen bzw. 2 Monaten der Tremor wiederkehrte. In den restlichen 6 Fällen waren die Symptome doppelseitig und bei dreien von ihnen stand eine Akinese und Rigidität derart im Vordergrund, daß die Patienten „wie zu Eis erstarrt" schienen. Diese 3 akinetischen Kranken sind einige Tage post operationem an den Folgen des Eingriffs gestorben, ohne daß ein besonderer Autopsiebefund erhoben werden konnte. Bei den 3 anderen Kranken wurde der Tremor der Gegenseite vollständig beseitigt, er blieb aber homolateral unbeeinflußt.

Durch die Benutzung eines temporalen Zuganges konnte FÉNÉLON (1950) das größere Risiko des transventrikulären Vorgehens von MEYERS' zur Durchschneidung der pallidofugalen Verbindungen herabsetzen. FÉNÉLON hat in 2 PARKINSON-Fällen die Ansa lenticularis und das pallidäre Bündel durchtrennt und damit angeblich nicht nur eine beachtliche Besserung der Tremorsymptome, sondern vor allem auch der Akinese und des muskulären Hypertonus erzielt. In einem von diesen beiden Fällen hat FÉNÉLON 4 Wochen nach der 1. Operation mit Erfolg denselben Eingriff auch auf der anderen Seite durchgeführt. Hervorzuheben ist, daß in FÉNÉLONs erstem Fall unmittelbar nach der Operation eine sofortige Verminderung der Starre homolateral zur Seite der Craniotomie eingetreten ist, dagegen nicht auf der Gegenseite. Erst in den folgenden Tagen und Wochen zeigte sich auch eine gewisse Besserung der Rigidität auf der Gegenseite, welche verzögert, aber fortschreitend eingetreten sein soll. Im zweiten Falle jedoch ist sofort nach der 1. Sitzung der Operation eine deutliche Besserung der muskulären Hypertonie, Akinese und Tremorsymptome auf der Gegenseite vorhanden gewesen, während homolateral der Tremor bestehen blieb. Nach der in einer zweiten Sitzung 4 Wochen später kontralateral ausgeführten Operation ist dann auch der persistierende Tremor der anderen Seite verschwunden und der Hypertonus und die Akinese vermindert gewesen. FÉNÉLON hat aber nicht versucht, für diese widersprechenden Reaktionen, nämlich daß einmal die Besserung der Erscheinungen homolateral zur Seite des Eingriffs und ein anderes Mal kontralateral eingetreten ist, eine plausible Erklärung zu geben.

Angeregt und ermutigt durch die Erfahrungen von MEYERS und von FÉNÉLON haben GUIOT und BRION (1952) versucht, durch eine *Zerstörung des inneren Pallidumgliedes* auf die unkontrollierten Bewegungen einzuwirken. In einem Zeitraum von 2 Jahren operierten sie 57 Patienten mit abnormen Bewegungen und teilten das Ergebnis der ersten 47 Eingriffe, darunter 40 PARKINSON-Syndrome und 7 choreoathetotische Bewegungsstörungen, mit. Von den 40 PARKINSON-*Kranken* wurden 17 mit sehr gutem Erfolg operiert, 9 zeigten eine Besserung und 9 wurden nicht beeinflußt, 2 zeigten eine Verschlechterung des Zustandes und 3 starben nach dem Eingriff. In den erfolgreichen Fällen waren Tremor und Hypertonus auf einer Seite sofort und definitiv beseitigt und mitunter wurde auch eine beidseitige Besserung beobachtet. Bei den einfachen Besserungen sind nach einem unmittelbar guten Operationsresultat in den folgenden Wochen und Monaten die Symptome bis zu einem gewissen Grad, jedoch niemals in vollem Umfang, wiedergekehrt. Die 2 Verschlechterungen des Zustandes glauben GUIOT und BRION einer fehlerhaften Operationstechnik zur Last legen zu können. Die Todesfälle gingen ursächlich in einem Falle auf eine tiefe intracerebrale Blutung, in einem anderen auf eine postoperative Hyperthermie und schließlich auf die ungewöhnliche Belastung einer in einer Sitzung durchgeführten doppelseitigen Operation zurück. — Unter den 7 *choreoathetotischen Syndromen* war diese chirurgische Intervention in 3 Fällen erfolgreich und in 4 Fällen ergebnislos. Nach Auffassung von GUIOT und BRION scheinen die choreatischen Bewegungen durch den Eingriff unterdrückt werden zu können, während die Bewegungen der Athetose nicht wesentlich zu beeinflussen sind. Zur Zerstörung des inneren Pallidumgliedes, der *Pallidotomie,* wählten GUIOT und BRION verschiedene Techniken, einmal einen frontalen Zugang, dann einen Zugang durch die eröffnete Fissura Sylvii und schließlich die Methode der gezielten Ausschaltung. Der Zugang durch die breit eröffnete Fissura Sylvii scheint der sicherste zu sein und die zuverlässigsten Resultate gegeben zu haben.

Die Operationstechnik wird im folgenden Abschnitt beschrieben.

Einen ganz neuen Weg, um Unterbrechungen an den subcorticalen extrapyramidalen Steuerungskreisen herbeizuführen, beschritten erstmals SPIEGEL und WYCIS (1947). Nachdem sie dem bis dahin nur in der Physiologie benutzten Stereoencephalotom nach einigen Abänderungen Eingang in die Klinik verschafft hatten, versuchten sie unter anderem den Hyperkinesen durch *gezielte elektrolytische Läsionen im Gebiet der Basalganglien und ihrer Verbindungen* beizukommen. Es ist vom pathophysiologischen Standpunkt aus interessant, das Ergebnis ihrer verschiedenen Ausschaltungsversuche zu verfolgen, bis es ihnen endlich gelang, eine permanente Besserung der unwillkürlichen Bewegungen zu erreichen.

Im Jahre 1948 behandelten SPIEGEL und WYCIS den ersten Patienten mit einer Hyperkinese mit ihrem Zielgerät. Als Zielpunkt wählten sie für die *choreoathetotischen*

*Bewegungen* zunächst den *dorsomedialen Kern des Thalamus*, von der Überlegung ausgehend, daß einerseits Läsionen des dorsomedialen Thalamuskernes emotionelle Reaktionen herabsetzen können und andererseits hier eine Unterbrechung der von PAPEZ (1942) beschriebenen thalamopallidären Faserverbindungen zu erreichen sein müsse.

Der von SPIEGEL und WYCIS zuerst behandelte Fall einer Hyperkinese war ein 53jähriger Mann mit bilateralen choreiformen Bewegungen. Als erstes setzten sie bei ihm einen gezielten elektrolytischen Schädigungsherd im linksseitigen dorsomedialen Thalamuskern und rechtsseitig injizierten sie gezielt einen Tropfen 50%igen Alkohol in das Gebiet des Globus pallidus. Anschließend war rechtsseitig vorübergehend eine Besserung der Bewegungsstörung eingetreten, während diese auf der linken Körperseite völlig unbeeinflußt blieb. Nach Verlauf von 6 Wochen bestand praktisch wieder der gleiche Zustand wie vor dem Eingriff. — Beim gleichen Patienten wurde nun in einer zweiten Sitzung 10 Monate nach der ersten Operation auf der rechten Seite der dorsomediale Kern durch Elektrolyse geschädigt. Diesmal fand sich postoperativ eine transitorische Besserung der Bewegungsstörung auf der linken Seite, welche sich allerdings nur in einer Frequenzverminderung der Automatismen äußerte und nicht länger als 3 Wochen lang angehalten hat. — Obgleich nach $^1/_2$ Jahr wieder ganz der gleiche Zustand wie vor den Eingriffen bestand, verdient das Fehlen irgendwelcher Nebenerscheinungen, insbesondere die völlig unbeeinflußt gebliebene Willkürmotorik, hervorgehoben zu werden.

In zwei weiteren Fällen einer HUNTINGTONschen Chorea blieben Läsionen des dorsomedialen Thalamuskernes ergebnislos und bei einem Jungen mit einer frühkindlichen Hemiparese und Athetose hat die Verminderung der unwillkürlichen Bewegungen nur einige Tage nach der auf der Gegenseite vorgenommenen Thalamotomie angehalten.

Den 4. Kranken, einen 68jährigen Neger mit einer familiären HUNTINGTON-Chorea haben SPIEGEL und WYCIS 3mal hintereinander im Abstand von etwa 3 Monaten mit weitaus besserem Endresultat gezielten Koagulationen unterzogen. In der ersten Sitzung wurden ausgedehnte Schädigungsherde im linken dorsomedialen Kern und dazu ein kleiner Herd in der vorderen Spitze des rechten Globus pallidus gesetzt ohne den geringsten Effekt auf die Bewegungsstörung. — In einer 2. Sitzung wurden ausgedehntere Herde im äußeren Glied des rechten Globus pallidus hinzugefügt, wonach die unwillkürlichen Bewegungen auf der linken, der Gegenseite, verschwanden und daneben eine diskrete linksseitige Parese in Erscheinung trat, welche aber nach 2 Wochen schon nahezu vollständig restituiert war. — In einer 3. Sitzung wurden nun nach dem vorausgegangenen Erfolg in der gleichen Weise ausgedehnte Koagulationsherde im äußeren Pallidumglied der linken Seite gesetzt, wodurch die choreiformen Bewegungen auch der rechten Seite, mit Ausnahme der Zehen, behoben gewesen sein sollen. Auch nach dem letzten Eingriff sei es lediglich zu einer vorübergehenden motorischen Schwäche der rechtsseitigen Gliedmaßen gekommen. Selbst 9 Monate nach diesen Eingriffen sollen die unkontrollierten Bewegungen nicht wiedergekehrt sein. Als einziges Restsymptom blieb eine leichte motorische Schwäche des linken Beines bestehen.

Es zeigte sich also, daß die *Thalamotomie*, d. h. eine Läsion im dorsomedialen Kern des Thalamus, nur zu einer vorübergehenden Besserung *choreoathetotischer Bewegungen* führt. Dagegen konnten durch eine *Pallidotomie*, d. h. durch eine ausgedehnte Schädigung des äußeren Pallidumgliedes, Bewegungsstörungen aus dem hyperkinetisch-hypotonen Formenkreis (Choreoathetose) dauerhaft und nahezu vollständig behoben werden, ohne daß dadurch gleichfalls die Willkürmotorik wesentlich in Mitleidenschaft gezogen wurde.

Zur Beeinflussung der *Tremorsymptome bei der Paralysis agitans* versuchten SPIEGEL und WYCIS drei verschiedene Ausschaltungsmodi.

1. Die *Mesencephalotomie*, eine Unterbrechung aufsteigender Leitungswege im Mittelhirndach, ist ergebnislos hinsichtlich der Tremorsymptome geblieben.

2. Die *Thalamotomie*, eine Unterbrechung der Impulsleitung vom Thalamus zum Striopallidum, hat meist nur eine vorübergehende Besserung des Tremors für die Dauer von einigen Tagen zur Folge gehabt.

3. Die *Ansotomie*, eine Unterbrechung der pallidofugalen Impulsleitung, zeigte eine deutliche und dauerhafte Besserung der Tremorsymptome. Durch die Ansotomie ist nach dem Bericht der Autoren definitiv der Tremor der Paralysis agitans an der kontralateralen Körperhälfte zu vermindern, ohne die Willkürbewegungen, die Oberflächen- und Tiefensensibilität zu beeinträchtigen. Der Muskeltonus wird ihrer Erfahrung nach nicht verändert.

In der Folgezeit sind weitere Erfahrungen mit gezielten Eingriffen an subcorticalen Strukturen gesammelt worden. So hat TALAIRACH zusammen mit PAILLAS und DAVID

(1950) einen Fall von *Hemiballismus* mitgeteilt, in welchem nach einem unzulänglichen Ergebnis mit einer präzentralen Cortectomie eine gezielte Koagulation mit Erfolg nachgeholt wurde. Sie setzten 6 Monate nach dem mißglückten corticalen Eingriff Koagulationsherde im *Verbindungsgebiet zwischen Putamen und Schwanzkern*, in der *Linsenkernschlinge* und im *vorderen Teil des Globus pallidus*. Die daraufhin eingetretene Besserung des hemiballistischen Syndroms ist nach den bisherigen Erfahrungen wohl im wesentlichen auf die Schädigung des pallidofugalen Systems zu beziehen. Ob die anfänglich gute Besserung der Symptome dauerhaft bestehen blieb, ist nicht hinreichend gesichert.

Beim PARKINSON-*Tremor* haben TALAIRACH und Mitarbeiter (1950) die gezielte Koagulation auf den Kopf des Nucleus caudatus und den vorderen Teil des Putamens, in Höhe der Verbindungsfasern zwischen Putamen und Schwanzkern, beschränkt. Der zunächst beseitigte Tremor ist aber bereits nach einigen Tagen wiedergekehrt.

Im Jahre 1952 machen FÉNÉLON und Mitarbeiter die Mitteilung über ein gutes Behandlungsergebnis bei 2 PARKINSON-Kranken, bei denen sie mit der stereotaxischen Ausschaltung im gleichen Kerngebiet eingegriffen haben, an welches sie 2 Jahre vorher bei zwei anderen Kranken durch eine große operative Freilegung von frontotemporal her gelangten. In allen 4 Fällen, ob durch operative Freilegung oder durch gezielte Ausschaltung, setzten sie eine umschriebene Schädigung in der Gegend unmittelbar unter dem Pallidum, wo die Dichte der pallidofugalen extrapyramidalen Neurone am größten ist. Die Hauptfasersysteme, der Fasciculus lenticularis und die Linsenkernschlinge, werden an dieser Stelle unterbrochen. Durch den Eingriff werden angeblich nicht nur die Tremorsymptome, sondern vor allem auch die Starre und der muskuläre Hypertonus permanent herabgesetzt. Die pyramidale Motorik wird dagegen nicht beeinträchtigt.

In Deutschland sind es RIECHERT und WOLFF (1952), welche mit einer eigenen Zielmethode begrenzte subcorticale Läsionen bei Hyperkinesen ausgeführt haben. Im Falle einer *Hemiathetose* schalteten sie nach dem Vorbild von MEYERS, FÉNÉLON und GUIOT das *innere Pallidumglied* aus und erreichten damit eine gute Besserung der Bewegungsstörung. Bei einem PARKINSON-*Kranken* versuchten sie eine gezielte Ausschaltung im *oralen Ventralkern des Thalamus*. Es sei während des Eingriffs sehr eindrucksvoll gewesen, wie der Tremor auf der Gegenseite unter der Ausschaltung geringer geworden sei, um schließlich vollständig zu sistieren. Wie lange dieser in einem Einzelfall erzielte günstige Behandlungseffekt angedauert hat ist noch abzuwarten.

Die *mittleren basalen Teile des Globus pallidus* hat nach einer persönlichen Mitteilung LEKSELL (1953) bei einer Hemichorea koaguliert. Er sah jedoch keinen Effekt auf die Bewegungsstörung, auch dann nicht, als er in einer 2. Sitzung den Globus pallidus fast vollständig zerstörte. Durch den Erfolg der gezielten Ansotomie von SPIEGEL und WYCIS angeregt, hat LEKSELL (1953) diese in 2 Fällen von Tremor versucht. In einem Falle ist 3—4 Wochen nach der Ausschaltung der Tremor wiedergekehrt und nach einem Vierteljahr war der Zustand wieder wie vor der Operation. Im anderen Falle waren die Tremorsymptome wesentlich gebessert und die willkürliche motorische Kraft nicht beeinträchtigt, doch kam es 3 Monate nach dem Eingriff unter emotionellen Affekten wieder zu einer Verstärkung der Tremorsymptome, während auf der anderen Seite der Ruhetremor beseitigt blieb.

## 1. Die operative Technik der subcorticalen Eingriffe.

1. Zum *Kopf des Schwanzkernes* und zum *vorderen Schenkel der inneren Kapsel* gelangt MEYERS durch ein transfrontales und transventrikuläres Vorgehen. Etwa an der Grenze zwischen Feld 6 und 8 wird von einer Rindenincision aus das Vorderhorn des Seitenventrikels eröffnet. Mit dem Sauger wird der lateral gelegene Kopf des Nucleus caudatus entfernt, bis die weißen Markfasern der inneren Kapsel sichtbar werden. Nun werden mit einem stumpfen Häkchen die im vorderen Schenkel der Capsula interna verlaufenden parapyramidalen corticopetalen Fasern durchtrennt. MEYERS hat daran

anschließend von hier aus in einigen Fällen auch das ventrale Drittel vom Putamen und vom Pallidum zerstört, deren Strukturen in dieser Höhe unmittelbar lateral vom vorderen Schenkel der inneren Kapsel gelegen sind. Die im hinteren Drittel des vorderen Schenkels der inneren Kapsel vorbeiziehenden Pyramidenfasern werden von MEYERS geschont, indem er die Durchschneidung vor Erreichen des Kapselknies unterbricht (s. Abb. 11 und 12).

2. Für die Durchschneidung der *pallidofugalen Verbindungen*, welche unmittelbar unterhalb des Striopallidum in horizontaler Verlaufsrichtung in einem dichten Bündel nach medial ziehen, benutzt MEYERS einen ähnlichen Zugang. Nahe der Mittellinie wird in der 1. Stirnwindung, etwa im vorderen Teil der Area 6, eine Rindenincision ausgeführt

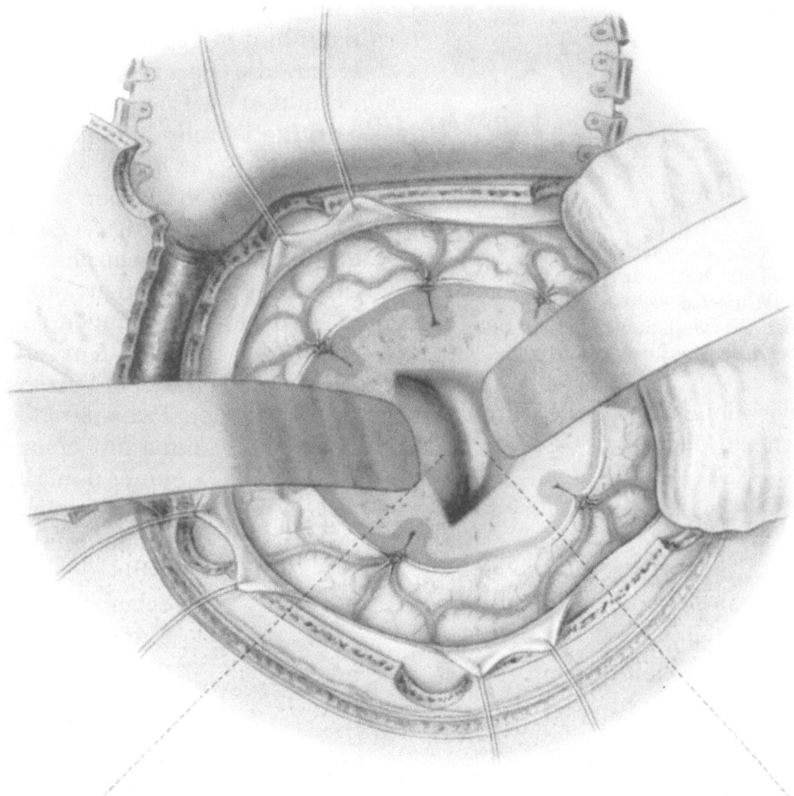


Abb. 11. Transventrikulärer Zugang zum linken Schwanzkernkopf, wie er von MEYERS und BROWDER benutzt wird.

und senkrecht in die Tiefe vorgegangen. Der Seitenventrikel wird durch die Balkenstrahlung hindurch eröffnet. Nun wird durch eine Incision an der tiefsten Stelle des Foramen Monroi, an der posterolateralen Seite des Fornix entlang, ein Spezialinstrument eingeführt, welches einem stumpfen Nervenhäkchen ähnelt, um die Ansa lenticularis sowie die pallidofugalen Fasern zu durchtrennen (s. Abb. 13 und 14).

Beim doppelseitigen PARKINSON-Syndrom soll es nicht schwer sein, durch das Septum pellucidum hindurch auch auf der Gegenseite die Unterbrechung der pallidofugalen Verbindungen durchzuführen.

3. Die *Capsulotomie* von BROWDER muß ebenfalls transventrikulär vorgenommen werden. BROWDER empfiehlt, das Vorderhorn des Seitenventrikels möglichst weit vorn zu eröffnen. Dazu wird eine etwa 2,5:3 cm große Rindenresektion im Bereich des hinteren Frontallappens, unmittelbar vor dem prämotorischen Feld und 3 cm von der Falx entfernt, durchgeführt. Nach der Ventrikeleröffnung muß mit dem Sauger oder Löffel

zuerst die vordere Hälfte des Schwanzkernkopfes entfernt werden, um die inneren Fasern des vorderen Schenkels der Capsula interna freizulegen. Die von diesen Fasern am weitesten vorn verlaufenden biegen bei ihrem Eintritt in die innere Kapsel in Form eines Regenbogens von vorn nach hinten. An dieser Stelle, das ist am vorderen Rand der inneren Kapsel auf der Höhe der Endigung der Corona radiata, beginnt die Durchschneidung. BROWDER benutzt dazu ein stumpfes, angelhakenförmiges Instrument, dessen Haken 8 mm lang ist. Nun werden schrittweise, von vorn nach hinten gegen das Knie der inneren Kapsel zu, die Fasern durchschnitten. An einem Punkt etwa 1,5—1 cm vor dem Kapselknie wird die Durchschneidung beendet, vorausgesetzt, daß bei dem während des Eingriffs beobachteten Patienten der Tremor kontralateral vollständig verschwunden ist. Als Merkmal, daß die Durchschneidung ausreicht und beendet werden kann, muß diese nach BROWDERs Erfahrungen so lange gegen das Knie der inneren Kapsel fortgeführt werden, bis neben dem Verschwinden des Tremors eine merkliche Parese der Hand erscheint, welche den Patienten lediglich noch zu einer schwachen Beugung der Finger befähigt. Nur dann könne mit einer bleibenden, einer dauerhaften Besserung gerechnet werden. Anderenfalls, d.h. bei fehlenden Lähmungserscheinungen, kehre der Tremor gewöhnlich nach einigen Wochen zurück (s. Abb. 11 und 12).

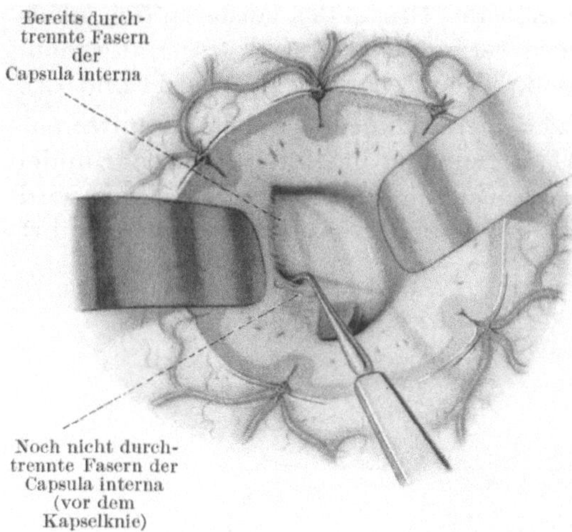


Abb. 12. Nachdem der Schwanzkernkopf abgetragen ist, werden die weißen Markfasern des vorderen Schenkels der Capsula interna sichtbar. Sie werden mit einem stumpfen Nervenhäkchen schrittweise von vorn nach hinten durchtrennt.

4. Zur *Durchschneidung der pallidofugalen Fasern* hat FÉNÉLON einen transtemporalen Zugangsweg gewählt, nachdem er vorher durch Ausmessungen an Leichenhirnen die Tiefe dieser Strukturen und ihre Entfernung von der Oberfläche des Schläfenlappens bestimmt hat. Bedauerlicherweise fehlen exakte Angaben zu den Messungen, welche an Frontalschnitten, 75 mm vom Frontalpol entfernt, ausgeführt wurden. FÉNÉLON hebt lediglich hervor, daß seine Messungen eine bemerkenswerte Konstanz der Lage der zentralen grauen Kerne gezeigt haben und daß die topographischen Abweichungen nur Millimeter betragen. Dann weist er auf die Gefahren hin, welche bei Benutzung einer hoch oder

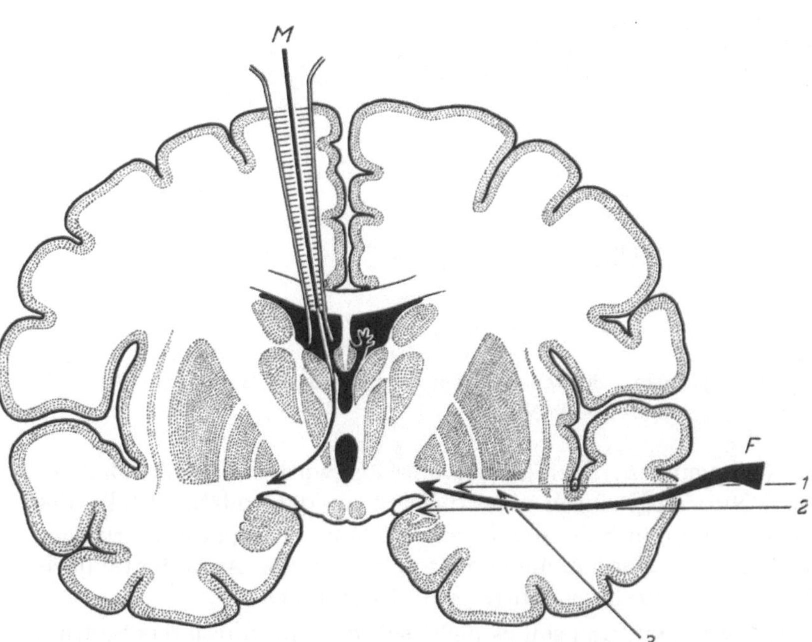


Abb. 13. Unterbrechung der pallidofugalen Faserverbindungen, links im Bild nach MEYERS (*M*), rechts im Bild nach FÉNÉLON (*F*) (s. Text).

einer tief angelegten horizontalen Schnittführung drohen. Beim hoch angelegten transtemporalen Horizontalschnitt ist eine Verletzung der unteren Gefäße der Fissura Sylvii und Insel zu fürchten (Schnittführung 1 in Abb. 13). Bei einem tiefer unten angelegten Horizontalschnitt (Schnittführung 2 in Abb. 13) besteht die Gefahr einer Läsion des

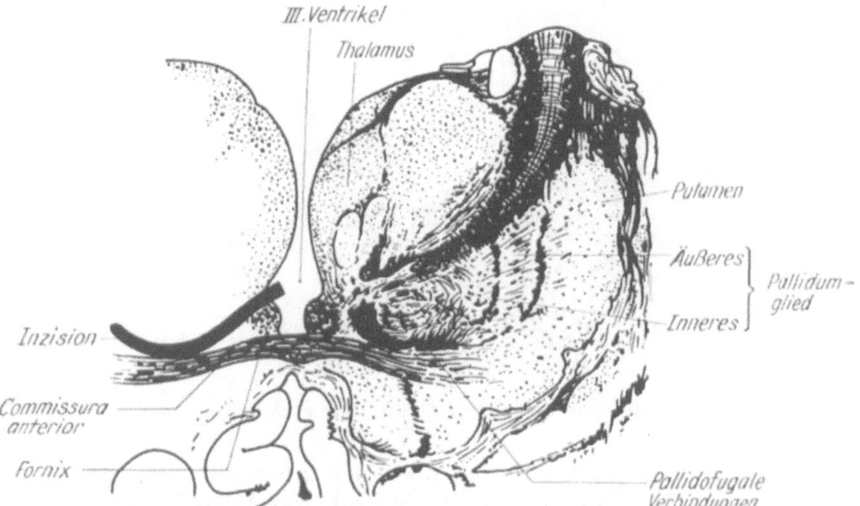


Abb. 14. Transventrikuläre Durchschneidung der pallidofugalen Verbindungen nach MEYERS (s. Text).

Tractus opticus und des Plexus chorioideus vom Unterhorn und schließlich würde ein schräg von basal her nach oben und medial gerichteter Schnitt nur einen kleinen Teil der stets ganz horizontal verlaufenden Fasern treffen (Schnittführung 3 in Abb. 13). Aus diesen Gründen gibt FÉNÉLON eine nach unten konvexe Schnittführung an, mit welcher man sich, von der 1./2. Schläfenwindung ausgehend, förmlich zwischen zwischen diesen beiden Gefahrenpunkten hindurchschlängeln muß. Zur Durchschneidung benutzt FÉNÉLON ein

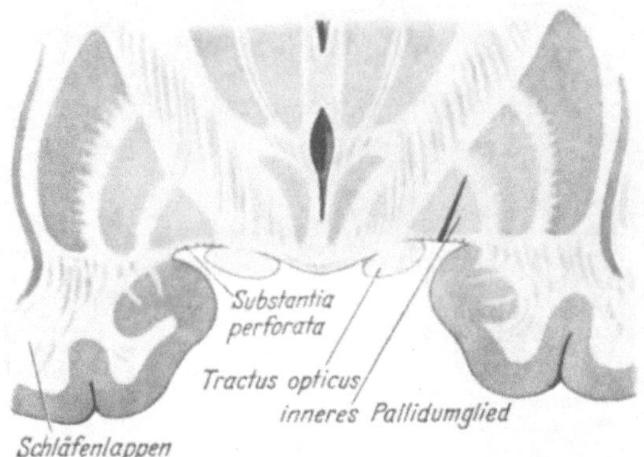


Abb. 15. Die Pallidotomie nach GUIOT und BRION (Frontalschnitt, schematisch).

dünnkalibriges biegsames Instrument. Wie aber ein derartiges Vorgehen im Dunkeln noch mit hinreichender Genauigkeit zu einer selektiven Ausschaltung nur der pallidofugalen Faserzüge führen soll, ist wenig einleuchtend. Doch FÉNÉLON behauptet sogar, daß eine Durchschneidung im rückwärtigen Teil des Bündels auf die Symptome der oberen Extremität und im vorn liegenden Teil auf die der unteren Extremität einwirke. Er selbst hat aber, wie oben ausgeführt wurde, widersprechende Ergebnisse in 2 Fällen mitgeteilt, in denen einmal die Besserung der PARKINSON-Symptome auf der Seite des Eingriffs und ein anderes Mal auf der Gegenseite gesehen wurde. Es wäre natürlich sehr interessant, in Erfahrung bringen zu können, welche Strukturen in Wirklichkeit geschädigt wurden (s. Abb. 13).

5. Bei der *Pallidotomie* nach Guiot und Brion wird das *innere Pallidumglied* durch Elektrokoagulation zerstört. Der Zugang kann auf verschiedene Weise, auf subfrontalem

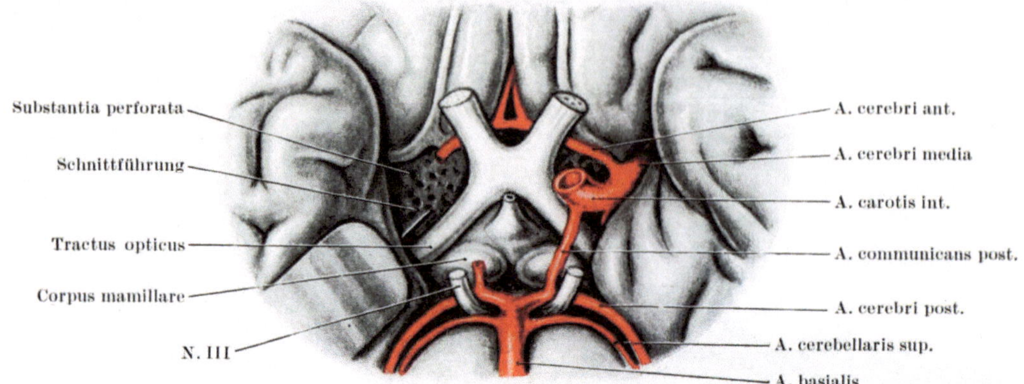


Abb. 16. Die Pallidotomie nach Guiot und Brion (Ansicht von der Basis).

Wege wie zur Hypophysenoperation oder über den kürzeren Weg durch die Fissura Sylvii, erreicht werden. Der letztere bietet die größeren Vorteile, so daß auf eine Beschreibung des subfrontalen Weges verzichtet werden kann.

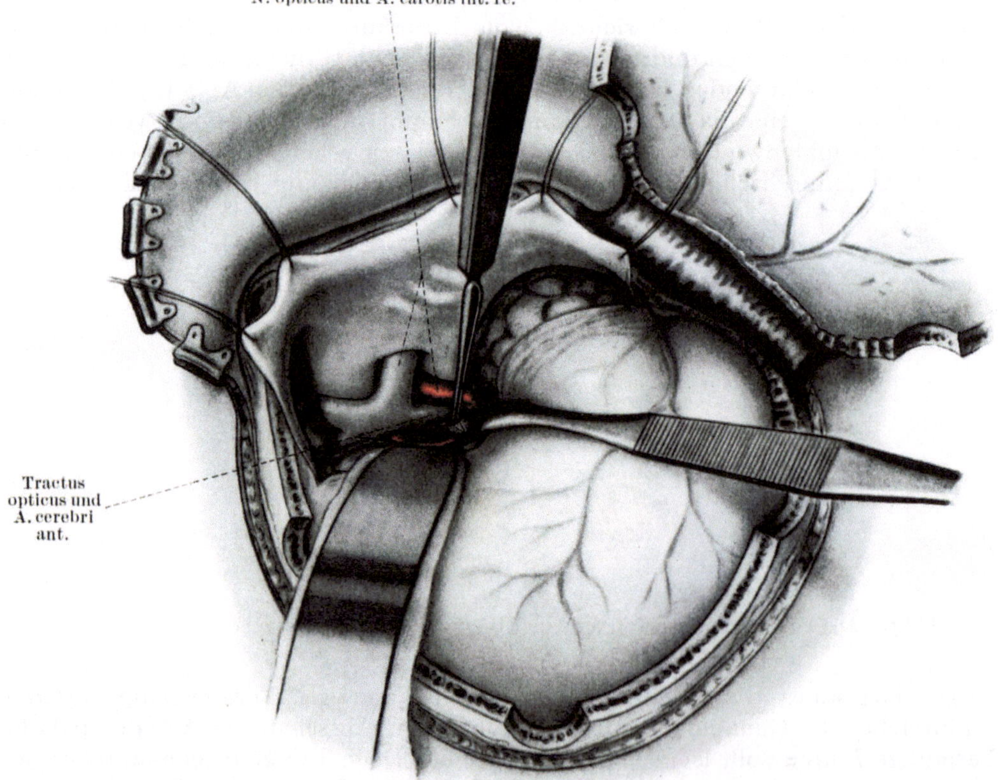


Abb. 17. Die Pallidotomie nach Guiot und Brion (Operationszugang von rechts, s. Text).

Zur Freilegung der Fissura Sylvii wird die übliche frontotemporale Craniotomie ausgeführt. Wichtig ist es, den Knochen bis zur Basis hin abzutragen und auch den lateralen

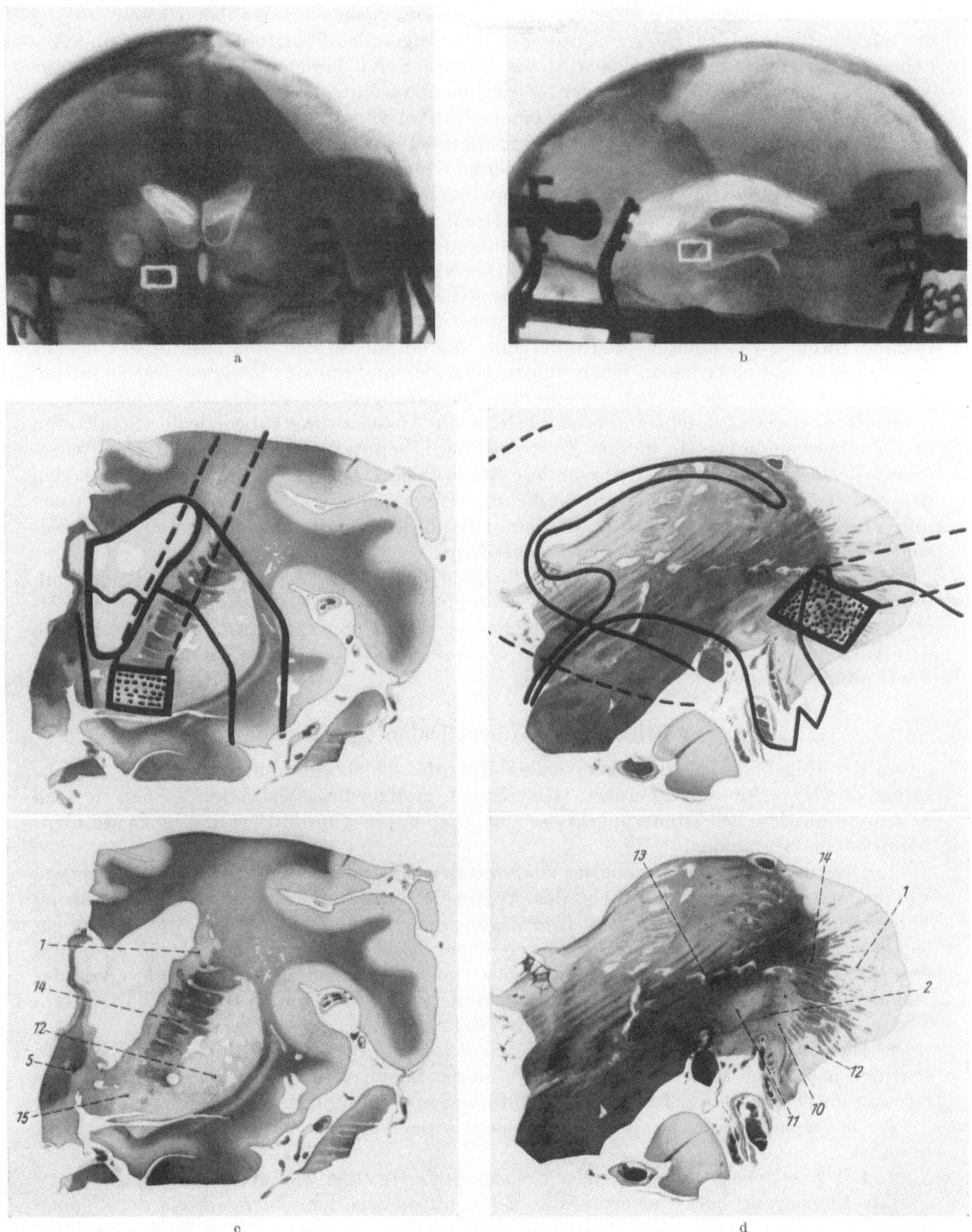


Abb. 18a—d. Ansotomie durch gezielte Ausschaltung. (Nach TALAIRACH.) a u. b. Lokalisation und Ausdehnung der gezielten Läsion auf dem Vorder- und Seitenbild. c u. d. Die Lage der Läsion im histologischen Schnitt (c Frontalschnitt, d Sagittalschnitt). *1* Schwanzkern; *2* Commissura ant.; *5* vorderer Pfeiler des Dreiecks vom Septum pallucidum; *10* äußeres Pallidumglied; *11* inneres Pallidumglied; *12* Putamen; *13* hinterer Schenkel d. Caps. int.; *14* vorderer Schenkel d. Caps. int.; *15* Stelle der Putamen-Caudatusverbindungen.

Teil des Keilbeinflügels zu entfernen, um sich das Vorgehen am Keilbeinrücken entlang und an der Basis zu erleichtern. Unter Zurückdrängen des Schläfenlappenpoles und Anheben des hinteren Stirnlappens wird die Fissura Sylvii breit eröffnet und nun bis zur Teilungsstelle der Carotis vorgegangen. Zwischen den behutsam etwas zur Seite gehaltenen Gefäßen wird mit einem stumpfen, in einem Winkel von 45$^{0}$ abgebogenen Häkchen die Substantia perforata anterior lateral und parallel zum Tractus opticus durchstoßen. Diese Stelle liegt etwa in Höhe des hinteren Chiasmawinkels und 3 mm lateral vom Tractus. Die Durchstoßung mit dem abgewinkelten Häkchen, welches eine Länge von 4 mm hat, geschieht unter einer leichten Drehung nach außen in einer Richtung nach oben hinten. Nun liegt das Häkchen im inneren Segment des Pallidum, etwa 4 mm tief. Durch Anwendung des gewöhnlichen Diathermiestromes ist dann eine Gewebsnekrose von einigen Millimetern im Umkreis zu erreichen, wobei wahrscheinlich nicht nur das innere Pallidumglied, sondern eben auch das subpallidäre Bündel, welches die pallidofugalen Impulse weiterleitet, zugrunde geht. Es empfiehlt sich, das Instrument bis zur Abwinkelung mit einer feinen Isolierung zu versehen und nur das Häkchen frei zu lassen, um Nebenschädigungen durch unbemerkte Berührungen des Stieles zu vermeiden.

6. Unter den Operationsmethoden, welche zur Ausschaltung subcorticaler Strukturen und Faserverbindungen in diesem Zusammenhang benutzt werden, nehmen die „*Stereotaxie*"-*Verfahren* zweifellos eine besondere Stellung ein. Die Technik einzelner Methoden der gezielten Hirnoperationen (Spiegel und Wycis, Talairach, Leksell, Riechert und Wolff) werden von Leksell in diesem Band des Handbuches behandelt, so daß es sich erübrigt, sie an dieser Stelle zu beschreiben[1].

Hier sollen lediglich zur Veranschaulichung dieser Art des Vorgehens einige Abbildungen von Talairach wiedergegeben werden, welche das Ausmaß einer gezielten Zerstörung im Gebiet des inneren Pallidumgliedes, der pallidofugalen Fasern einschließlich der Ansa lenticularis und der zwischen Putamen und Nucleus caudatus bestehenden Verbindungen zeigen (s. Abb. 18a—d).

## 2. Epikrise zu den subcorticalen Operationen.

In der Regel werden die subcorticalen Eingriffe gleichfalls kontralateral zur Lokalisation der Hyperkinese ausgeführt. Gewöhnlich greifen diese Methoden an den inneren extrapyramidalen Rücksteuerungskreisen an und lassen eine Mitläsion des Pyramidenbahnsystems vermeiden.

1. Die zuverlässigsten Ergebnisse sind von den Eingriffen zu erwarten, welche es gestatten, unter unbehinderter Sicht des Auges die Struktur, an welcher die Zerstörung vorgenommen werden soll, direkt freizulegen, oder welche es erlauben, durch ein geeignetes Zielverfahren diese exakt zu erreichen. Diese Bedingungen werden zum Teil von Meyers' Eingriffen, von der *Capsulotomie* nach Browder und insbesondere von der *Pallidotomie* nach Guiot bzw. von den bekannten *gezielten Operationen* erfüllt (Spiegel-Wycis, Talairach, Leksell, Riechert-Wolff).

2. Die *Ansotomie* und *subpallidäre Fasciculotomie* nach Meyers oder nach Fénélon scheinen in ihrem Ergebnis zu unsicher, da deren Schnittführung auf eine zu weite Entfernung im Dunkeln ausgeführt werden muß, um noch hinreichend exakt sein zu können.

3. Die *Mesencephalotomie* und *Thalamotomie* nach Spiegel-Wycis haben sich nicht bewährt.

4. Die *Resektion des Caput nuclei caudati* nach Meyers war ebenfalls erfolglos.

Zur Beseitigung oder Besserung der Bewegungen aus dem Formenkreis der *Choreoathetosen* scheinen herdförmige Ausschaltungen im äußeren Segment des Globus pallidus als auch im Gebiet des inneren Pallidumgliedes mit Unterbrechung der pallidofugalen Impulsleitung eine gewisse Aussicht auf Erfolg zu haben. Die Pallidotomie nach Guiot

---

[1] Ein zusammengefaßter Überblick über die Methoden der gezielten subcorticalen Ausschaltungen zu diesem Thema wurde von mir in einem Übersichtsreferat gegeben [Zbl. Neurochir. **13**, 223 (1953)].

scheint nach den bisherigen Erfahrungen des Autors einen noch unbestimmten günstigen Einfluß auf die choreatischen Bewegungsautomatismen auszuüben, die athetotischen Symptome dagegen unbeeinflußt zu lassen. Auch MEYERS hat schon angegeben, daß seine Durchschneidung der pallidofugalen Faserverbindungen ohne den geringsten Effekt auf die athetotischen Bewegungsstörungen geblieben ist. Über die Anwendung von BROWDERs Capsulotomia anterior bei den unkontrollierten Bewegungen der Choreoathetosen ist bisher nichts bekannt geworden.

Man sieht, daß die Resultate nach Eingriffen an den subcorticalen Kernstrukturen und Faserverbindungen bei den Choreoathetosen noch sehr umstritten sind. Sie haben bisher in der Mehrzahl der Fälle enttäuscht.

Aussichtsreicher sind die subcorticalen chirurgischen Maßnahmen bei den Erscheinungen der PARKINSON-*Erkrankungen* gewesen, wie die bisherigen Erfahrungen gezeigt haben. Mit einer Ausschaltung der Erregungen, welche ihren Weg über die Ansa lenticularis, das subpallidäre Bündel und die pallidofugalen Verbindungen nehmen, scheint es ebenso gut wie mit einer Zerstörung des inneren Pallidumgliedes möglich zu sein, nicht nur die Tremorsymptome, sondern auch die Starre und Bewegungsarmut günstig beeinflussen zu können. Die pyramidale Willkürmotorik wird hierbei entweder überhaupt nicht oder nur unbedeutend in Mitleidenschaft gezogen. Der transventrikulären vorderen Capsulotomie von BROWDER kommt demgegenüber sicher eine geringere Bedeutung zu, einerseits wegen des ungleich größeren Operationsrisikos und andererseits wegen der obligat notwendigen Erzeugung einer Pyramidenbahnschädigung (Hemiparese), da sonst der Eingriff wirkungslos bleibt. Unter den verschiedenen Techniken ist zur Zeit wohl dem Zielverfahren und der Operation von GUIOT der Vorzug zu geben.

Trotz des bisher Erreichten muß jedoch zugegeben werden, daß die heutigen Erfahrungen keineswegs ausreichen, selbst wenn sie reich an physiologischen Erkenntnissen gewesen sind, ein endgültiges Urteil über den Wert der Eingriffe an den subcorticalen Strukturen und Erregungskreisen zu fällen. Nicht allein, daß vorläufig noch jeder Operateur seinen eigenen Zugang oder sein eigenes Zielverfahren mit einer mehr oder minder exakten Lokalisationsmöglichkeit der Elektroden benutzt, sondern insbesondere die Verschiedenartigkeit der gewählten Schädigungsorte, nach welchen Besserungen der Bewegungsstörungen gesehen wurden, läßt das Experimentierstadium erkennen, in welchem die subcorticalen chirurgischen Maßnahmen einschließlich der stereotaxischen Methoden sich zur Zeit noch befinden. Schließlich kann es schwerlich befriedigen, wenn wir heute feststellen müssen, daß die gewagten Operationen an den Stammganglien von MEYERS, PUTNAM, HAMBY, FÉNÉLON oder GUIOT, welche zu ausreichend massiven Schädigungen eines oder mehrerer Kern- und Schaltungssysteme führen, vorerst noch hinsichtlich der Behandlungsresultate gegenüber den weitaus beschränkteren und weniger belastenden gezielten Läsionen überlegen zu sein scheinen. Immerhin lassen sich durch weitere Fortschritte mit den Zielverfahren, unter Umständen schon allein mit ausgedehnteren Läsionsherden, in Zukunft günstigere Heilungsaussichten erhoffen.

Soweit sich bisher abschätzen läßt, sind möglicherweise für den Erfolg subcorticalen Eingreifens zwei Dinge entscheidend. Erstens dürfte es von größter Bedeutung sein, daß die Impulsleitung gerade unterhalb des Ortes unterbrochen wird, von dem man annimmt, daß dort die krankhaften Erregungen entstehen und ihren Ausgang nehmen. Zweitens dürfte für den Erfolg aber auch das Quantum der durchschnittenen Fasern, welche der Impulsleitung dienen, eine nicht zu unterschätzende Rolle spielen. Nun scheint es ja, daß man durch ausreichende Zerstörungen im Gebiet des pallidofugalen Systems beiden Faktoren gerecht wird. Einerseits wird die Weiterleitung und Verbreitung der im Striopallidum entstehenden krankhaften Impulse zu den darunter gelegenen wichtigen Zentren (Corpus subthalamicum Luysi, ventromedialer Kern des Thalamus, Substantia nigra, Nucleus ruber) unterbrochen. Andererseits ist im Gebiet des pallidofugalen Systems die Faserdichte der ableitenden Wege wohl am größten, so daß durch eine Ausschaltung in diesem Bereich auch die größte Gewähr dafür besteht, daß eine genügend große Anzahl ableitender extrapyramidaler Neurone getroffen wird. Denn offenbar scheint es zur Herstellung eines gewissen Gleichgewichtes notwendig, daß eine bestimmte Anzahl zu tiefergelegenen Zentren ableitender Bahnen ausgeschaltet werden muß. Das ist nun innerhalb der subcorticalen Rücksteuerungsverbindungen am sichersten dort zu erreichen, wo ihre Dichte am größten ist.

*Vorteile der subcorticalen Eingriffe.* Hier ist zwischen den umschriebenen gezielten Ausschaltungen mit einem geeigneten Zielverfahren und den großen operativen Freilegungen zu unterscheiden. An gemeinsamen Vorteilen sind zu nennen:

1. Bei richtiger Wahl des Schädigungsortes wird anscheinend ein günstiger Einfluß nicht nur auf die Zittererscheinungen (Tremor), sondern auch auf die Muskeltonusstörungen (Rigidität und Hypertonus) des Parkinson-Syndroms ausgeübt.

2. Läsionen des pyramidalen motorischen Systems (Hemiparesen) lassen sich in der Regel umgehen.

Darüber hinaus bieten die gezielten Eingriffe noch weitere Vorteile:

a) Minimum an Nebenschädigungen durch Läsionen benachbarter Strukturen.

b) Minimum an Operationsbelastung, so daß bei nicht ausreichendem Resultat der Eingriff fast beliebig oft wiederholt und der Läsionsherd weiter ausgedehnt werden kann.

c) Auch ältere Patienten können einer solchen Prozedur unterzogen werden.

*Nachteile der subcorticalen Eingriffe.*

1. Die Nachteile sind einerseits in unserer bislang noch mangelhaften Kenntnis der physiologischen und pathophysiologischen Zusammenhänge der normalen und gestörten motorischen Funktion begründet, welche die richtige Auswahl und Ausdehnung des Ausschaltungsmodus zur Verminderung störender Impulse erschwert bzw. sogar verhindert. Hierin kann die Zukunft vielleicht in absehbarer Zeit eine Änderung bringen.

2. Das transventrikuläre Vorgehen ist mit einer, wie uns scheinen will, untragbaren Operationsgefährdung verbunden.

3. Bei den großen Operationen sind eine Anzahl unangenehmer Nebenerscheinungen zu fürchten, wie eine Verminderung der motorischen Kraft, eine Dyspraxie, Epilepsie oder auch eine Herabsetzung der geistigen Leistungsfähigkeit (Meyers). Guiot sah manchmal während der Operationen Atemstörungen, nach der Operation in einem Drittel der Fälle transitorisch eine Hyperthermie (einmal jedoch mit tödlichem Ausgang), häufig vorübergehende psychische Alterationen und Gewichtszunahmen, welche mit einem Verlust der Libido verbunden waren.

Die *Mortalität* ist mit Ausnahme der gezielten Operationsmethoden ungewöhnlich hoch, sie liegt um 20%. Meyers hatte eine Mortalität von 16% und Browder bei seinen Kapseloperationen 24%. Bei Hamby betrug die Zahl der postoperativen Todesfälle sogar 41% (!). In einer Gesamtserie von 17 Fällen verlor Hamby 3 Patienten nach einer doppelseitigen Durchschneidung der pallidofugalen Verbindungen, 3 Patienten nach einer einseitigen Kapseloperation und einen Patienten nach einer in 2 Sitzungen bilateral ausgeführten vorderen Capsulotomie. Dagegen hatte Guiot unter 47 Pallidotomien nur 3 Todesfälle (6,4%).

Die geringe Operationsmortalität bei den gezielten Hirnoperationen wurde bereits hervorgehoben. In ihrer ersten Serie von 35 Stereoencephalotomien, allerdings aus den verschiedensten Indikationen heraus, hatten Spiegel und Wycis 2 Sterbefälle (5,7%), und Riechert hatte unter 14 derartigen Eingriffen keinen tödlichen Ausgang.

## 3. Die Ligatur der Arteria chorioidea anterior.

Diese meines Wissens jüngste Methode in der chirurgischen Behandlung der Parkinson-*Erscheinungen* hat einem Zufall ihre Übernahme in die Klinik zu verdanken, wie Cooper 1953 auf der Jahresversammlung der American Neurological Association bekanntgab. Als Cooper bei einem 39jährigen Mann, welcher an einem rechtsseitigen Hemiparkinsonismus litt, eine Pedunkulotomie nach Walker auf der linken Seite durchführen wollte, kam es zu einer ungewollten Verletzung der A. chorioidea anterior. Die Blutung wurde durch Verschluß des Gefäßes mit einem Silberclip gestillt. Da COOPER nicht die Folgen dieser Gefäßligatur übersah, unterließ er die geplante Durchschneidung am Hirnschenkelfuß. Über den postoperativen Krankheitsverlauf war man dann sehr überrascht, denn der Ruhetremor des rechten Armes und Beines waren verschwunden und es fehlte die geringste Bewegungsschwäche. Als dieser Zustand auch 9 Monate nach dem Eingriff noch unverändert geblieben war, der Patient inzwischen wieder arbeitete und „Geld verdienen konnte", entschloß sich COOPER, mit der Unterbindung der A. chorioidea anterior bei PARKINSON-Kranken empirisch Erfahrungen zu sammeln.

Unter den 30 bis heute von COOPER operierten PARKINSON-Erkrankungen ereigneten sich 4 Todesfälle. Zwei davon wurden der arteriosklerotischen Form zugerechnet, welche man zukünftig mit den senilen Formen von diesem Eingriff ausschließen sollte. Bei der Mehrzahl der Patienten soll ein postencephalitischer Parkinsonismus vorgelegen haben und das Resultat überraschend gut gewesen sein, besser auch als bei der idiopathischen Form. Insbesondere wird von COOPER als das beständigste und bedeutsamste Ergebnis der Gefäßligatur die dauerhafte Besserung der chronischen invalidisierenden *Starre* hervorgehoben, welche selbst unbewegliche und ans Bett gefesselte hilflose Kranke wieder gehfähig und unabhängig von fremder Hilfe hätte werden lassen. In einem Falle hätte der Patient nach der Operation seit Jahren das erste Wort schreiben können. In 9 von 11 postencephalitischen Fällen wäre es darüber hinaus zu einer Besserung oder zum völligen Verschwinden des *alternierenden Ruhetremors* gekommen, während der ataktische bzw. *Intentionstremor* stets unbeeinflußt geblieben sei. Die Katamnesen reichen allerdings nur 7 Monate bis längstens 1 Jahr zurück. Als Indikationskriterien verlangt COOPER jetzt das Vorliegen überaus chronischer und weit fortgeschrittener Krankheitsbilder der postencephalitischen und idiopathischen Form des Parkinsonismus, in denen die Krankheit bereits zu Erwerbsunfähigkeit und Pflegebedürftigkeit geführt habe.

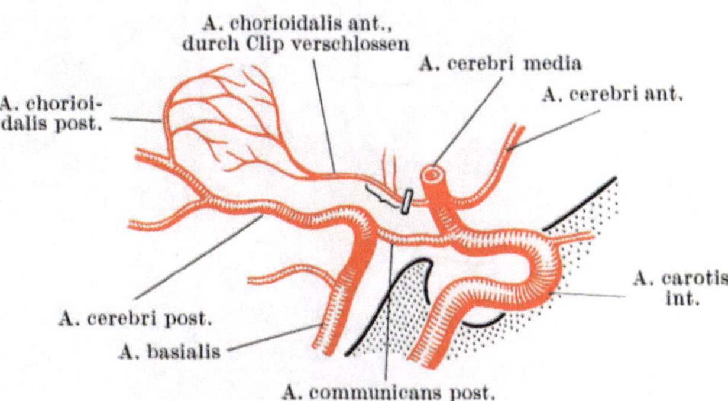


Abb. 19. Schematische Darstellung des Ursprungs und Verlaufs der vorderen Chorioidalarterie und ihrer kollateralen Verbindungen mit der hinteren Chorioidalarterie. (Die Klammer zeigt die Strecke des Gefäßes an, welche koaguliert werden muß, um eine retrograde Versorgung über die Anastomosen der hinteren Chorioidalarterie zu verhindern).

**Anatomisches.** Die A. chorioidea anterior kommt aus der A. carotis interna, und zwar zwischen A. cerebri media und A. communicans posterior. Die letzte ist am tiefsten und weitesten medial gelegen und die A. chorioidea anterior liegt in der Mitte zwischen jener und der weiter lateral und höher gelegenen mittleren Hirnarterie. Die A. chorioidea anterior wendet sich in ihrem Verlauf nach mediodorsal, an der Außenseite des Tractus opticus entlang, und endigt über dem Corpus geniculatum laterale. Hier bestehen Anastomosen mit der A. chorioidea posterior, weshalb es nach COOPERs Ligatur anscheinend nicht zu homonymen Gesichtsfeldausfällen kommen kann. Bald nach ihrem Abgang von der Carotis interna gibt die A. chorioidea anterior Äste ab, welche Endarterien ohne Kollateralen sind, und welche regelmäßig vor allem zu den medialen und intermediären Segmenten des Globus pallidus, zur Ansa lenticularis und auch zum retrolentikulären Teil der Capsula interna und zum Hippocampus führen. Da aber Anastomosen der vorderen mit der hinteren Chorioidalarterie über das Corpus geniculatum laterale bestehen, muß die Unterbindung des Gefäßes vor und hinter dem Abgang des tiefen Astes zur Versorgung des Pallidum durchgeführt werden, um einen möglichen kollateralen Blutzufluß über diese Anastomosen zu verhindern. Übrigens soll das Vorkommen und der pallidäre

Versorgungsbereich der vorderen Chorioidalarterie nach den Untersuchungen von Abbie und Alexander außerordentlich konstant sein (Abb. 19 und 20).

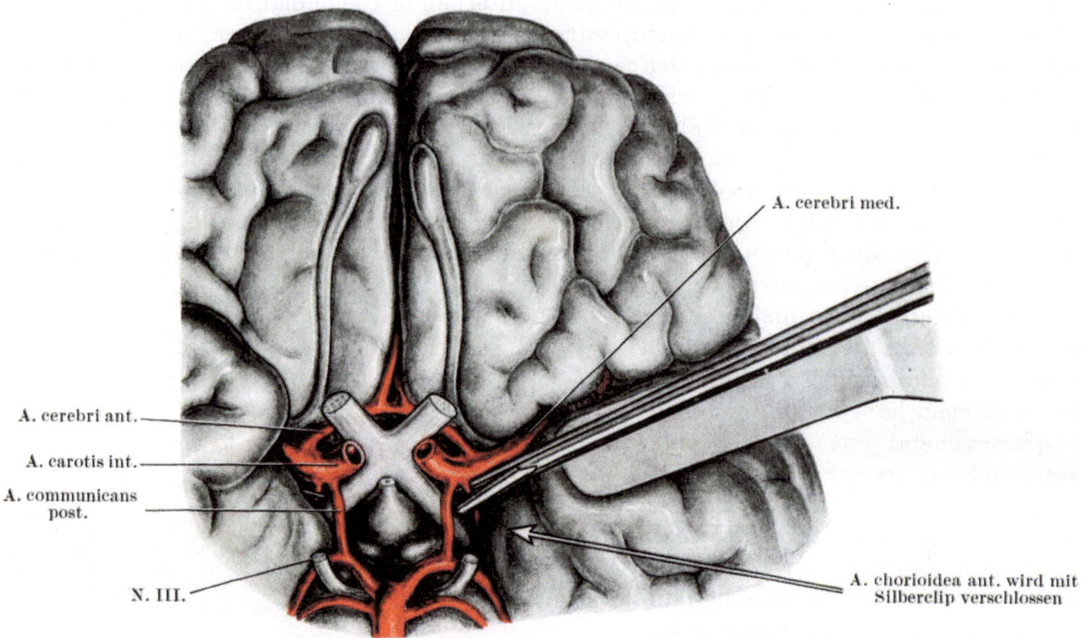


Abb. 20. Die Ligatur der A. chorioidalis ant. (schematische Darstellung der Anatomie an der Hirnbasis).

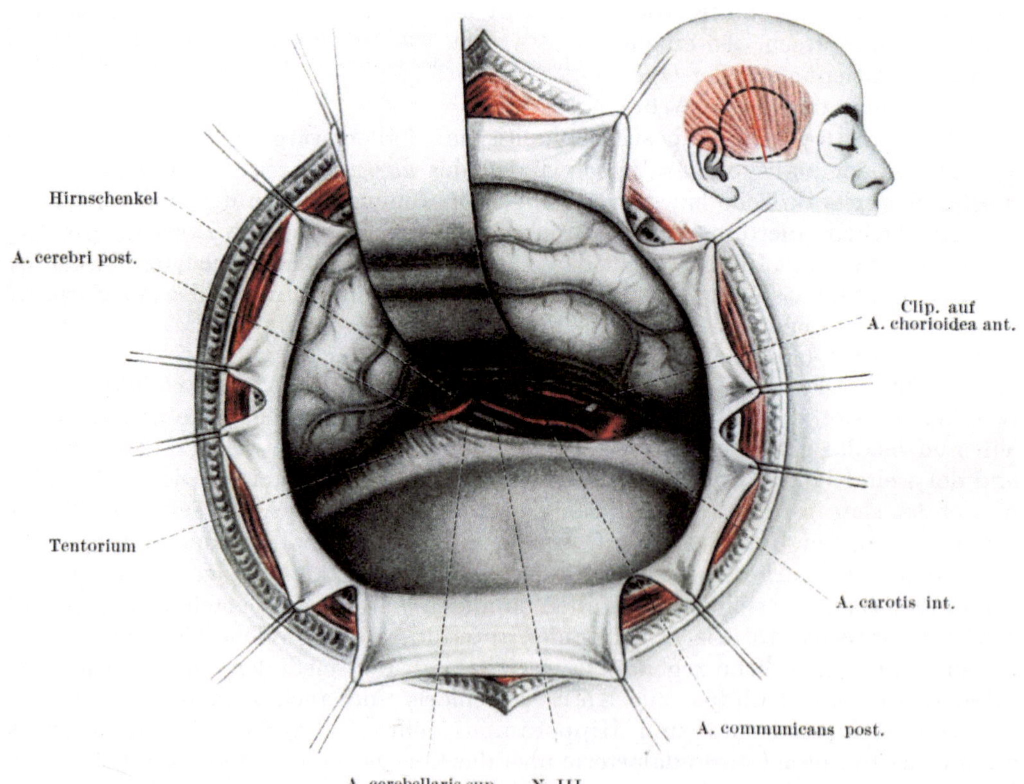


Abb. 21. Die Ligatur der A. chorioidalis ant. (Operationsskizze).

**Technik der Gefäßligatur.** Vor der Operation wird die Durchführung einer doppelseitigen Arteriographie zur Feststellung des Gefäßverlaufes und zum Ausschluß von Anomalien im Circulus arteriosus Willisi empfohlen.

Die Operation wird jetzt, nachdem COOPER den früheren Weg einer großen osteoplastischen frontotemporalen Kraniotomie mit Zugang entlang des Keilbeinrückens wieder verlassen hat, in Seitenlage von einem temporalen Vertikalschnitt aus vorgenommen. Ein leichtes Herabhängen des Kopfes auf der Stütze des Operationstisches erleichtert das Anheben des Schläfenlappens bis zur Darstellung des freien Randes vom Tentorium. Nun wird die Arachnoidalmembran der basalen Cisterne eröffnet und der Liquor abgesaugt, wodurch auch mehr Platz gewonnen wird. Der N. oculomotorius und die A. carotis interna mit ihren Ästen sind jetzt gut zu sehen. Man folgt den beiden benachbarten Gefäßen, der A. communicans posterior und der A. chorioidea anterior, bis zu ihrem Abgang an der Carotis interna. Die A. chorioidea anterior wird nun möglichst nahe an ihrem Ursprung von der Carotis mit einem Silberclip unterbunden. Anschließend muß das Gefäß noch wenigstens auf eine Länge von 1 cm in seinem Verlauf nach dorsal koaguliert werden, um einerseits mit Sicherheit einen vollständigen Verschluß des Lumens zu erreichen und andererseits, um das Gefäß über die Stelle hinaus zu unterbinden, von welcher der tiefe Ast zur Versorgung des Pallidum abgeht, wodurch die Möglichkeit einer retrograden Versorgung über die Anastomosen der hinteren Chorioidalarterie verhindert wird. — Auf diese Elektrokoagulation legt COOPER neuerdings besonders großen Wert, da in zwei frühen Fällen seiner Serie, in denen das Gefäß lediglich geclipt worden war, die günstige Wirkung auf den gegenseitigen Tremor und Rigor ausblieb. Die postoperative arteriographische Kontrolle hat dann gezeigt, daß das Gefäß durchgängig geblieben war, und erst die Nachoperation mit erreichtem vollständigem Verschluß der A. chorioidea anterior war angeblich prompt von einem Nachlassen des Tremors und der Starre gefolgt (Abb. 21 und 22).

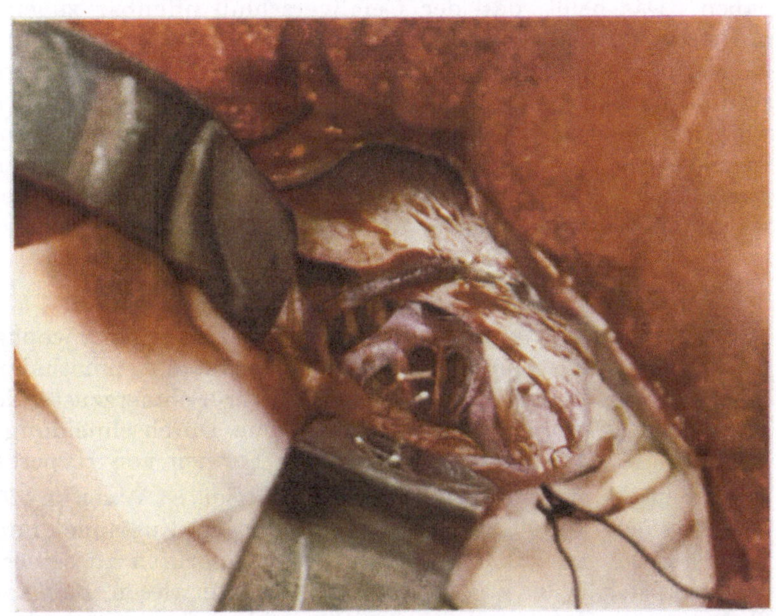

Abb. 22. Operationsphoto von COOPERS Gefäßligatur beim Parkinsonismus. Der rechte Schläfenlappen ist angehoben, die basale Cisterne eröffnet und die vordere Chorioidalarterie durch 2 Silberclipse unterbunden[1]. (Oben im Bild ist die Basis der mittleren Schädelgrube und daran anschließend nach mediodorsal der freie Rand des Tentoriums zu erkennen.)

Zum Schluß weist COOPER darauf hin, daß diese Patienten während der Nachbehandlung besonders zu betreuen seien, da sie zu gewissen neurovegetativen Störungen neigen. Wegen des vermehrten Speichelflusses mit erhöhter Aspirationsgefahr ließ sich in einigen Fällen die Tracheotomie rechtfertigen. Eine fast regelmäßige Folge sind Bewußtseinsstörungen verschiedenen Grades, welche gewöhnlich nach der ersten Woche abklingen.

**Die Mortalität** betrug 13,3% unter 30 Fällen. An erheblichen Nebenerscheinungen trat zweimal postoperativ die Komplikation einer kompletten Hemiplegie auf, welche in einem autoptisch gesicherten Fall ursächlich auf einen Infarkt im Versorgungsgebiet der

[1] Herrn Prof. TÖNNIS ist für die Überlassung der Abb. 22 besonders zu danken.

mittleren Hirnarterie zurückzuführen war, für den man gern durch die Gefäßligatur hervorgerufene Spasmen angeschuldigt hätte.

Der endgültige praktische Wert einer Ligatur der A. chorioidea anterior beim Parkinsonismus läßt sich heute gewiß noch nicht beurteilen. Wenn die noch nachzuprüfenden Angaben COOPERs zutreffen, müßte man annehmen, daß mit einem Verschluß dieses Gefäßes über eine bestimmte Strecke eine ischämische Nekrose gerade der Strukturen und Faserverbindungen zustande käme, nach deren direkter Zerstörung MEYERS, FÉNÉLON, GUIOT u. a. eine Besserung der PARKINSON-Erscheinungen wie Tremor und Starre ohne ein damit verbundenes Defizit der willkürlichen motorischen Funktion gesehen haben. Das heißt, daß der Gefäßverschluß offenbar zu einem selektiven Ausfall der medialen Portion des Pallidum (inneres Segment) und seiner efferenten Verbindungen zum Corpus subthalamicum Luysi, zum ventrolateralen Kern des Thalamus, zur Substantia nigra und zum Nucleus ruber, also der pallidofugalen und subpallidären Bahnen, wie Ansa lenticularis, führt. Es ist sehr zu bedauern, daß COOPER gerade zu dieser Frage, welche Strukturen in seinen autoptisch untersuchten Fällen von der Erweichung betroffen waren, keine Stellung nimmt. Zur Klärung der neurophysiologischen Zusammenhänge wären diese Befunde doch von unschätzbarem Wert gewesen.

## 4. Die Pedunkulotomie.

Nachdem A. E. WALKER im Jahre 1942 seine „Mesencephalotomie“ oder Mittelhirntraktotomie, eine Durchschneidung des Tractus spinothalamicus in Höhe der Hirnschenkel, zur Beseitigung unbeeinflußbarer Schmerzzustände angegeben hat, teilte er 1949 seine „*Cerebral Pedunkulotomy*“, eine Durchschneidung der Pyramidenbahnen im Hirnschenkel, zur Therapie bestimmter Formen von Hyperkinesen mit.

Wie die Mehrzahl der Autoren zu dieser Zeit ist WALKER offenbar von den Ergebnissen der physiologischen Untersuchungen über das Zustandekommen des *Tremors* und von den Erfahrungen mit den chirurgischen Eingriffen zu seiner Beseitigung ausgegangen. Es hatte sich ja bis dahin verschiedentlich erwiesen, daß zur sicheren Beseitigung des Tremors eine Unterbrechung der Pyramidenbahn an irgendeiner Stelle — cortical, kapsulär oder cervical — erforderlich zu sein schien. Auf Grund seiner relativ isolierten und oberflächlichen anatomischen Lage im Hirnschenkel hielt WALKER den Pyramidenstrang an dieser Stelle chirurgisch für besonders zugänglich, vor allem hinsichtlich der verminderten Gefahr einer Nebenschädigung anderer Strukturen. WALKER sah noch einen weiteren Vorteil, insbesondere für das Erhaltenbleiben einer gewissen Willkürmotorik, in einer durch dieses Vorgehen ermöglichten Schonung vieler *nicht* durch den Hirnschenkel verlaufender extrapyramidal-motorischer Bahnen, über welche manche Bewegungsfunktion wiederkehren könne (Abb. 23).

Zuerst wurde von WALKER diese Operation nicht beim PARKINSON-Tremor, sondern in einem Fall von *Hemiballismus* mit einem angeblich ausgezeichneten Ergebnis ausgeführt. Beim PARKINSON-*Tremor* faßt WALKER seine an 10 Fällen gemachten Erfahrungen dahingehend zusammen, daß der Tremor vorübergehend oder vollständig durch den Eingriff beseitigt werden kann, was sich verständlicherweise auch zum Teil nach dem Grad der postoperativen kontralateralen Parese richtet. Darüber hinaus sei mitunter ein nach der Operation wiedergekehrter Tremor einer medikamentösen Therapie zugänglicher geworden. Andere Symptome des Parkinsonismus aber, wie die Rigidität und Bewegungsarmut u. a., werden kaum beeinflußt. Die Erfahrungen stützen sich, das muß betont werden, auf mehrjährige Fallbeobachtungen.

Über gleichfalls gute Resultate mit der Pedunkulotomie berichten GUIOT und PECKER (1949), welche diese in 2 Fällen von *Hemiparkinsonismus* angewandt haben. Der Tremor verschwand in einem Falle vollständig und konnte im anderen beträchtlich vermindert werden. Sie bestätigen die Unbeeinflußbarkeit der Starre und Akinese durch den Hirnschenkelschnitt. Zur Zeit ihrer Veröffentlichung hat die postoperative Beobachtungszeit

1 Jahr betragen. Als Folge des Eingriffs heben GUIOT und PECKER eine pyramidale Hemiplegie mit Neigung zu Spastik und Kontrakturbildung hervor. Die Lähmungserscheinungen scheinen faciobrachial betont zu sein.

**Technik der lateralen Pedunkulotomie.** Der Eingriff wird kontralateral zur Seite der Hyperkinese ausgeführt. Gegenüber dem occipitodorsalen transtentoriellen Zugang ist dem subtemporalen Weg der Vorzug zu geben. In Seitenlage des Patienten wird von einem senkrechten Schnitt über dem Schläfenbein aus, welcher vor dem vorderen Ohransatz endet, eine etwa 5×5 cm große Knochenlücke geschaffen (Abb. 24). In leichter Kopfhängelage wird nach Eröffnung der Dura der Temporallappen angehoben und an der Basis der mittleren Schädelgrube bis zur Darstellung des freien Randes vom Tentorium vorgegangen. Nun wird die basale Cisterne eröffnet, wonach der N. trochlearis, der N. oculomotorius und an Gefäßen die A. cerebellaris superior zu sehen sind. Der N. trochlearis und die obere Kleinhirnarterie müssen gewöhnlich etwas beiseite gehalten werden, um den Einschnitt in den Hirnschenkel gefahrlos durchführen zu können. Hierzu ist es unter Umständen auch erforderlich, den Rand vom Tentorium etwas einzukerben, was sich nach Anheben des Randes mit einem stumpfen Häkchen leicht durchführen läßt. Wenn man sich so den Hirnschenkelfuß übersichtlich dargestellt hat, werden die äußeren Zweidrittel bis Dreiviertel mit einem in einem Winkel von 45° abgebogenen Chordotom durchschnitten. Die Tiefe der Incision beträgt etwa 6—7 mm. Zur Sicherheit kann durch eine elektrische Reizung die Pyramidenbahn vor der Durchschneidung lokalisiert werden. Die Incision ist dann an der Stelle auszuführen, von welcher durch die Reizung eine schwache Muskelkontraktion am Arm oder im Gesicht hervorgerufen werden kann. Vor der Durchschneidung kann außerdem zur Vermeidung von Blutungen aus den kleinen Gefäßen der Pia eine vorsichtige Oberflächenkoagulation vorgenommen werden (Abb. 25 und 26).

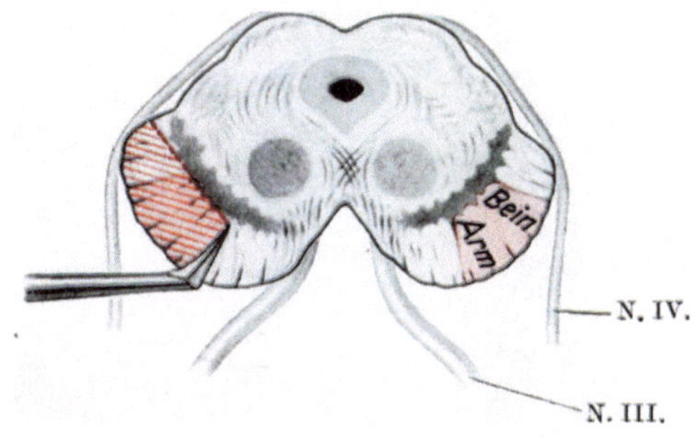

Abb. 23. Die laterale Pedunkulotomie nach WALKER (Ausdehnung des Einschnittes auf dem Querschnitt).

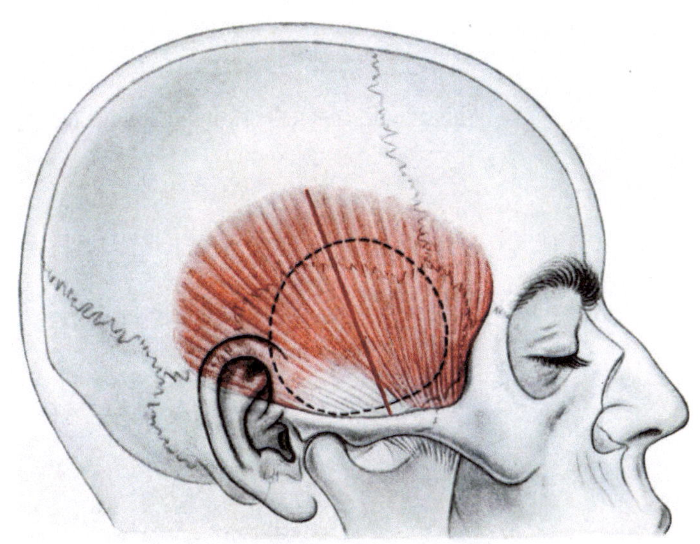
Abb. 24. Schnittführung bei der lateralen Pedunkulotomie nach WALKER.

Die technische Durchführung der Operation ist einfach und die Gefahr der Nebenschädigungen gering.

**Epikrise.** Mit hinreichender Sicherheit lassen sich durch diesen Eingriff offenbar die *Tremorsymptome* der Paralysis agitans beseitigen oder zumindest verringern, wenn es sich lohnt, dafür eine pyramidale Parese einzutauschen, deren Grad sich vorher schwer bestimmen läßt. Da die übrigen Symptome des Parkinsonismus, wie Starre, Hypokinese und Hypertonus nicht beeinflußt werden, würden sich demnach hierfür nur halbseitige Syndrome eignen, in denen der Schütteltremor das hervorstechendste Merkmal der Erkrankung ist.

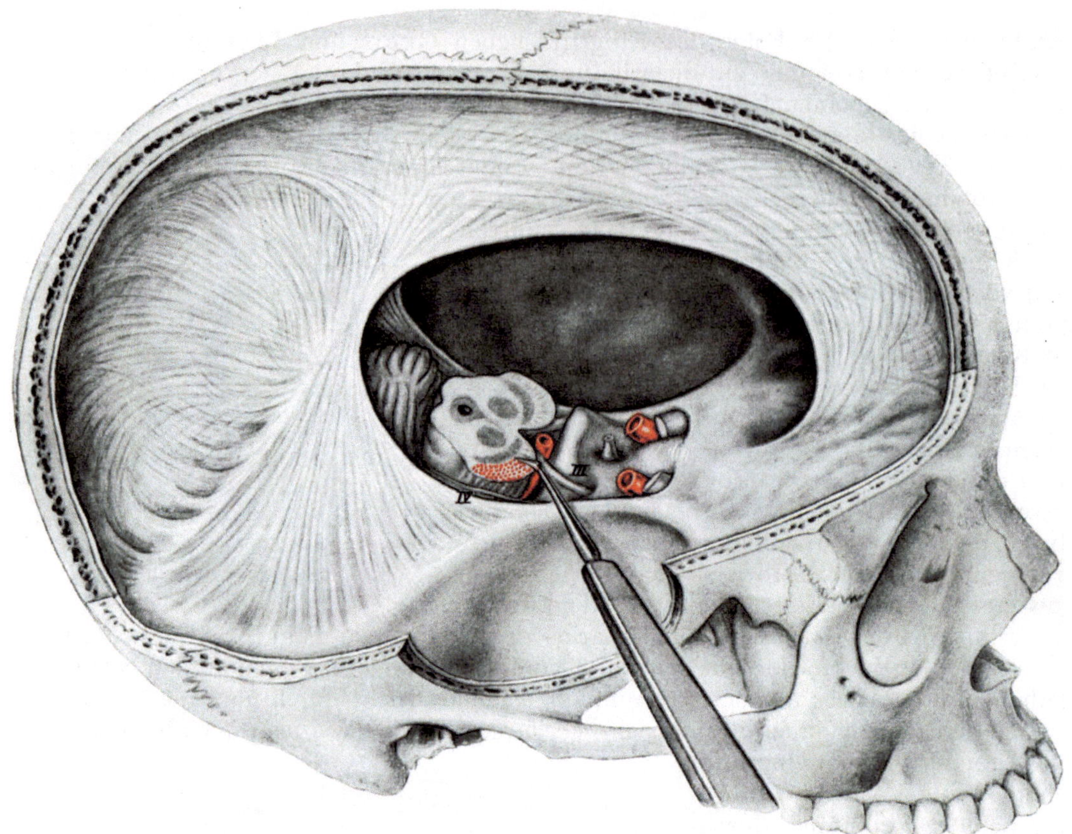


Abb. 25. Die laterale Pedunkulotomie (topographische Situation).

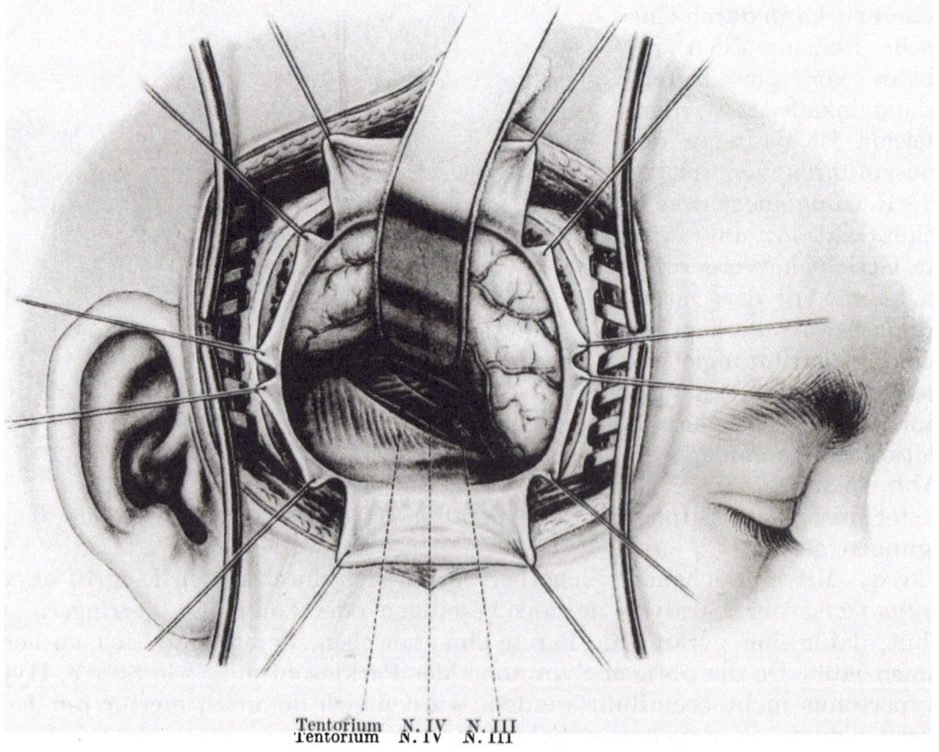


Abb. 26. Die laterale Pedunkulotomie (Operationsskizze mit eingezeichnetem Hirnschenkelschnitt).

Beim *Hemiballismus* scheint die Pedunkulotomie erfolgversprechend zu sein.

Bei den *Choreoathetosen* müßten mit dieser Operation noch Erfahrungen gesammelt werden. Jedenfalls schließt sich ihre Anwendung bei bilateralen Formen von selbst aus, da das Risiko einer doppelseitigen Parese nicht tragbar ist. Wir versuchten die Pedunkulotomie bei diesem Krankheitsbild und beschränkten die Durchschneidung auf $^1/_3$—$^1/_2$ des äußeren Teiles vom Hirnschenkelfuß, um das Ausmaß der postoperativen Lähmung möglichst gering zu halten. Obschon die Hyperkinese unmittelbar nach der Operation ohne wesentliches Defizit der Gliedmaßenbeweglichkeit gut gebessert war, bestand bereits nach 3—4 Wochen wieder der alte Zustand. Man wird also unbedingt den Tractus corticospinalis vollständig durchtrennen müssen, wenn man ein dauerhaftes Resultat erhalten will. Dann allerdings ist eine postoperative Hemiplegie die Folge, welche man aber nur bei einer schweren Hemichorea für die Beseitigung der Bewegungsstörung in Kauf nehmen wird. Ein anderes Mal haben wir bei einer solchen Indikation mindestens $^2/_3$—$^3/_4$ durchschnitten mit dem Erfolg eines vollständigen Sistierens der Hyperkinese, aber auch der Folge einer kompletten Hemiparese, welche allerdings eine gewisse Rückbildung zeigte.

*Vorteile der Pedunkulotomie.* Es ist ein technisch einfacher und wenig belastender Eingriff, welcher mit einem Minimum an Nebenschädigungen die Pyramidenbahnen sicher und praktisch vollständig ausschalten läßt.

*Nachteile der Pedunkulotomie.*

1. Der wesentlichste Nachteil ist darin zu sehen, daß mit diesem Verfahren die Beseitigung oder Besserung einer Hyperkinese nur gegen den Eintausch einer mehr oder weniger schweren Hemiparese zu erreichen ist.

2. Der Grad der postoperativen Lähmungserscheinungen ist schwer vorauszusagen.

3. Der Grad der erreichten Besserung geht etwa parallel mit der Schwere der postoperativen Parese.

4. Daher kann der Eingriff nur halbseitigen und sehr erheblichen Störungsformen, welche ohnehin schon zu einer Unbrauchbarkeit der Gliedmaßen der betroffenen Seite geführt haben, vorbehalten bleiben.

5. Ein „Rezidiv" ist ziemlich sicher, wenn die Pyramidenbahn nur unvollständig durchtrennt wurde.

Die *Mortalität* ist sicher unbedeutend. Bisher ist jedenfalls kein tödlicher Ausgang bekannt geworden.

## III. Die cervicospinalen Eingriffe.

Den Operationen im Bereich der Halsnervenwurzeln und insbesondere des Halsmarkes selbst sind gleichfalls eine Reihe experimenteller Untersuchungen und klinischer Erfahrungen vorausgegangen, ehe sich die eine oder andere Methode abhob, von deren Durchführung eine gewisse Wirkung auf bestimmte Formen unwillkürlicher Bewegungen erwartet werden durfte.

**Historisches.** Die *Durchschneidung der spinalen Wurzeln* zur Besserung spastischer Zustände ist schon sehr früh von KEEN (1891) empfohlen worden. Offenbar waren WINSLOW und SPEAR (1912) die ersten, welche nur die *hinteren Wurzeln* durchschnitten haben und hierdurch die Besserung einer Athetose in der unteren Extremität gesehen haben wollen. Aber heute wird man sich fragen dürfen, ob nicht die Erscheinungen in ihrem Falle einzig und allein die Manifestation einer Spastik gewesen sind, da weder FRAZIER (1918) noch FOERSTER (1921) imstande gewesen sind, die Symptome der Choreoathetose durch eine Hinterwurzeldurchschneidung zu bessern. Gleichfalls ist der Tremor der Paralysis agitans durch die Hinterwurzeldurchschneidung nicht beeinflußt worden, wie FOERSTER (1927), POLLOCK und DAVIS (1930) und PUUSEPP (1930) mitgeteilt haben. Allerdings wurde von ihnen hiernach eine gewisse Verminderung der Rigidität und Starre gesehen. Ohne Erfolg wurde beim Schütteltremor auch die *Durchschneidung der Hinterstränge* von PUUSEPP (1930) und von RIZZATTI und MORENO (1936) versucht, wodurch jedoch eine gewisse Besserung der Muskelrigidität zustande gekommen sein soll.

Nach Einführung der Chordotomie des Tractus spinothalamicus in die Chirurgie des Schmerzes vor mehr als 40 Jahren (1911/12)[1] ist diesem Eingriff auch in seinen Beziehungen zum Muskeltonus und zur motorischen Funktion viel Beachtung geschenkt worden.

Nachdem sich die Unwirksamkeit der ausgedehnten extraduralen Wurzeldurchschneidungen zur Beeinflussung choreoathetotischer und parkinsonistischer Krankheitsbilder erwiesen hatte, versuchte FOERSTER (1927) im Falle einer rechtsseitigen Hemiparalysis agitans luischer Genese die *Vorderseitenstrangdurchschneidung.* Er hatte kurz zuvor ohne Erfolg beim gleichen Patienten eine hintere Rhizotomie von $C_4$—$D_2$ rechts ausgeführt, nach welcher der Rigor der oberen Extremität nahezu beseitigt, aber der Tremor nicht verändert worden sei. Die bald darauf angeschlossene Vorderseitenstrangchordotomie wurde in Höhe des oberen Randes vom 6. Cervicalsegment vorgenommen, und, obschon unmittelbar nach dieser Operation der Tremor fast vollständig sistierte, so war doch dies anfänglich erfreuliche Ergebnis nur von kurzer Dauer. Innerhalb weniger Wochen waren die Tremorsymptome in praktisch vollem Umfang zurückgekehrt, aber FOERSTER hat daraufhin noch nicht aufgegeben. Er versuchte kurze Zeit später beim gleichen Kranken auf derselben Seite nochmals eine Vorderseitenstrangchordotomie, diesmal ein Segment höher ($C_5$). Jedoch konnte auch hierdurch nur vorübergehend geholfen werden, denn das zunächst gute Resultat hat nicht lange angedauert. Der Tremor, welcher tatsächlich unmittelbar nach dem letzten Eingriff verschwunden war, ist später gleichfalls in vollem Umfang wiedergekehrt, ebenso wie sich die anfangs gelinderte Starre langsam zunehmend wieder eingestellt hat.

Offenbar ließ FOERSTER sich in seinem Vorgehen von der Vorstellung leiten, daß mit einer Durchschneidung des Vorderseitenstranges die abnormen efferenten (motorischen) Impulse und die afferenten (sensorischen) Muskeldehnungsreflexe durch eine teilweise Unterbrechung ihrer Leitungsbahnen ausgeschaltet werden können. FOERSTER hat jedoch an dem unzureichenden Ergebnis dieser Strangdurchschneidung sofort folgerichtig erkannt, daß *nicht genügend efferente und afferente Leitungswege* hiermit erfaßt werden.

*Physiologisches.* Schließlich begann man sich auch wieder für die frühen tierexperimentellen Studien ROTHMANNS und seiner Mitarbeiter (1902/03) zu interessieren. ROTHMANN hatte in Versuchen an Katzen und Hunden die bedeutsame Feststellung gemacht, daß eine *völlige Ausschaltung der beiden lateralen Pyramidenbahnen,* sei es in der Medulla oblongata oder in der Decussatio, keineswegs von einer andauernden Störung der motorischen Funktion gefolgt sein mußte. Daraufhin hat ROTHMANN seine Untersuchungen zur spinalen Leitungsphysiologie der Motorik an Affen fortgesetzt, da wegen der nicht wesentlichen Differenz im anatomischen Aufbau des Rückenmarks die an Affen gewonnenen Untersuchungsergebnisse eher auf die menschlichen Verhältnisse bezogen werden konnten als die nach den Versuchen an Hunden und Katzen erhaltenen Resultate.

Es ist sicher lohnend, von ROTHMANNS zahlreichen und einschlägigen Untersuchungen einige in diesem Zusammenhang wichtig erscheinende herauszugreifen. In Höhe des 3. Cervicalsegmentes wurde einmal der Pyramidenseitenstrang, ein anderes Mal der Tractus rubrospinalis, dann wieder einmal der ganze Seitenstrang in seiner vollständigen Ausdehnung, zusätzlich auch in Verbindung mit dem Vorderstrang, zerstört. Die Tiere, welche mehrere Wochen nach einem solchen Eingriff beobachtet wurden, zeigten nach *völligem Ausfall der lateralen Pyramidenbahn* keinen wesentlichen Ausfall der motorischen Funktion, ebensowenig nach einer alleinigen *Zerstörung des Tractus rubrospinalis.* Eine *gemeinsame Zerstörung von Pyramidenbahn und Tractus rubrospinalis* setzte die Kraft und Geschicklichkeit des ipsilateralen Armes herab und hat auch in den ersten Tagen nach der Operation eine Hemiparese nach sich ziehen können, welche aber in der Folgezeit bis auf einen geringen Rest ausgeglichen wurde. Die leichtere Störung der motorischen Funktion des Beines war in der Regel schon innerhalb weniger Tage vollkommen restituiert. Die *vollständige Zerstörung einer ganzen Markhälfte* (Hemisektion) mit Ausnahme des Hinterstranges führte zu einer vorübergehenden vollständigen Lähmung, deren Restitution am Bein bereits nach 4 Tagen und am Arm nach 8 Tagen einsetzte. Die Rückbildung der Lähmungserscheinungen an der unteren Extremität soll so schnell fortgeschritten sein, daß nach 14 Tagen nur noch eine geringe Abweichung von der Norm bestand, während die Motorik der oberen Extremität erheblicher geschädigt blieb und auch nach 3 Wochen nicht mehr als Massenbewegungen erlaubte. Selbst bei einer *doppelseitigen Ausschaltung beider Seitenstränge,* also beider Pyramidenseitenstränge und beider Rubrospinalbahnen, soll es ebenfalls zu einer weitgehenden Restitution der motorischen Funktion gekommen sein, obgleich ihr zur Leitung ja nur mehr die efferenten Vorderstrangsysteme zur Verfügung stehen konnten.

Die Erkenntnisse aus ROTHMANNS neurophysiologischen Untersuchungen über die Leistung cervicospinaler Leitungseinheiten haben vermutlich nicht allein bei der Chordotomie des Tractus spinothalamicus, zu deren Durchführung er ja 1912 in Breslau TIETZE und FOERSTER angeregt hat, Pate gestanden. Sie dürften auch die Einführung der cervicospinalen Operationsmethoden in die Chirurgie der extrapyramidalen Bewegungs-

[1] Die „klassische" Schmerzchordotomie wurde zuerst von SPILLER und MARTIN (1911) in Philadelphia, und, unabhängig von ihnen, von TIETZE und FOERSTER (1912) in Breslau auf Anregung von ROTHMANN und SCHÜLLER durchgeführt.

störungen grundlegend beeinflußt haben. Es ist allerdings zu berücksichtigen, daß den Hyperkinesen ein pathologischer Zustand am motorischen System zugrunde liegt, während bei den experimentellen Untersuchungen ROTHMANNs vor den Operationen keine Störung der motorischen Funktion vorgelegen hat. Man hat auf Grund seiner Ergebnisse immerhin schließen dürfen, daß selbst nach ausgedehnten Markdurchschneidungen, welche zu einer vollständigen Leitungsunterbrechung efferenter Bahnensysteme führten, offenbar andere absteigende Bahnen vikariierend für eine weitgehende Erhaltung der Willkürmotorik eintreten können.

## 1. Die cervicale Vorderstrangdurchschneidung (Extrapyramidotomie).

Die ersten mit dauerhaftem Erfolg ausgeführten Halsmarkeinschneidungen bei unwillkürlichen Bewegungen gehen auf TRACY J. PUTNAM (1933 und 1938) zurück.

Im Jahre 1933 stellte PUTNAM fest, daß die unkontrollierten Bewegungen der *Choreoathetosen* mit einer Durchschneidung bzw. elektrochirurgischen Zerstörung der im Vorderstrang des Halsmarkes absteigenden extrapyramidalen Neuronensysteme gut zu vermindern waren. Ein Einfluß auf den rhythmischen *Tremor* konnte mit diesem Eingriff jedoch ebensowenig wie mit der Vorderseitenstrangchordotomie erzielt werden (FOERSTER, PUTNAM, OLDBERG).

Bei der mit „*Extrapyramidotomie*" bezeichneten Vorderstrangdurchschneidung kommt es im wesentlichen auf eine Unterbrechung des Tractus vestibulospinalis, reticulospinalis und tectospinalis in Höhe des 2.—3. Cervicalsegmentes an. Dadurch, daß mit diesem Vorgehen die Willkürmotorik so gut wie gar nicht beeinträchtigt wird, kann die Durchschneidung doppelseitig ausgeführt werden. PUTNAMs Operation hat daher insbesondere bei den doppelseitigen choreoathetotischen Bewegungsstörungen, bei der „*Athétose double*", eine größere Bedeutung erlangen können (s. Abb. 27).

Bei insgesamt 42 Kranken hat PUTNAM 53mal die Extrapyramidotomie ausgeführt und in mehr als der Hälfte der Fälle eine dauerhafte Besserung der Bewegungsstörungen gesehen, wobei der Autor über mehrjährige Katamnesen verfügte (1939, 1940 und 1942). In der ersten Serie von 27 Operierten soll sogar in 20 Fällen eine beachtliche Besserung erzielt worden sein, so daß unter anderem 4 Kranke ihre früher aufgegebene Berufsarbeit wieder hätten aufnehmen können.

Unsere eigenen Erfahrungen mit der doppelseitigen Vorderstrangdurchschneidung stützen sich auf das Ergebnis von 45 operierten Fällen. Die ersten an 6 Fällen erzielten Resultate haben wir 1949 und das Spätergebnis an 33 Fällen haben wir 1952 veröffentlicht. Unter den 33 bis dahin operierten Kranken hatten wir diesen Eingriff nicht allein den unwillkürlichen Bewegungen der *Athétose double* vorbehalten, sondern hatten ihn bewußt auch bei den *paraspastischen, diplegischen Erscheinungsbildern der* LITTLE*schen Krankheit* und selbst bei der *Torsionsdystonie* versucht. Das spätere Ergebnis, welches sich auf die 2—4 Jahre nach der Operation durchgeführten Nachuntersuchungen stützt, hat entsprechend der verschiedenen Indikation ganz erhebliche Differenzen gezeigt (SCHÜRMANN 1952).

Bemerkenswert ist die *unmittelbar nach der Operation* vorhandene völlige Erschlaffung der gesamten Gliedmaßen- und Rumpfmuskulatur, welche fast obligat in *allen* Fällen — gleich welcher Störungsform zugehörig — eintritt. Es besteht also zunächst eine hochgradige muskuläre Hypotonie mit abnormer passiver Beweglichkeit der Gelenke und eine Verminderung der groben Kraft bei aktiven Bewegungen. Die unwillkürlichen Bewegungsabläufe sind anfangs wie ausgelöscht. Sowohl die pyramidalen als auch die extrapyramidalen Zustandsbilder zeigen demnach sofort nach dem Eingriff ein ziemlich einheitliches, einförmiges Syndrom muskulärer Hypotonie und artikulärer Hyperflexibilität, welches in der Regel 1—3 Wochen (selten auch einmal länger) bestehen bleibt. Nach dieser Zeit kehrt der Muskeltonus und die motorische Funktion schrittweise zurück. Bei den präoperativ *rein spastischen Formen* kann bereits nach 1—2 Monaten der alte Zustand in vollem Umfang zurückgekehrt sein (in etwa 50%). In der anderen Hälfte der Fälle ist der Muskeltonus selbst nach einem Jahr noch nicht vollständig wiedergekehrt, so daß von einer gewissen Besserung gesprochen werden könnte, wenn diese nicht auf Kosten der groben Kraft und der Ausdauer ginge. Diese waren in allen diesen Fällen herabgesetzt und sind es auch trotz intensiver heilgymnastischer Übungen geblieben, wenn später nicht doch noch eine weitere Zunahme der Spastik eintrat. Selbst nach 1—2 Jahren ist in einigen Fällen diese Tonussteigerung langsam fortschreitend noch eingetreten, so daß in *13 von 15 operierten diplegischen paraspastischen* LITTLE-*Syndromen* nach 3—4 Jahren praktisch wieder der alte Zustand bestand, wie er vor der Operation gewesen ist (Tabelle 1).

Tabelle 1. *Operationsergebnis nach* PUTNAMS *Extrapyramidotomie bei der Diplegia spastica infantilis.*

| Alter<br>Jahre | Anzahl | Ergebnis bis zu 1 Jahr nach der Operation | | | Ergebnis nach 2—4 Jahren nach der Operation | | |
|---|---|---|---|---|---|---|---|
| | | gut | befriedigend | unbefriedigend | gut | befriedigend | unbefriedigend |
| 3— 6 | 3 | — | 2 | 1 | — | 1 | 2 |
| 7—12 | 6 | — | 2 | 4 | — | — | 6 |
| 13—20 | 2 | — | 1 | 1 | — | — | 2 |
| 21—35 | 4 | — | 2 | 2 | — | 1 | 3 |
| | 15 | — | 7 | 8 | — | 2 | 13 |

Viel hoffnungsvoller sind die Ergebnisse bei den vorwiegend extrapyramidalen Störungsformen, insbesondere bei der reinen *Athétose double.* In diesen Fällen besteht postoperativ zunächst, wie bei allen mit der bilateralen Extrapyramidotomie behandelten Patienten, das mehr oder weniger gleichförmige Bild einer allgemeinen Muskelerschlaffung. Die unkontrollierten wurmförmigen Bewegungsabläufe sind anfangs entweder ganz erloschen oder doch so weitgehend vermindert, daß sie in erheblich abgeschwächter Form und nur unter emotionellen Affekten noch in Erscheinung treten. Im wesentlichen scheint das hypotone hyperkinetische Syndrom sofort nach dem Eingriff in ein rein hypotones Syndrom umgewandelt worden zu sein. Spontanbewegungen sind mit herabgeminderter Kraft erhalten. Im Verlauf der nächsten 2—4 Wochen nimmt fortlaufend der Muskeltonus wieder etwas zu, so daß die Willkürbewegungen zunehmend kräftiger werden. Im Idealfall würden die Bewegungsautomatismen für immer vollständig beseitigt bleiben und auch nach Jahren nicht zurückkehren, was aber bedauerlicherweise, wenn auch verständlicherweise, mit diesem Vorgehen niemals zu erreichen sein wird. Immerhin konnten wir in 6 von 15 derartigen Fällen (= 40 %) ein nahezu „ideales" Resultat erzielen, d. h., daß die unwillkürlichen Bewegungen der *Athétose double* so vollständig beseitigt waren, daß sie nur unter emotionellen Affekten in milder Form in Erscheinung getreten sind. Nur als befriedigend ließ sich das Dauerergebnis in 5 von 15 Fällen (= $33^1/_3$ %) bezeichnen, in denen eine gewisse Wiederkehr der unwillkürlichen Bewegungen eingetreten ist. In 2 Fällen war das Spätergebnis nach 2—4 Jahren völlig unzureichend, da in beiden Fällen die athetotischen Bewegungen nahezu ihre frühere Intensität wieder erreicht hatten. Zwei postoperative Todesfälle erlebten wir bei Kindern unterhalb des 5. Lebensjahres, weshalb Kinder unter 5 Jahren zukünftig besser von der Operation auszuschließen sind (Tabelle 2).

Tabelle 2. *Operationsergebnis nach* PUTNAMS *Extrapyramidotomie bei der Athétose double und extra pyramidalparaspastischen Mischformen.* (Mischbilder: striär > pyramidal).

| Alter<br>Jahre | Anzahl | Ergebnis bis zu 1 Jahr nach der Operation | | | Ergebnis nach 2—4 Jahren nach der Operation | | |
|---|---|---|---|---|---|---|---|
| | | gut | befriedigend | unbefriedigend | gut | befriedigend | unbefriedigend |
| 3— 6 | 4 | 2 | — | †† | 2 | — | — |
| 7—12 | 7 | 5 | 2 | — | 3 | 3 | 1 |
| 13—20 | 2 | 2 | — | — | 1 | 1 | — |
| 21—35 | 2 | 1 | 1 | — | — | 1 | 1 |
| | 15 | 10 | 3 | 2† | 6 | 5 | 2(+2†) |

Den Versuch, diesen Eingriff auch bei der *Torsionsdystonie* anzuwenden, mußten wir bald wieder aufgeben. Ausgewählt wurden 3 Fälle, bei denen die dystonischen Verkrampfungen in der Hauptsache auf die Muskulatur des Halses, des Nackens, der Schultergürtel und der oberen Extremität sowie der proximalen Rumpfhälfte beschränkt waren. Von vornherein war also mit einer nur für den Torticollis bestimmten FOERSTER-DANDYschen Operation, d. h. mit einer Durchschneidung der spinalen Accessoriuswurzeln und der motorischen Wurzeln von $C_1$—$C_3$, nicht auszukommen. So wurde in diesen 3 Fällen die FOERSTER-DANDYsche Operation mit der Vorderstrangdurchschneidung kombiniert. Mit Ausnahme der zu erwartenden dauerhaften Besserung in den nach FOERSTER-DANDY denervierten Hals- und Nackenmuskeln haben sich in allen 3 Fällen bereits nach 3—4 Monaten — nach Abklingen der postoperativen allgemeinen Muskelerschlaffung — die Verkrampfungen in den übrigen Muskelgebieten, wie im Bereich der Schultergürtel, der oberen Extremitäten und oberen Rumpfpartie in vollem Umfang wieder eingestellt (Tabelle 3).

Tabelle 3. *Operationsergebnis nach* PUTNAMS *Extrapyramidotomie bei der Torsionsdystonie.*

| Alter<br>Jahre | Anzahl | Ergebnis bis zu 1 Jahr nach der Operation | | | Ergebnis nach 2—4 Jahren nach der Operation | | |
|---|---|---|---|---|---|---|---|
| | | gut | befriedigend | unbefriedigend | gut | befriedigend | unbefriedigend |
| 10 | 1 | 1 | — | — | — | 1 | — |
| über 30 | 2 | — | 1 | 1 | — | — | 2 |
| | 3 | 1 | 1 | 1 | — | 1 | 2 |

Die übrigen 12 Patienten unseres Krankengutes von 45 Fällen sind entweder noch nicht nachuntersucht oder die Nachuntersuchung liegt noch keine 2 Jahre zurück, so daß keine endgültige Beurteilung des Spätresultates möglich ist. Immerhin lassen die schriftlichen Rückfragen darauf schließen, daß die bisherigen Erfahrungen ihre Bestätigung finden werden.

Eine kurze Zusammenfassung der eigenen Erfahrungen mit der bilateralen Extrapyramidotomie läßt folgendes aussagen:

1. Die *Willkürmotorik* wird auf die Dauer praktisch nicht beeinträchtigt.

2. Bei den rein *pyramidalen paraspastischen Formen der* LITTLE*schen Krankheit* hält eine durch den Eingriff erzielte Lockerung der Spasmen gewöhnlich nur einige Wochen an. Nach spätestens 1—2 Jahren besteht in der Regel der gleiche Zustand wie vor der Operation.

3. Bei der *Athétose double* und auch bei den *Mischformen*, in denen Pyramidenbahnsymptome und striäre Bewegungsautomatismen nebeneinander vorkommen, ist eine zufriedenstellende und permanente Besserung der Bewegungsstörung in nahezu der Hälfte der Fälle zu erreichen. In den übrigen Fällen muß mit einer Wiederkehr der unwillkürlichen Bewegungen in verminderter Stärke oder auch in vollem Umfang gerechnet werden. Die Vermutung (SCHÜRMANN 1949), daß offenbar bei Kindern und Jugendlichen das Spätergebnis besser als bei Erwachsenen ist, scheint sich am eigenen Material zu bestätigen; sie ist auch bislang unwidersprochen geblieben.

4. Die unkontrollierten Bewegungen der *Torsionsdystonie* sind nicht dauerhaft zu beeinflussen, da nach längstens 3—4 Monaten die Bewegungsstörung in ihrem vollen Umfang wieder vorhanden ist.

5. An *postoperativen Komplikationen* sind transitorische zentrale Atemstörungen, an denen wir einen Patienten verloren haben, und unter Umständen eine zentrale Hyperthermie zu beachten, welche in 2 Fällen sofort nach dem Eingriff auftrat und anderntags wieder abklang.

## Technik der cervicalen Vorderstrangdurchschneidung (Extrapyramidotomie).

Die Extrapyramidotomie wird gleichseitig zur Lokalisation der Hyperkinese, meist jedoch doppelseitig in verschiedener Segmenthöhe, bei $C_2$ und $C_3$ ausgeführt.

In der üblichen Weise wird von einem Mittelschnitt im Nacken aus eine Laminektomie im Gebiet des 2.—4. Halswirbels vorgenommen. Es empfiehlt sich in diesen Fällen, die betreffenden Wirbelbögen so weit als möglich nach lateral fortzunehmen, um auf diese Weise für die später erfolgende Markeinschneidung an den Seiten ausreichend Platz zu gewinnen. Nach Eröffnung der Dura durch einen Längsschnitt wird auf der einen Seite die Vorderstrangchordotomie in Höhe des 2. und auf der anderen Seite in Höhe des 3. Cervicalsegmentes durchgeführt, also in einem Abstand von etwa einer Segmenthöhe. Hierzu wird nun das Lig. denticulatum von der Durainnenfläche abgetrennt, und, indem das Mark am Lig. denticulatum um seine Längsachse leicht gedreht wird, macht man sich die Seitenfläche des Markes mit der Austrittsstelle der motorischen Wurzel zugänglich. Es ist von Vorteil ein Chordotom mit einer doppelschneidigen Klinge zu benutzen, dessen Klingenlänge 5—6 mm beträgt und dessen Klinge um etwa $45^0$ abgewinkelt ist. — Die Klingenspitze wird nun nahezu rechtwinklig an einem Punkt eingestochen, welcher in der Mitte zwischen der Insertion des Lig. denticulatum am seitlichen Längsmeridian des Markes und dem Austritt der Vorderwurzel gelegen ist (Abb. 27a und b). Die vollständige Einführung der Chordotomklinge geschieht in Richtung auf die Fissura mediana anterior. Bei einer Tiefe von 5 mm werden anschließend die *vor* der ventralen Klingenschneide gelegenen extrapyramidal-motorischen Leitungssysteme durchtrennt, indem der Chordotomschaft behutsam nach hinten geschwenkt wird unter gleichzeitigem Herausziehen der Klinge. Gewöhnlich spürt man hierbei von innen her den etwas derberen elastischen Widerstand der Pia mater, welche gewissermaßen als Führung für die Klingenspitze dienen kann. Das heißt mit anderen Worten, daß die Chordotomklinge bei diesem Schnitt in ständiger Fühlungnahme mit der Innenseite der ventralen Pia mater bleiben kann, wenn man hierbei die erforderliche Sorgfalt beachtet und entsprechend behutsam vorgeht. — Verletzungen der kleinen Pialgefäße können im allgemeinen vermieden werden, zudem sind Blutungen aus ihnen leicht mit Muskelstückchen oder Fibrinschwämmchen, welche anschließend wieder entfernt werden, zu stillen. — Die Dura sollte man durch eine fortlaufende Naht dicht schließen.

Bei einem solchen Vorgehen hat man nicht allein die Gewähr, die betreffenden Bahnen (Tractus vestibulospinalis, reticulospinalis und tectospinalis) mit einer großen Sicherheit vollständig durchtrennt zu haben, sondern verringert insbesondere weitgehend die Gefahr einer Verletzung der A. spinalis anterior, deren vollständiger Ausfall ein Zugrundegehen der infraläsionellen Vorderhornsäulen mit einer konsekutiven schlaffen Tetraplegie zu bedeuten hätte.

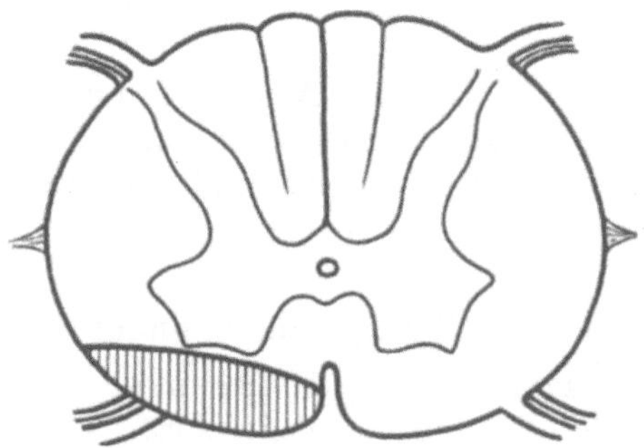

Abb. 27a. Die cervicale Extrapyramidotomie. (Nach PUTNAM.)

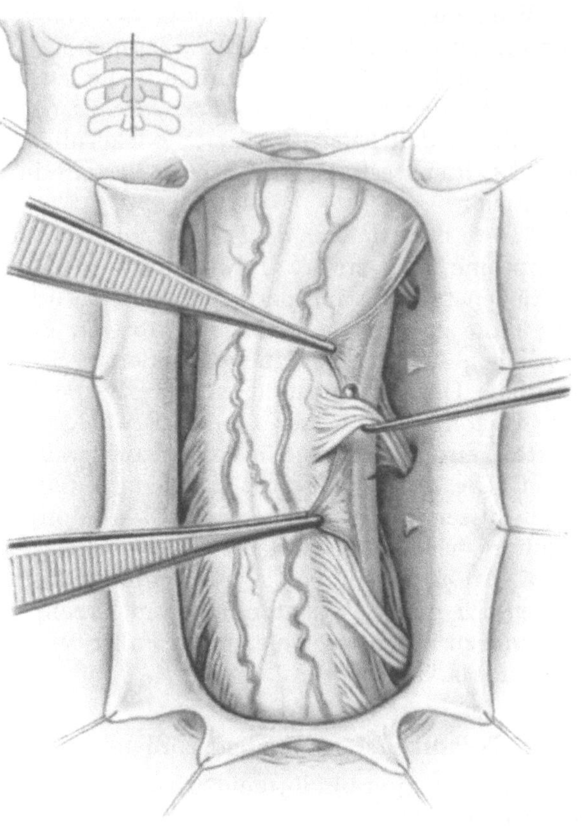

Abb. 27b. Die cervicale Extrapyramidotomie nach PUTNAM (Operationszugang mit eingezeichnetem Markeinschnitt).

Ebenso ist bei der bilateralen Ausführung des Eingriffs der Gefahr eines flüchtigen Querschnittsyndroms, unter Umständen verbunden mit ernsthaften Atemstörungen, dadurch am besten zu begegnen, indem die Durchschneidung der Vorderstränge in verschiedener Segmenthöhe ausgeführt wird. Hierdurch verringert sich die Gefährdung, welche infolge eines stärkeren postoperativen kollateralen Wundödems in dieser Höhe des Halsmarkes zu fürchten ist.

## 2. Die cervicale Durchschneidung des Pyramidenseitenstranges (laterale Pyramidotomie).

Dieser Eingriff wurde im Jahre 1938 von PUTNAM zur chirurgischen Behandlung des *einseitigen* PARKINSON-*Tremors* angegeben, nachdem sich bei diesem Leiden die Erfolglosigkeit der cervicalen Durchschneidung des Vorderstranges herausgestellt hatte.

Der *Mißerfolg der Extrapyramidotomie beim* PARKINSON-*Tremor* hat die auf Grund von tierexperimentellen Untersuchungen und an Hand der klinischen Erfahrungen mit der Cortectomie gewonnene Erkenntnis bestätigt, daß das Bestehen der Tremorsymptome offenbar an die Integrität des pyramidalen motorischen Systems gebunden ist. Das hat aber konsequenterweise zu bedeuten, daß der Tremor durch eine cervicale Chordotomie nur dann zu beeinflussen ist, wenn die pyramidalen Leitungswege ausreichend geschädigt werden.

Nun glaubte PUTNAM auf Grund der experimentellen Beobachtungen ROTHMANNS an Affen (1903), daß eine Durchschneidung des Pyramidenseitenstranges auch vom Menschen ohne erheblichen motorischen Funktionsausfall vertragen werden müsse. — Nach einigem Bemühen ließ sich ein geeignet erscheinender Fall finden. Ausgesucht wurde eine 32 Jahre alte Frau mit einem seit 16 Jahren bestehenden schweren *Hemiparkinsonismus* der rechten Körperseite. Die erheblichen Tremorsymptome hatten inzwischen zu einer Unbrauchbarkeit der betroffenen Gliedmaßen geführt, so daß eine *Durchschneidung der gleichseitigen lateralen Pyramidenbahn* gewagt werden konnte. Nach der Durchschneidung im 4. Cervicalsegment, deren Technik später besprochen wird, bestand sofort eine ipsilaterale Hemiplegie. Es konnten lediglich geringfügige Bewegungen der Finger ausgeführt werden. Die motorische Kraft kehrte aber sehr schnell in die betroffenen Gliedmaßen zurück. Bereits am 18. Tage nach der Operation war die Patientin wieder zum Gehen fähig und konnte auch ihre Hand zum Trinken und Schreiben gebrauchen. Zunächst wurde kein Ruhetremor mehr beobachtet, aber bei intendierten Bewegungen erschien wieder ein leichter Tremor. Der Muskeltonus soll nicht verändert gewesen sein. Im Laufe von 4 Monaten kehrte aber auch der Ruhetremor, etwa zur Hälfte seiner Originalstärke, wieder zurück. PUTNAM entschloß sich daher zu einem radikaleren Vorgehen. Die Patientin wurde relaminektomiert. Während PUTNAM in der 1. Sitzung lediglich das Chordotom am Austritt der Hinterwurzel in einem Winkel von 15° zur Senkrechten 4 mm tief in den Hinterseitenstrang eingestochen und dann wieder herausgezogen hat, vervollständigte er jetzt in der 2. Sitzung die Durchschneidung im Seitenstrang. Diesmal hat er nach dem 4 mm tiefen Einstich am Eintritt der Hinterwurzel die Chordotomspitze nach außen bis zum horizontalen Meridian des Markes geschwenkt. Hierdurch war ein dreieckiger Bezirk durchschnitten worden, dessen Seiten durch das Hinterhorn einerseits und durch die Senkrechte vom Lig. denticulatum aus andererseits, begrenzt waren. Das Längenmaß dieser Seiten betrug je 4 mm. — Noch 1 Jahr nach der 2. Operation fehlte in Ruhe der Tremor vollständig, er machte sich aber bei Willkürbewegungen wieder leicht bemerkbar. Der Gang blieb hemiparetisch und auch die motorische Kraft der oberen Extremität blieb um etwa die Hälfte vermindert (Abb. 28).

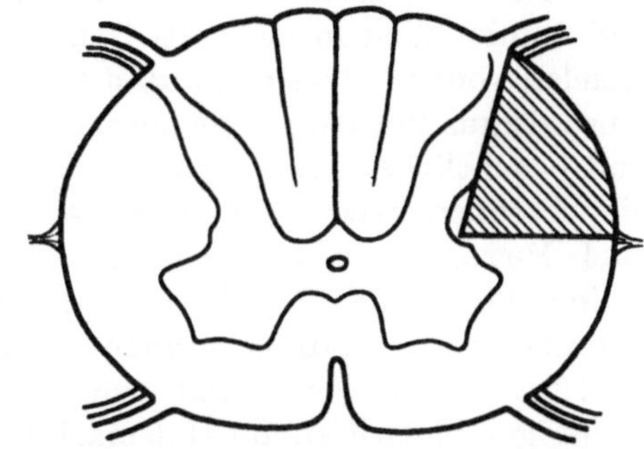

Abb. 28. Die laterale cervicale Pyramidotomie nach PUTNAM.

Ermutigt durch den Erfolg der *vollständigen Durchschneidung der Pyramidenseitenstrangbahn* beim PARKINSON-Tremor hat PUTNAM nachfolgend diesen Eingriff an insgesamt 22 Kranken ausgeführt. Zusammen mit HERZ gibt er im Jahre 1950 einen Erfahrungsbericht, welcher sich auf das Ergebnis von Nachuntersuchungen stützt, die mehrere Jahre nach der Operation erhoben wurden. — Das *Früh*resultat unmittelbar nach der Operation war in allen Fällen ausgezeichnet, denn bei 20 Kranken war der Tremor vollständig verschwunden und bei den restlichen 2 Kranken war dieser erheblich vermindert. Sofort nach dem Eingriff bestand allerdings bei 11 Patienten eine komplette Hemiplegie, stets am Arm und den proximalen Abschnitten der oberen Extremität stärker ausgeprägt. Das *Spät*resultat war erwartungsgemäß weniger gut. In etwa $^1/_3$ der Fälle blieb der Tremor dauerhaft und vollständig beseitigt. In einem weiteren Drittel war der Tremor auch nach 1 Jahr und länger noch wesentlich gebessert und im letzten Drittel war nach etwa 1 Jahr keine Besserung der Tremorsymptome mehr festzustellen. Nach dieser Zeit war die Willkürmotorik in einem wesentlichen Grad nur in 5 Fällen beeinträchtigt. In 4 Fällen wurde lediglich eine leichte Verminderung der motorischen Kraft festgestellt und in mehr als der Hälfte der Fälle (13 Patienten) war keine nachweisbare Störung der willkürlichen motorischen Funktion mehr vorhanden.

PUTNAM beschränkt die laterale Pyramidotomie auf jene Kranke mit einem *schweren einseitigen alternierenden Tremor*, wenn die Symptome der Akinese und Starre von untergeordneter Bedeutung sind (Beschreibung der Operationstechnik S. 112).

Im Jahre 1949 hat OLIVER über seine Erfahrungen mit PUTNAMs lateraler Pyramidotomie an Hand einer Serie von 48 Fällen von PARKINSON-*Tremor* berichtet. Er bestätigt, daß diese Operation in sorgfältig ausgewählten Fällen gute Aussichten für eine Besserung der Tremorsymptome bietet, daß die Ergebnisse aber bei *den* Patienten besser gewesen seien, welche nach der Operation analgetische Bezirke auf der Gegenseite zeigen, als Folge einer Beteiligung des Tractus spinothalamicus. Diese Beobachtung veranlaßte OLIVER zu dem Versuch, die Resultate mit einer ausgedehnteren Markincision als nach PUTNAMs

Originalmethode zu verbessern. Dazu wurde von ihm die *Seitenstrangchordotomie einfach etwas radikaler* ausgeführt, indem er die Tiefe der Markincision von 4 mm auf 5 mm ausdehnte, so daß jedesmal eine komplette Analgesie der kontralateralen Körperseite die Folge war. Es ist jedoch wahrscheinlich, daß bei Olivers Modifikation auch Teile des Tractus rubrospinalis mit durchschnitten werden. Der Eingriff wurde von ihm in Höhe des 2.—3. Cervicalsegmentes durchgeführt. — Schon 1 Jahr später war Oliver (1950) in der Lage, über ein Erfahrungsgut von 79 operierten einseitigen Parkinson-Fällen zu berichten. In den letzten 18 Fällen hat er sogar eine *totale Durchschneidung des Seitenstranges* vorgenommen und hiermit offensichtlich die besten Resultate erhalten, da 17 Patienten anschließend keinen Tremor mehr gezeigt hatten (94 % !). Eine vollständige dauerhafte Beseitigung der Tremorsymptome hatte er vorher, auch mit seiner radikaleren Pyramidotomie, nicht in mehr als 12,5 % und eine Besserung in nicht mehr als 37,5 % der Fälle erzielen können. Das heißt, daß erst die *totale Seitenstrangdurchschneidung* beim Hemiparkinsonismus mit einiger Sicherheit in mehr als nur 50 % der Fälle eine wirklich dauerhafte und beachtliche Besserung erreichen läßt. Selbstverständlich sind nach Olivers Vorgehen die postoperativen Hemiplegien sehr viel erheblicher und weniger rückbildungsfähig als nach Putnams einfacher Pyramidotomie. Trotzdem kommt es zu einer gewissen Restitution der motorischen Funktion, während der kontralaterale Verlust der Schmerz- und Temperaturempfindung permanent ist (Beschreibung der Operationstechnik S. 112).

Etwa zur gleichen Zeit wurde von Ebin (1949) eine andere Modifikation zu den bisherigen Eingriffen am Halsmark für die Behandlung des *einseitigen Tremors* mitgeteilt, die *kombinierte laterale und ventrale Pyramidotomie*. Ebin hatte sich gefragt, weshalb mit der lateralen Pyramidotomie von Putnam gewöhnlich nicht mehr als ein teilweises Verschwinden des Tremors erreicht werden konnte. Den Grund hierfür schrieb er dem Umstand zu, daß durch die laterale Pyramidotomie nicht alle Fasern der Pyramidenbahnen, welche von den großen Betzschen Zellen der Area 4 $\gamma$ kommen, zu unterbrechen sind. Im Hinblick auf die Erfahrungen Bucys mit der Exstirpation der Area 4 $\gamma$ müßte also der Nachteil der bis dahin verwandten cervicalen Methoden darin gesehen werden, daß diese nicht auch den ungekreuzten Pyramidenvorderstrang erfaßten. Eine vollständigere Besserung der Tremorsymptome schien Ebin demnach mit einer Durchschneidung der gleichseitigen Pyramidenseitenstrangbahn in Verbindung mit einer Durchschneidung der gegenseitigen Pyramidenvorderstrangbahn möglich. Da entgegen der technisch einfachen Durchtrennung des Pyramidenseitenstranges die selektive Unterbrechung des Pyramidenvorderstranges auf der Gegenseite auf Grund seiner Lage längs des Sulcus medialis schwierig ist, hat Ebin eine kreuzende Incision von der Gegenseite her vorgeschlagen. Diese erlaubt es, den Pyramidenseitenstrang der einen und den Pyramidenvorderstrang der anderen Seite gleichzeitig durch eine einzige Incision, vom Eintritt der Hinterwurzel ins Mark aus — etwa in Höhe des 4.—5. Cervicalsegmentes — zu durchschneiden (s. Abb. 29).

Unter 26 von Ebin operierten Parkinson-Fällen war der Tremor in 23 Fällen das dominierende Symptom. Die postoperative Beobachtungszeit erstreckte sich über 7 Monate bis zu 4 Jahren. Im *Früh*resultat unmittelbar nach der Operation war der Tremor sofort in 19 Fällen (82 %) erheblich und in 4 Fällen (18 %) leicht vermindert, also in all *den* Fällen gebessert, in denen er das hervorstechende Symptom gewesen ist. In der Regel fehlte der Ruhetremor vollständig, aber kam es noch zu einem schwachen Intentionstremor bei willkürlichen Bewegungen und emotionellen Affekten. Das *Spät*resultat läßt Ebins Vorgehen in weniger günstigem Licht erscheinen. Danach waren die Tremorsymptome nur noch bei 10 Patienten gebessert (38,4 %), in 7 Fällen war der Zustand unverändert (26,9 %), in weiteren 7 Fällen war der Zustand weiter fortgeschritten (26,9 %) und in 2 Fällen ist 3 Monate nach der Operation außerhalb der Klinik der Tod eingetreten (6,6 %). In allen Fällen hat postoperativ auf der Seite des Eingriffes eine mehr oder weniger stark ausgeprägte Hemiparese bestanden, deren gute Tendenz zur Rückbildung aber hervorgehoben wird. Auch die Symptome der Starre sollen etwas gebessert worden sein, was jedoch nach den bisherigen Erfahrungen mit den Pyramidotomien zweifelhaft erscheinen muß. — Verständlicherweise sind auch für dieses Vorgehen die *einseitigen Tremorsyndrome* vorzuziehen, obgleich EBIN seinen Eingriff auch doppelseitig ausgeführt hat (Beschreibung der Operationstechnik S. 112).

Die jüngst vom Verfasser (SCHÜRMANN 1952) mitgeteilte Modifikation cervicaler Operationsmethoden, die *kombinierte Hinterseiten-Vorderstrangdurchschneidung* oder „Traktotomia posterolateralis et ventralis", hat die Unterbrechung *aller* efferenten Bahnensysteme, welche Fasern für die betroffene Körperseite führen, zum Ziele. Diese wird erreicht mit der Durchschneidung des gleichseitigen Pyramidenseitenstranges, des Tractus rubrospinalis und des Vorderstranges und der Durchschneidung des gegenseitigen Pyramidenvorderstranges. Der Eingriff, gewissermaßen eine *kombinierte Pyramido-Extrapyramidotomie*, wird in einer Sitzung und zwar in Höhe des 1.—2. Cervicalsegmentes vorgenommen (Abb. 30). Durch die hiermit erstrebte vollständige „Des-Efferenzierung" der betroffenen Körperseite ist mit einer bisher nicht erreichten Sicherheit die Wiederkehr der abnormen motorischen Impulse über irgendwelche sonst erhalten gebliebenen absteigenden Bahnen praktisch unmöglich gemacht worden. Man ist hierdurch gegen „Rezidive" gewissermaßen absolut gesichert. Maßgebend für ein solch radikales Vorgehen ist für den Verfasser die nach der allgemeinen und eigenen Erfahrung nicht seltene Wiederkehr der abnormen Bewegungen gewesen, ob nun die Pyramidenbahnen oder die extrapyramidalen Bahnen durchschnitten wurden. Die relativ häufige Wiederkehr der unkontrollierten Bewegungen aber läßt darauf schließen, daß praktisch *alle* absteigenden Bahnen zur Leitung der abnormen extrapyramidalen Impulse befähigt sein müssen. Die abnormen Erregungen können demnach, vorausgesetzt, daß sie in ausreichender Stärke wirksam sind, auch auf quantitativ verringerten efferenten Wegen ankommen. Deshalb empfiehlt es sich gerade bei den *schwersten Formen halbseitiger Hyperkinesen*, die abnormen Impulse ihrer efferenten Leitungsbahnen möglichst total zu berauben, um ihre Wiederkehr hinreichend sicher zu verhindern.

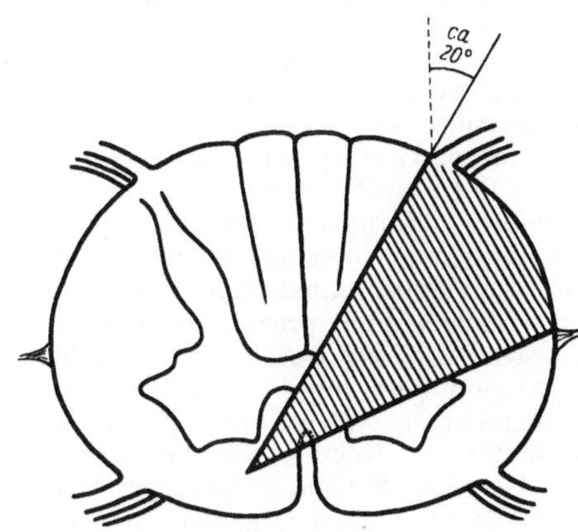


Abb. 29. EBINS kombinierte ventrale und laterale Pyramidotomie.

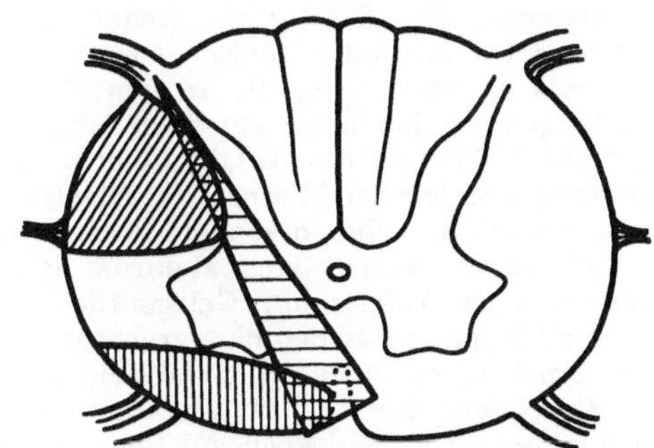

Abb. 30. Die kombinierte Pyramido-Extrapyramidotomie.

Bei leichteren Störungsformen dagegen kann unter Umständen allein eine quantitative Verminderung der efferenten Wege bereits für eine dauerhafte Besserung der unwillkürlichen Bewegungen genügen.

Die radikale cervicale Traktotomie des Verfassers ist nur bei *sehr schweren halbseitigen Hyperkinesen*, aber hier wirklich mit großem Vorteil und zum Segen des Kranken anzuwenden, wie die folgenden Beispiele zeigen mögen. Stets ist eine spastische Hemiparese auf der Seite des Eingriffes und eine Hemianalgesie und -thermanaesthesie auf der Körpergegenseite die Folge. Bisher in 4 Fällen angewandt, hat der Verfasser für die *kombinierte Pyramido-Extrapyramidotomie* schwere Formen einer *Hemichoreoathetose mit torsionsdystonischen Elementen* oder die quälende *halbseitige Torsionsdystonie* ausgewählt (Beschreibung der Operationstechnik S. 112).

**Fall 1.** Josef K., 33 Jahre[1]. *Schwere Hemichoreoathetose rechts mit Torsionen und mit Anfallcharakter der Hyperkinese.*

[1] Herrn Privatdozent Dr. H. TELLENBACH, Oberarzt an der Universitätsnervenklinik München, gebührt für die freundliche Überlassung der Untersuchungsbefunde besonderer Dank.

Familienanamnese o. B. — Eigene Anamnese: Angeblich normale Geburt. Im Anschluß an eine frühkindliche Encephalitis im 3. Lebensjahr entwickeln sich rechtsseitige Hyperkinesen. Das Kind war damals auffällig verändert, klagte eine Zeitlang über heftige Kopfschmerzen, war abnorm erregbar und neigte zu zornmütigen Impulshandlungen. Störungen des Schlafes und Appetits fielen auf. Im 4. Lebensjahr zeigte sich eine Schwäche der rechten Seite. Hinzu kamen anfallsartig auftretende Verkrampfungen der rechten Gliedmaßen ohne Bewußtseinsverlust, die zwischen dem 5. und 17. Lebensjahr etwas seltener wurden. Auch die psychischen Veränderungen des akuten Krankheitsstadiums gingen zurück. Die zunächst kurzen Krampfzustände traten auf bei Intention *rascher* Bewegungen oder bei *unvermitteltem* Kontakt mit unvertrauten Personen. In unmittelbaren Zuständen, wie Spielen, unbeobachteter körperlicher Betätigung usw. traten keine Krämpfe auf. — In der Schule Auffassungs- und Konzentrationsstörungen, hat zweimal repetiert. Mit 17 Jahren erneut Häufung und Intensivierung der krampfartig auftretenden Hyperkinesen, auch seelisch wieder labiler. — Keine Berufsausbildung. Ein Jahr vor der Aufnahme gedecktes commotionelles Trauma mit 4stündiger Bewußtlosigkeit. Danach Entwicklung eines charakteristischen postcommotionellen Syndroms mit häufigem Erbrechen, welches mehrere Monate anhielt. Seit dem Unfall waren bei den geringsten Anlässen länger anhaltende Krampfzustände in der rechten Körperseite zu beobachten, wodurch das Handeln und Sprechen noch weiter behindert wurden. Durch eine starke sexuelle Betätigung, insbesondere aber durch einen erheblichen Alkoholkonsum sollen die quälenden Verkrampfungen etwas gemildert worden sein. Unter den üblichen Bedingungen war eine Arbeit oder Berufsausübung nicht möglich. Zuletzt geriet K. in einen Zustand zunehmender Verzweiflung mit ernsthaften Suicidabsichten. — Keine cerebralen Krampfanfälle.

*Aus dem Befund.* 33jähriger Mann ohne krankhaften Befund an Körperbedeckung, Schleimhäuten und inneren Organen. RR 125/90 mm Hg.

*Neurologisch.* Leichtes Rechtsabweichen der Zunge. Gaumensegelschwäche rechts. Die linke Körperseite ohne krankhaften Befund. Die rechte Körperseite weist eine mäßige Hypotrophie mit gleichmäßiger Verkürzung der Gliedmaßen auf. Geringe Halbseitenparese rechts mit positiven Pyramidenzeichen. Ein differenzierter Befund ist wegen der ständig einschießenden Hyperkinesen nicht zu erheben.

*Die Hyperkinesen.* Der rechtsseitige Krampfzustand tritt bei geringsten Anlässen auf, er ist schmerzlos und dauert meist einige Minuten. Es kommt hierbei zu heftigen Kontraktionen der rechten Gesichtsmuskeln, zu Spontanbewegungen der Zunge. Beim Versuch zu sprechen, werden einzelne ungeformte Laute zustande gebracht. Die Atmung ist stoßweise, die rechte Schulter wird ruckartig hochgezogen. An den Extremitäten beginnt die Verkrampfung mit einem blitzartig einschießenden Hypertonus. Der Arm geht in Flexion, die Finger in Bajonettstellung, das Bein in Hyperextension, die Großzehe in Babinskistellung. Agonisten und Antagonisten sind gleichzeitig angespannt. Die Glieder, die weder aktiv noch passiv bewegt werden können, bleiben in diesem Zustand für Sekunden tonisch fixiert. In der Folge kommt es in blitzartigem Wechsel zu enorm vertrackten Stellungen, die an den Fingern mit unlösbarem Faustschluß abwechseln. Die Gliedstellungen werden unterschiedlich lang beibehalten; dabei werden die Gliedmaßen oftmals leicht gedreht. Während des Anfalls können äußere Reize die Muskelspannung steigern oder einen rasch aufeinanderfolgenden Wechsel der Gliedstellungen bewirken. Die Verkrampfung endet meist plötzlich und hinterläßt keine besondere Ermüdung oder gar Lähmung (Abb. 31).

*Psychisch* besteht eine abnorme Reizbarkeit, eine Merk- und Konzentrationsschwäche, eine verlangsamte Auffassung. Gelegentlich kommt es zu Zwangslachen. Auffällig langes Anhalten des Heiterkeitsausdrucks bei inkongruenter Gemütslage. Grundstimmung düster, verzweifelt, hoffnungslos; ernst zu nehmende Suicidabsichten.

*Operation.* Kombinierte Pyramido-Extrapyramidotomie des Verfassers in Höhe des 2. Cervicalsegmentes rechts. — Noch auf dem Operationstisch wird ein Dauerkatheter in die Harnblase eingeführt und über ein Zweiwegesystem mit einer Spülvorrichtung verbunden, welche der Patient selbständig stundenweise bedienen kann.

*Verlauf nach der Operation.* Ungestörte postoperative Wundheilung. Unmittelbar nach der Operation bestand eine schlaffe Lähmung der rechtsseitigen Gliedmaßen. Vollständiges Sistieren der Hyperkinesen bis auf die in der rechten Gesichtshälfte und rechten Halsseite. Auf der Gegenseite intakte Motorik, aber Thermanaesthesie und Analgesie. Blase und Mastdarm waren zunächst gelähmt. Vom 7.—8. Tage ab nahm der Muskeltonus im rechten Bein langsam zu. Gleichzeitig wurden Beugereflexe auslösbar. Der rechte Arm blieb bis etwa zum 10.—12. Tag völlig schlaff. Am 12. Tag bestand im Bein eine deutliche spastische Tonuserhöhung. Eine aktive Bewegung war allerdings noch nicht möglich. Der Babinski konnte von der Fußsohle und vom Oberschenkel her ausgelöst werden. Am 14.—15. Tag konnte das Bein erstmals ein wenig aktiv bewegt werden. Zu dieser Zeit begann auch der Muskeltonus des rechten Armes anzusteigen. Die Blasen-Mastdarmlähmung war noch vorhanden. In der weiteren Folge setzte nun eine rasche Restitution der Willkürmotorik des rechten Beines ein. Am Übergang der 3. zur 4. Woche konnte der Patient selbständig aufstehen und einige Schritte gehen. Am rechten Arm hatte der Muskeltonus weiter zugenommen, aber es war aktiv zunächst nur eine einfache Beugung im Ellbogengelenk möglich. Die Blasen-Mastdarmfunktion hatte sich zu dieser Zeit wieder zur Genüge eingespielt, so daß der Dauerkatheter entfernt werden konnte. Der

Restharn war noch 3—5 Tage etwas erhöht, dann nicht mehr. Zwischen der 4. und 5. Woche konnte der Patient schon längere Strecken gehen. Der rechte Arm war vorerst nur zu synergistischen Massenbewegungen fähig.

*Nachuntersuchungsbefund 3 Monate p. op.* Persistenz der Hyperkinese im Gebiet der Hirnnerven und obersten Halsnervenwurzeln. Darüber hinaus sind keine Hyperkinesen mehr in den rechten Gliedmaßen und im rechten Schultergürtel vorhanden. Es besteht ein cervicales BROWN-SÉQUARD-Syndrom mit typischer spinaler Hemiplegie rechts und Thermanaesthesie und Analgesie links. Die

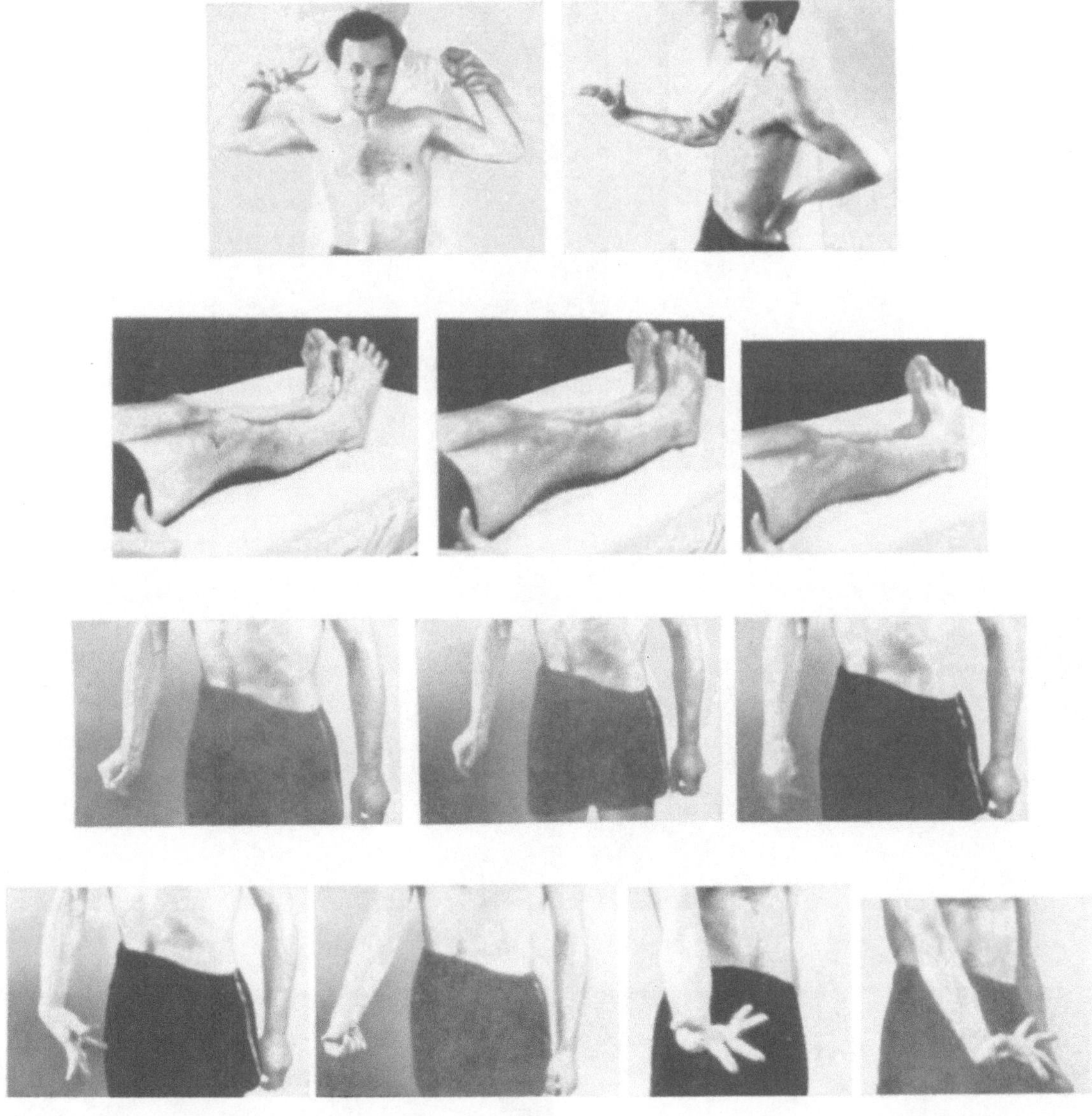

Abb. 31. Fall 1. 33jähriger Mann mit einer rechtsseitigen Hemichoreoathetose und anfallsartigen Torsionen. Zustand *vor* der Operation.

Paresen sind am rechten Arm, vor allem distal, stärker ausgebildet als am Bein. Anaesthesie für alle Qualitäten im Gebiet der Nn. supraclaviculares, welche vermutlich auf eine segmentale Hinterwurzelläsion zurückgeht. Am rechten Bein können zum Teil schon gut isolierte Bewegungen ausgeführt werden. Die Fußmuskulatur ist indessen noch nahezu paralytisch. — *Psychisch* ist der Patient nun ausgeglichener. Er hat neuen Lebensmut gefaßt und hat es durch intensive Übungen soweit gebracht, daß er kleinere Bergausflüge unternehmen und eine leichtere Arbeit annehmen konnte. Die postcommotionellen Störungen haben sich, möglicherweise durch die mehr oder weniger „unfreiwillige Liegekur", völlig verloren.

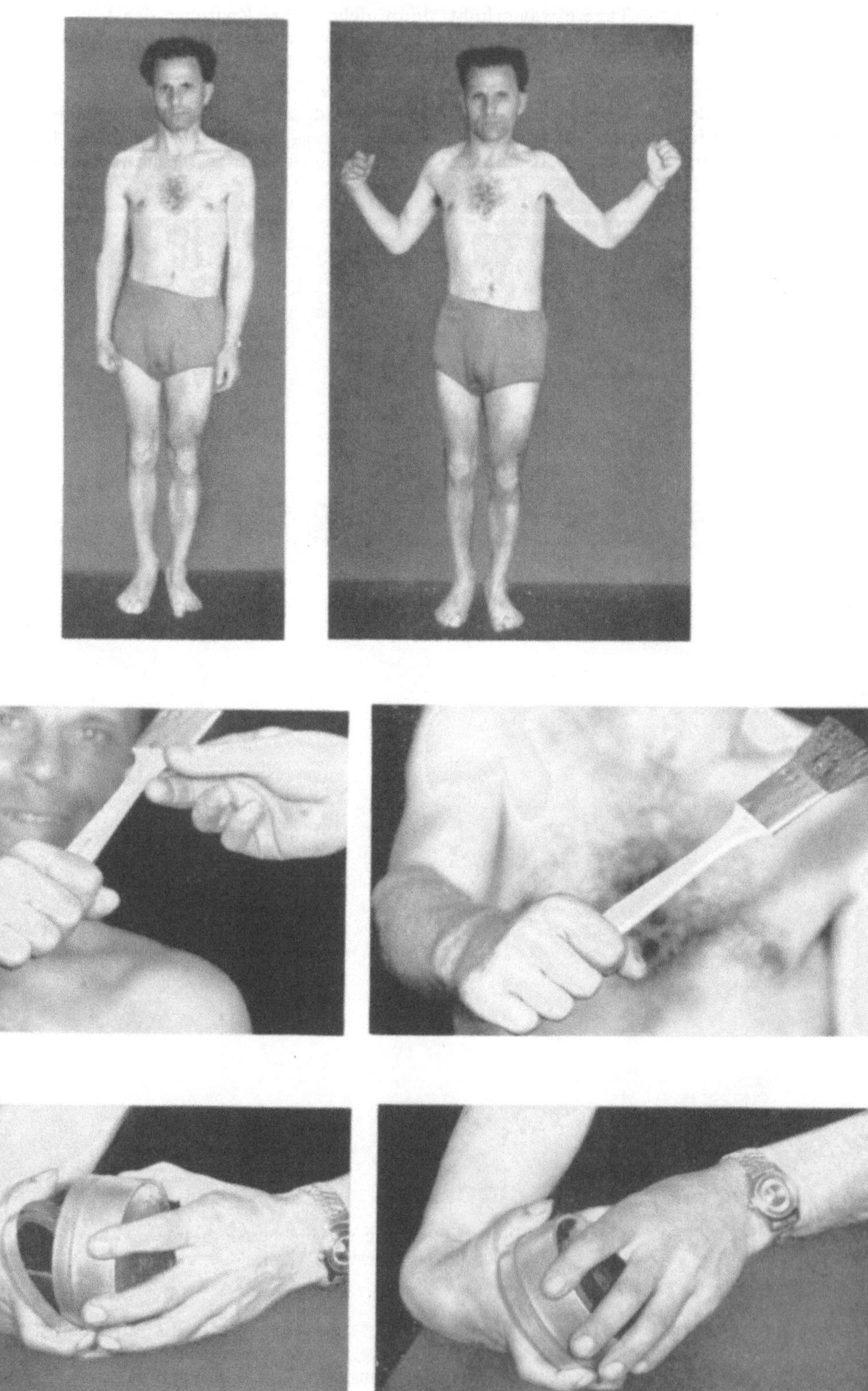

Abb. 32. Fall 1. 33jähriger Mann mit einer schweren rechtsseitigen Hemichoreoathetose und anfallsartigen Torsionen. Zustand $2^1/_2$ Jahre *nach* einer cervicalen kombinierten Pyramido-Extrapyramidotomie. Die Hyperkinesen sind beseitigt; isolierte Bewegungen der Finger sind nicht möglich, sondern nur Massenbewegungen.

*Nachuntersuchungsbefund 1 Jahr p. op.* K. spürt gelegentlich — ohne besonderen Anlaß — ein nur sekundenlang auftretendes Gefühl des Vibrierens im rechten Arm und Bein. Äußerlich ist dabei eine Bewegung an den Gliedmaßen nicht zu sehen. Die anfallsartigen Verkrampfungen der rechten Körperseite sind nicht mehr aufgetreten, mit Ausnahme an der rechten Gesichts- und Halsseite. — Die Beweglichkeit des rechten Beines hat sich wesentlich gebessert und ist kraftvoller geworden. — Im 11. Monat nach der Operation in 6 Std Aufstieg von Kufstein auf das Stripsenjoch (etwa 2000 m). — Heben des rechten Armes und Ellenbeugung weiter gebessert und kräftiger. Dagegen keine Besserung der Fingerbeweglichkeit (zu einer regelmäßigen heilgymnastischen Nachbehandlung war der Patient leider nicht zu bewegen). Die Empfindungsstörung auf der linken Seite ist unverändert.

*Nachuntersuchungsbefund $2^1/_2$ Jahre p. op.* Im wesentlichen unveränderter Zustand gegenüber dem Nachuntersuchungsbefund vor $1^1/_2$ Jahren. Allerdings hat sich inzwischen die willkürliche Beweglichkeit der rechtsseitigen Gliedmaßen weiterhin etwas gebessert.

*Einzelheiten aus dem Befund.* Leichte spontane Kopfschiefhaltung nach links und Kopfdrehung nach rechts. Anfallsweise Dyskinesien im rechten Facialisgebiet, die in vereinzelten Zuckungen auf den Clavicularanteil des Trapezius, Sternocleido und Platysma übergreifen. Zunge und Gaumensegel weichen etwas nach rechts ab. *Im übrigen keinerlei Hyperkinesen mehr.* Rechter Arm: Hypotrophie der Muskulatur des rechten Schultergürtels und Armes. Fast fehlende Behaarung, leichte Atrophie der Haut. Spastisches Paresesyndrom. Hand in Beugestellung leicht kontrahiert, Finger spastisch kontrahiert und nur gegen Widerstand streckbar. Nach passiver Fingerstreckung ist Halten von Gegenständen und aktiver Faustschluß möglich, aktives Öffnen der geschlossenen Faust ist dagegen nur mit Hilfe der gesunden linken Hand möglich. Die aktive Beweglichkeit im Deltoideus, Teres minor und major ist nur mäßig eingeschränkt. Die Kraftentfaltung im Biceps und Triceps ist gut. Die Pronation des Unterarmes geschieht ausgiebig, dagegen ist die Supination eingeschränkt. Die Beugung im Handgelenk ist kräftig und nur wenig eingeschränkt, dagegen ist die Dorsalflexion der Hand erheblich eingeschränkt. Bis auf einen kräftigen Faustschluß sind isolierte Fingerbewegungen aktiv praktisch unmöglich. *Rechtes Bein:* Gleichmäßige Hypotrophie, leichte Verkürzung, Spitzfußstellung und Supination des Fußes. Mäßige Tonuserhöhung. Ausreichende Kraft in der Oberschenkelmuskulatur. Fuß- und Zehenmuskeln bis auf geringe Innervationsmöglichkeit im Tibialis anterior isoliert nicht zu innervieren. Die Sehnenreflexe sind gesteigert. Pyramidenzeichen fehlen. — Die *Tiefensensibilität* ist beiderseits ungestört. In der *Oberflächensensibilität* findet sich links eine ganz geringe taktile Hypästhesie ab $C_3$, eine Hypalgesie links von $C_3$—$C_5$, und eine Analgesie links ab $C_6$. Eine Thermhypästhesie besteht links von $C_3$—$D_3$ und eine Thermanaesthesie links ab $D_4$. Darüber hinaus besteht auf der rechten Seite eine leichte Herabsetzung für alle Empfindungsqualitäten im Gebiet von $C_3$. — *Psychisch* ist der Patient auch weiter leicht reizbar und erregbar. Die jetzige körperliche Situation wird gegenüber der früheren als Erlösung empfunden. Der Patient hat sich mit seiner Umwelt und Mitwelt ins Gleichgewicht gesetzt und ist um eine Berufsausübung bemüht.

**Fall 2.** Matthias H., 19 Jahre. — *Schwere einseitige Torsionsdystonie rechts mit choreoathetotischen Hyperkinesen* an den Gliedmaßenenden.

Familienanamnese o. B. — Eigene Anamnese: Angeblich normale Geburt nach einer 8 Monate langen Schwangerschaft. Normale frühkindliche Entwicklung, keine Paresen, zu normaler Zeit Sitzen, Laufen und Sprechen gelernt. Im 5. Lebensjahr toxische Diphtherie durchgemacht, welche eine mehrwöchige Krankenhausbehandlung erforderte und in deren Verlauf es nach etwa 5 Wochen zur Beobachtung einer Schwäche der rechtsseitigen Gliedmaßen mit unwillkürlichen Zuckungen gekommen sei. In den darauffolgenden Jahren trotz verschiedener Behandlungsversuche keine Besserung der Halbseitenlähmung und Zunahme der unwillkürlichen Verdrehungen und Verkrampfungen der rechten Körperseite. Die rechtsseitigen Gliedmaßen seien im Wachstum zurückgeblieben. Im 13. Lebensjahr Aufnahme in der orthopädischen Klinik der Universität Köln (Prof. M. Hackenbroch)[1]. Nach dem dortigen Bericht erfolgte die Behandlung des Jungen wegen der Folgen einer spastischen Hemiplegie rechts, die zu einer Flexions-Adduktionskontraktur des rechten Hüftgelenkes, einer Beugekontraktur des Kniegelenkes und einer nicht ausgleichbaren Spitzfußstellung geführt hatte. Der Gang war schwerstens gestört, der Junge bewegte sich auf dem linken Bein hüpfend vorwärts. Im rechten Schultergelenk fand sich eine Einrollungs- und Heranführungsstellung bei einer Beugekontraktur von Ellenbogen- und Handgelenk mit athetotischer Bewegungsunruhe der Finger. Durch die Torsionsspasmen wurde der rechte Arm in eine sehr quälende Zwangshaltung gezwungen, in welcher Unterarm und Hand auf dem Rücken zu liegen kamen. — Man war bestrebt, die Gelenkkontrakturen zu beheben, wobei im einzelnen eine Achillotenotomie, eine Einkerbung des Latissimus dorsi, eine z-förmige Verlängerung der Bizepssehne rechts und eine Resektion des rechtsseitigen Nervus obturatorius nach Selig durchgeführt wurden. Hierdurch konnten die Gelenkfehlstellungen gebessert werden. Eine Einschulung und Berufsausbildung wurde möglich. In der Folgezeit zeigte sich, insbesondere hinsichtlich der Stellung des Hüftgelenkes, ein volles Rezidiv mit erneuter extremer Flexions-Adduktionskontraktur. Außerdem war es zu einer fortschreitenden Entwicklung der Torsionsspasmen und unwillkürlichen Bewegungen der rechten Körperseite, vor allem des rechten Armes gekommen. Keine cerebralen Krampfanfälle.

[1] Herrn Dr. Kirsch von der orthopädischen Universitätsklinik Köln gebührt für die freundliche Überlassung der dort erhobenen Untersuchungsbefunde besonderer Dank.

*Aus dem Aufnahmebefund.* 19jähriger Mann ohne krankhaften Befund an den inneren Organen. Comedonenacne an der Gesichts- und Rückenhaut.

*Neurologisch.* Asymmetrie des Gesichts durch rechtsseitige Facialiszuckungen vorgetäuscht, keine Facialisparese. Gaumensegelschwäche rechts und leichtes Rechtsabweichen der Zunge. Die linke Körperseite weist keinen krankhaften Befund auf. Die rechte Körperseite zeigt eine durchgehende Hypotrophie und Verkürzung der Gliedmaßen von 8 cm an der oberen und 9 cm an der unteren

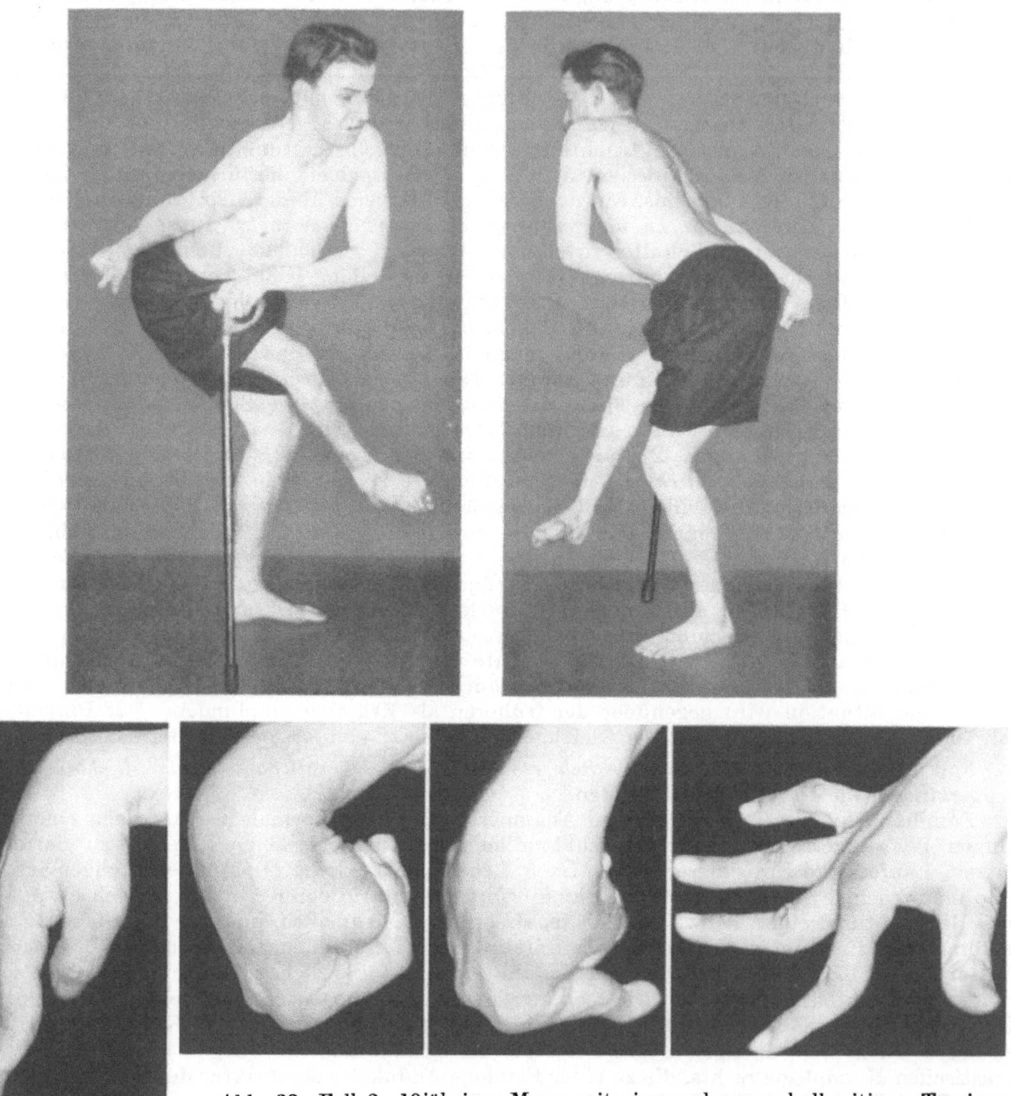

Abb. 33. Fall 2. 19jähriger Mann mit einer schweren halbseitigen Torsionsdystotonie und choreoathetotischen Bewegungselementen auf der rechten Seite. Zustand *vor* der Operation.

Extremität. Schwere rechtsseitige Hemiparese mit erheblichen Torsionen und Jaktationen, welche eine differenzierte Untersuchung der Reflexe unmöglich machen.

*Die Hyperkinesen.* Die unwillkürlichen Bewegungen, welche sich ausschließlich an der rechten Körperseite zeigen, haben geradezu einen grotesken Charakter. Sie sind nicht ständig vorhanden, treten aber bei geringsten äußeren Anlässen verstärkt in Erscheinung. Es kommt zu nichtrhythmischen, grimassierenden Verziehungen der rechten Gesichtshälfte. Der rechte Arm, der beinahe schlaff am Körper herunterhängen kann, wird durch einen unvermittelt auftretenden muskulären Krampf aus der Schulter heraus nach einwärts rotiert und, unter torquierenden ziehend-drehenden Bewegungen des Rumpfes, in einer Schleuderbewegung auf den Rücken gebracht, wo er in einem längerdauernden quälenden Beuge- und Innenrotationskrampf in seiner Lage verharrt. An den Fingern laufen in diesem minutenlangen Haltungskrampf des Armes langsam wurmförmige athetotische Bewegungen ab.

Diese führen zu extremen Überstreckungen und Beugestellungen der Finger. Der Beuge- und Innenrotationskrampf des Armes löst sich nur langsam und schrittweise. Der Patient ist nun aber bemüht, den Arm in der beschriebenen Stellung auf dem Rücken zu halten, da er den nächsten, in wenigen Minuten kommenden Krampfzustand fürchtet. Diesem begegnet er damit, daß der rechte Arm sich bereits in der Endstellung des Krampfes befindet, so daß sich der Krampfzustand nur noch an der verkürzten Muskulatur abspielen kann. Durch diesen „Kunstgriff" vermeidet der Patient sehr geschickt die wirklich grotesk wirkenden, weit ausfahrenden Schleuderbewegungen des Armes und der rechtsseitige Torsionskrampf muß sich gewissermaßen „auf der Stelle" abspielen. Hierbei bleibt die Rumpfverdrehung allerdings noch bizarr genug. — Am rechten Bein besteht eine tendinös und artikulär fixierte Beuge- und Adduktionskontraktur im Hüftgelenk und leichter Beugekontraktur im Hüftgelenk. Athetotisches Bewegungsspiel der Zehen, welche sich an den rechtsseitigen Torsions-

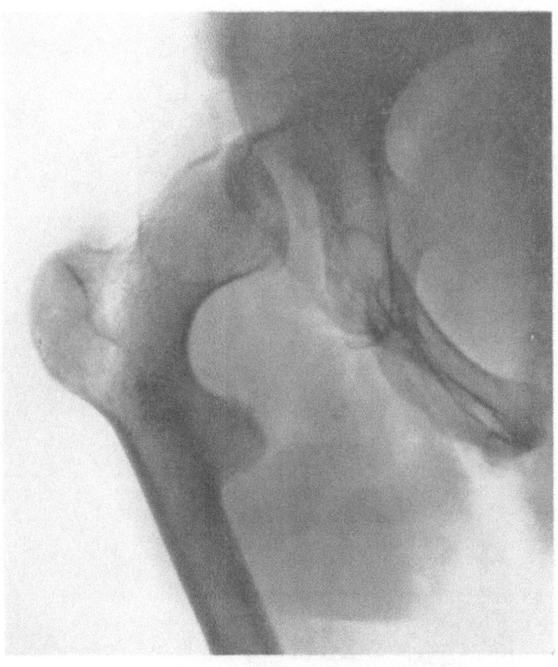

a

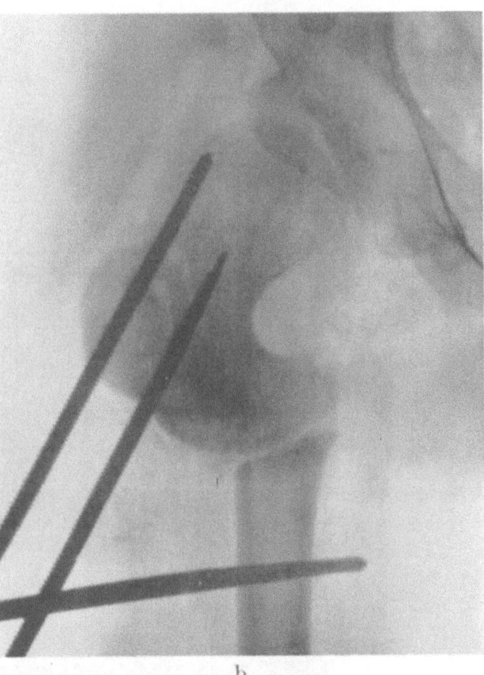

b

Abb. 34a u. b. Fall 2. Die als Folge des schweren Torsionsspasmus mit Beuge- und Adduktionskontraktur der unteren Extremität entstandene erhebliche und längst fixierte Fehlhaltung des rechten Hüftgelenkes. a *vor* und b *nach* der blutigen Stellungskorrektur des rechten Oberschenkelknochens mit Hilfe einer subtrochanteren Osteotomie (Prof. HACKENBROCH).

krämpfen mit einem Beugekrampf, der Fuß mit einem Supinationskrampf beteiligen. Das im Hüftgelenk gebeugte und nach innen adduzierte Bein kann nicht auf den Boden gesetzt werden. Indem es in der genannten Stellung förmlich vorangetragen wird, kann sich der Patient nur auf dem gesunden Bein hüpfend fortbewegen. Die rechtsseitigen Extremitäten sind zu keiner normalen willkürlichen Funktion fähig, sie sind selbst nicht zu den geringsten zweckvollen Bewegungen zu gebrauchen. Die rechte Hand kann nicht greifen, sie kann keinen Gegenstand halten; das rechte Bein kann weder als Standbein, noch zum Gehen benutzt werden. — *Psychisch* beherrscht eine nicht unbegründete Hoffnungslosigkeit das Bild. Der intelligente und willensstarke junge Mann hat es zum Abschluß einer kaufmännischen Lehre gebracht. Er scheut sich aber vor der Öffentlichkeit, da er bisher überall wegen der grotesken Erscheinungen seiner Bewegungsstörung Aufsehen erregt hat. Zu einer regelmäßigen Berufsausübung ist es deshalb nicht gekommen, mit Ausnahme einer Aushilfetätigkeit in der Kanzlei eines Krüppelheimes (s. Abb. 33).

*EEG.* Wegen starker Überlagerung von Muskelpotentialen nicht zu beurteilen.

*Operation.* Kombinierte Pyramido-Extrapyramidotomie des Verfassers in einer Höhe zwischen dem 1. und 2. Cervicalsegment. Nach beendeter Operation wird prophylaktisch eine suprapubische Harnfistel angelegt.

*Verlauf nach der Operation.* Am Abend des Operationstages ansprechbar, Temperatur 39,5°. Die Temperatursteigerung fällt nach Injektion einer „lytischen Mischung" (1 $cm^3$ Megaphen, 1 $cm^3$ Atosil, 1 $cm^3$ Dolantin) innerhalb von 2—3 Std auf 37,5° ab. Im übrigen glatter Heilungsverlauf. — Unmittelbar nach der Operation völlige schlaffe Lähmung der rechtsseitigen Gliedmaßen bis auf die arthrogene Beugefixation des rechten Hüftgelenkes. Die Hyperkinesen sind vollständig verschwunden. Eine halbautomatische Blasenspülung kann vom Patienten selbständig stundenweise betätigt werden. Am Ende der ersten Woche kann nach längerem Abklemmen des suprapubischen Blasenkatheters auf natürlichem Wege die Blase entleert werden. Der Katheter wird entfernt. — In der zweiten Woche wird mit Massagen und passiven Bewegungsübungen der rechten Körperseite eingesetzt,

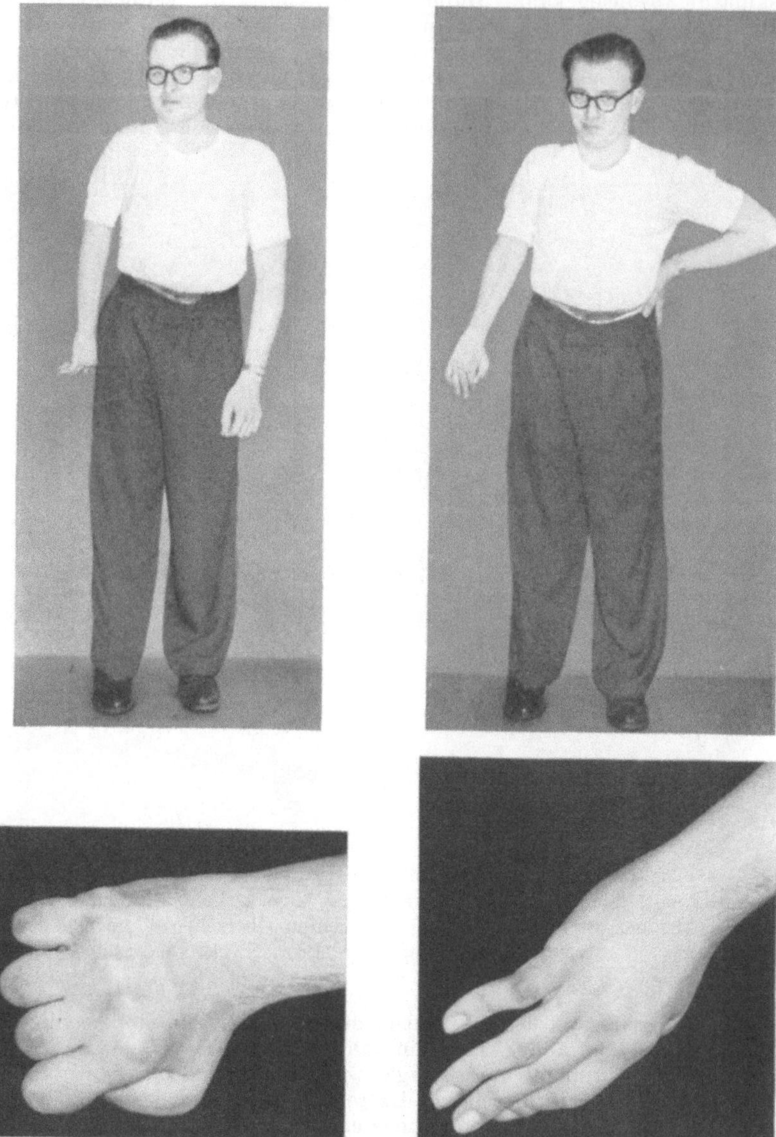

Abb. 35. Fall 2. Zustand $1^1/_2$ Jahre *nach* einer cervicalen kombinierten Pyramido-Extrapyramidotomie und subtrochanteren Osteotomie mit Stellungskorrektur des rechten Oberschenkelknochens. Die Hyperkinesen sind beseitigt. Feinere und isolierte Bewegungen an den distalen Gliedmaßenabschnitten sind nicht möglich. (Die angeborene Hemiatrophie der rechten Körperseite ist nun deutlicher erkennbar.)

wobei sich zeigt, daß trotz der nun vorhandenen Atonie der Muskulatur die arthrogene Hüftgelenksversteifung nicht zu überwinden ist. Gegen Ende der 2. und mit Beginn der 3. Woche beginnt der Tonus der Muskulatur zurückzukehren, zuerst im rechten Bein, dann auch im rechten Arm. In der 4. Woche besteht eine Halbseitenspastik rechts, die zu Streckstellungen der Gelenke neigt. Die arthrogene Hüftgelenkskontraktur rechts macht eine zusätzliche orthopädische Versorgung notwendig.

*Orthopädische Nachbehandlung* (6 Wochen nach dem neurochirurgischen Eingriff) in der orthopädischen Klinik der Universität Köln (Prof. M. Hackenbroch): „Die ungewöhnlich starke Fehlstellung des rechten Hüftgelenkes ist aus dem Röntgenbild vor Durchführung der Plastik zu ersehen

(Abb. 34a). Es zeigt, daß das rechte Hüftbein insgesamt hypoplastisch ist. Die rechte Hüftpfanne ist mangelhaft ausgebildet, flach und steilstehend. Der rechte Oberschenkelknochen zeigt außer der extremen Flexions-Adduktionskontraktur einen verminderten Schenkelhalsschaftwinkel. Der rechte Femurkopf findet sich in einer Luxationsstellung und hat nur geringen Kontakt mit der Pfanne. — Klinisch zeigt außerdem das rechte Kniegelenk eine Beugekontraktur. Nachdem durch eine zunächst versuchte *Extensionsbehandlung* keine wesentliche Beeinflussung der tendinösen und artikulären Schrumpfungskontrakturen möglich war, wurde eine ***subtrochantere Osteotomie mit Stellungskorrektur des rechten Oberschenkelknochens*** durchgeführt. Um einer Abdrehung von Schenkelhals und Trochantermassiv durch spastischen Muskelzug entgegenzuwirken, wurden in den Schenkelhals 2 SCHANZsche Schrauben eingeführt. Die durch diesen Eingriff gewonnene Situation zeigt das Röntgenbild unmittelbar nach der Operation (Abb. 34b). Es gelang, mit dieser Gelenkkorrektur die Coxa-vara-Stellung und die Flexions-Adduktionskontraktur zu beseitigen. Postoperativ erfolgte eine längere Fixation in einem Beckenbeingipsverband. Trotz der Gipsfixation und der Schraubenfixierung zeigte sich später eine gewisse Neigung zur Antekurvation, die aber zu keinen weiteren Maßnahmen Veranlassung gab, da eine Stützwirkung gegeben schien. Die knöcherne Konsolidation war gegenüber sonstigen subtrochanteren Osteotomien um etwa die Hälfte der Zeit verlängert. Die artikuläre Beugekontraktur des Kniegelenkes konnte durch Etappengipsredressement völlig beseitigt werden. — Nach Abschluß der Gipsbehandlung zeigte sich, daß infolge einer mangelhaften Muskelführung von Knie- und Fußgelenk eine Apparateversorgung nötig war, wobei zur Verhütung einer Veränderung in der erreichten Stellung des Hüftgelenkes die vorübergehende Anbringung eines Beckenkorbes ratsam schien. — Die Situation des rechten Armes wurde durch die vorläufige Anbringung einer Ledermanschette mit Steifstellung des Ellenbogengelenkes gebessert. — Später soll hier, bei unverändert bleibenden muskulären Ausfallserscheinungen die Frage einer Athrodese erwogen werden. Der Patient kann, da noch eine aktive Beweglichkeit im rechten Schultergelenk besteht, durch die Ledermanschette die rechte Hand beim Greifen als Gegenhalt und als Klemme benutzen.

*Nachuntersuchungsbefund $1^1/_2$ Jahre p. op.* Persistierende Hyperkinese im rechten Facialisgebiet. Keine Hyperkinese der rechtsseitigen Gliedmaßen und der rechtsseitigen Rumpfmuskulatur, auch nicht im rechten Schultergürtel. Darüber hinaus fehlen Torsionsbewegungen der Wirbelsäule, welche gerade und aufrecht gehalten wird. Es besteht eine spastische Hemiparese der rechten Körperseite. Durch die oben geschilderten zusätzlichen orthopädischen Maßnahmen konnte ein annähernd normaler, d. h. spastisch-circumducierender Gang eines Hemiplegikers erzielt werden. Die Beinverkürzung wurde durch einen orthopädischen Schuh ausgeglichen. Die Gebrauchsfähigkeit des rechten Armes ist soweit gebessert, daß er zum einfachen Gegenhalten benutzt werden kann. Isolierte Fingerbewegungen sind nicht möglich. Bemerkenswert ist, daß im Gegensatz zur spastischen Tonuserhöhung der rechtsseitigen Gliedmaßenmuskulatur die Finger noch eine vorwiegend schlaffe Lähmung zeigen. — Die Sensibilität zeigt eine deutliche Herabsetzung der Schmerz- und Temperaturempfindung auf der kontralateralen linken Körperseite von $C_2$ nach distal (BROWN-SÉQUARD). Die Berührungsempfindung und Tiefensensibilität ist auf beiden Seiten erhalten, wenn eine leichte segmentäre Herabsetzung für alle Empfindungsqualitäten in $C_2$ rechts nicht zu berücksichtigen wäre. *Psychisch* ist der Patient deutlich aufgelebt. Er ist glücklich, daß er das Leben in der Öffentlichkeit nicht mehr zu scheuen braucht. Dadurch ist er kontaktfähiger und selbstbewußter geworden. Er kann sich nun im Leben selbst weiterhelfen, er ist im kaufmännischen Beruf tätig. Durch fleißiges Training im Schreibmaschineschreiben mit der gesunden Hand hat er es bis zu 150 Anschlägen je Minute gebracht und hofft, eine noch bessere Fertigkeit darin zu erlangen (Abb. 35).

Dieser Fall mag als ein gutes Beispiel dafür gelten, was durch eine zweckgerichtete Zusammenarbeit von Neurochirurgie und Orthopädie selbst in hoffnungslos erscheinenden Syndromen zu erreichen ist.

**Fall 3.** Helga R., 12 Jahre. — *Schwere einseitige Torsionsdystonie rechts, mit athetotischen Hyperkinesen* an den Gliedmaßenenden.

Familienanamnese o. B. — Eigene Anamnese: Normale Geburt und normale frühkindliche Entwicklung. Im 4. Lebensjahr durch Unvorsichtigkeit beim Spiel linksseitige offene Hirnverletzung. Ein älterer Junge legte „zum Spaß“ mit einer Schrotflinte auf das Kind an. Die Flinte war geladen und die Schrotladung drang dem Mädchen durch das linke Stirnbein in die Schädelhöhle ein. Das Mädchen war sofort bewußtlos und rechtsseitig gelähmt. Nach 4 Tagen sei es aufgewacht, eine operative Wundversorgung sei weder sofort noch später erfolgt. In der Folgezeit seien die Gliedmaßen rechts im Wachstum etwas zurückgeblieben und es hätten sich eigenartige vertrackte Bewegungen mit Verdrehungen der rechten Körperseite eingestellt, welche später eher noch zugenommen hätten. — Mit 7 Jahren Schulbeginn, jedoch schlecht mitgekommen. Einmal repetiert und dann trotz unterdurchschnittlicher Leistungen immer wieder aus Rücksicht versetzt worden. Beim Spielen nicht auffällig, verhalte sich wie andere Kinder. Menarche: vor $^1/_2$ Jahr (12. Lebensjahr). Menses: regelmäßig alle 4 Wochen. Keine cerebralen Krampfanfälle.

*Aus dem Befund.* 12jähriges, normal entwickeltes Mädchen ohne krankhaften Befund an Haut, Schleimhäuten und inneren Organen.

*Lokal.* Über dem linken äußeren oberen Orbitalrand etwa einmarkstückgroße, pulsierende Knochenlücke mit reizloser Narbendecke.

*Neurologisch.* Die linke Körperseite ist ohne krankhaften Befund. Die rechte Körperseite weist eine durchgehende gleichmäßige Hypotrophie mit einer Verkürzung der Gliedmaßen von 3—4 cm auf. Geringe Halbseitenparese rechts mit brachiofacialer Betonung. Soweit die Hyperkinesen eine Untersuchung zulassen, sind eine Hyperreflexie und positive Pyramidenzeichen rechts festzustellen.

*Die Hyperkinesen.* Diese sind nach Lokalisation und Intensität von unterschiedlichem Charakter. Am erheblichsten ist die rechte obere Extremität betroffen, dann die rechte Gesichtsseite und am wenigsten das rechte Bein. In der rechten Gesichtshälfte kommt es, insbesondere unter affektbetonten Situationen, zu einseitigen grimassenhaften Verziehungen, unregelmäßigem Lidaugenschluß, halbseitigem grimassierendem Lächeln. An der oberen Extremität treten bei geringsten Anlässen torquierende, ziehend-drehende Bewegungen auf, welche durch plötzliche Schleuderbewegungen zeitweise unterbrochen werden. Während der unwillkürliche torquierende Bewegungsablauf an den proximalen Extremitätenmuskeln langsam und wurmförmig vor sich geht, kommt es distal zu blitzartigen vertrackten Stellungsveränderungen, vor allem der Finger, welche dem choreoathetotischen Bewegungssyndrom am nächsten stehen. Isolierte Fingerbewegungen sind nicht möglich, im Gegenteil, je ernsthafter der Versuch zu willkürlichen Einzelbewegungen gemacht wird, um so groteskere unwillkürliche Bewegungsbilder mit übermäßigen Beuge- und Streckstellungen sind die Folge. Die Torsionen erfolgen eigentümlicherweise aus Schulter und Oberarm, die Rumpf- und Wirbelsäulenmuskulatur bleibt praktisch unbeteiligt. Im rechten Bein kommt es zu häufigem unregelmäßigen Tonuswechsel, aber zu keinen eigentlichen Hyperkinesen, von vereinzelten arhythmischen muskulären Fasciculationen abgesehen. Es herrscht hier ein pyramidaler Hypertonus mit Neigung zu Streckkontraktur (Spitzfußbildung) vor (Abb. 36).

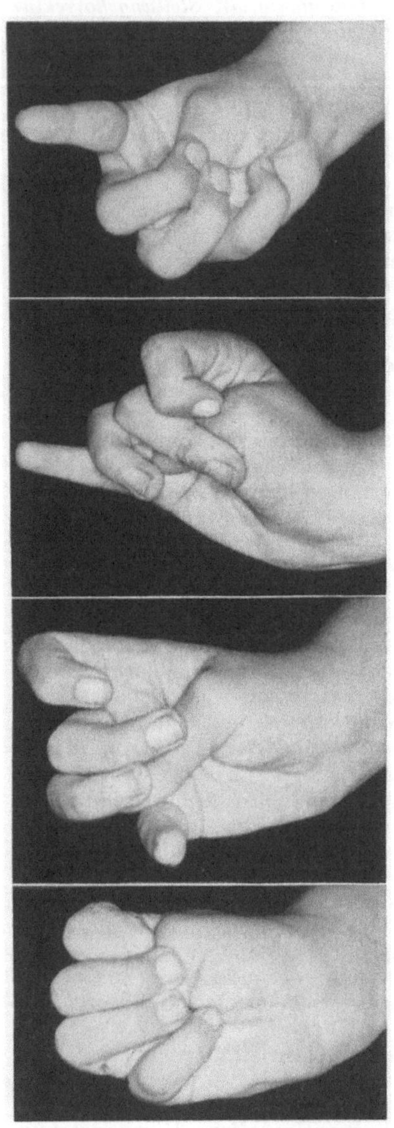

Abb. 36. Fall 3. 12jähriges Mädchen mit einer halbseitigen Torsionsdystonie rechts und athetotischen Hyperkinesen an den Gliedmaßenenden. Zustand *vor* der Operation.

*Psychisch* besteht eine deutliche Herabsetzung der geistigen Hirnleistung. Vorzeitige Ermüdung beim Lesen (übrigens fehlen aphasische Symptome!). Die Auffassung ist verlangsamt. Die Schulleistungen liegen weit unter dem Durchschnitt.

*EEG.* Allgemeinverändertes Hirnstrombild mit Betonung über linksseitig vorderen Punkten, kein $\delta$-Wellenherd, keine Krampfstrompotentiale.

*Operation.* Kombinierte Pyramido-Extrapyramidotomie des Verfassers in Höhe des 1. Cervicalsegmentes rechts (Laminektomie $C_1$—$C_2$), welche wegen der geringeren Bewegungsstörung weniger radikal ausgeführt wird.

*Verlauf nach der Operation.* Ungestörte Wundheilung. Unmittelbar nach der Operation bestand eine schlaffe rechtsseitige Hemiplegie. Am Abend des Operationstages Fieberanstieg auf 39,8$^0$, in der darauffolgenden Nacht Absinken auf 37,5$^0$. Vollständiges Sistieren der Hyperkinesen, ausgenommen im Facialisgebiet rechts. Ungestörte Willkürmotorik auf der Gegenseite, aber Thermanaesthesie und Analgesie ab $C_2$—$C_3$ links. Blasen- und Mastdarmfunktion waren zunächst gestört. — Nach 1 Woche Einsetzen einer fortschreitenden Tonuserhöhung, zuerst der Muskulatur des rechten Beines und 3—4 Tage später auch des rechten Armes. Unter Massagen und heilgymnastischen Übungen rasche Wiederkehr einer gewissen motorischen Funktion, so daß das Mädchen in der 2. Woche nach der Operation erstmalig aufstehen kann. Die ersten Gehversuche werden mit Unterstützung durch eine Hilfsperson ausgeführt. — Anfangs mußte die Harnblase durch Katheterisieren entleert werden. Vom 6. Tage an spontane Urinentleerung (Restharn 33 cm$^3$). Einige Tage später kein Restharn mehr. Mit Glycerineinläufen regelmäßige Stuhlentleerung. — Ende der 2. Woche p. op. kann die Patientin selbständig laufen. Mit dem rechten Arm sind vorerst nur Massenbewegungen möglich. Die Hyperkinesen sind vollständig beseitigt.

*Nachuntersuchung $1^1/_2$ Jahre nach der Operation.* Persistenz der geringen Hyperkinese im rechten Facialisgebiet. Die Hyperkinesen der rechten Körperseite sind vollständig beseitigt. Es besteht eine nicht sehr erhebliche spastische Hemiparese rechts, welche beim Gehen kaum auffällt. Der rechte Arm kann im Schulter- und Ellenbogengelenk mit herabgesetzter Kraft fast normal ausgiebig bewegt werden. Im rechten Handgelenk zeigt sich die Neigung zu einer Beugekontraktur, die zunächst passiv noch gut, aber aktiv schon nicht mehr zur Streckstellung überwunden werden kann. Ebenso ist eine beginnende Beugekontraktur der Finger festzustellen. Der Faustschluß ist kräftig und reicht zum Greifen und Festhalten von Gegenständen. Dagegen ist ein willkürliches Öffnen der geschlossenen Faust sehr erschwert, es geschieht unter Zuhilfenahme der gesunden linken Hand. Isolierte Fingerbewegungen sind rechts nicht möglich. Das rechte Bein ist in der Hüfte und im Kniegelenk nahezu uneingeschränkt zu bewegen, wenn auch mit verminderter Kraft. Am rechten Fußgelenk macht sich eine leichte Spitzfußstellung bemerkbar. Die willkürliche Dorsalflexion des Fußes gelingt gerade noch bis zu einem rechten Winkel, die Plantarflexion ist dagegen sehr kräftig und normal ausgiebig. Isolierte Zehenbewegungen sind nicht möglich. Hinsichtlich der Sensibilität findet sich in diesem Falle erst von $D_1$—$D_2$ an abwärts auf der Gegenseite (links) eine Hemihypalgesie und Thermhypaesthesie. Darüber hinaus ist die

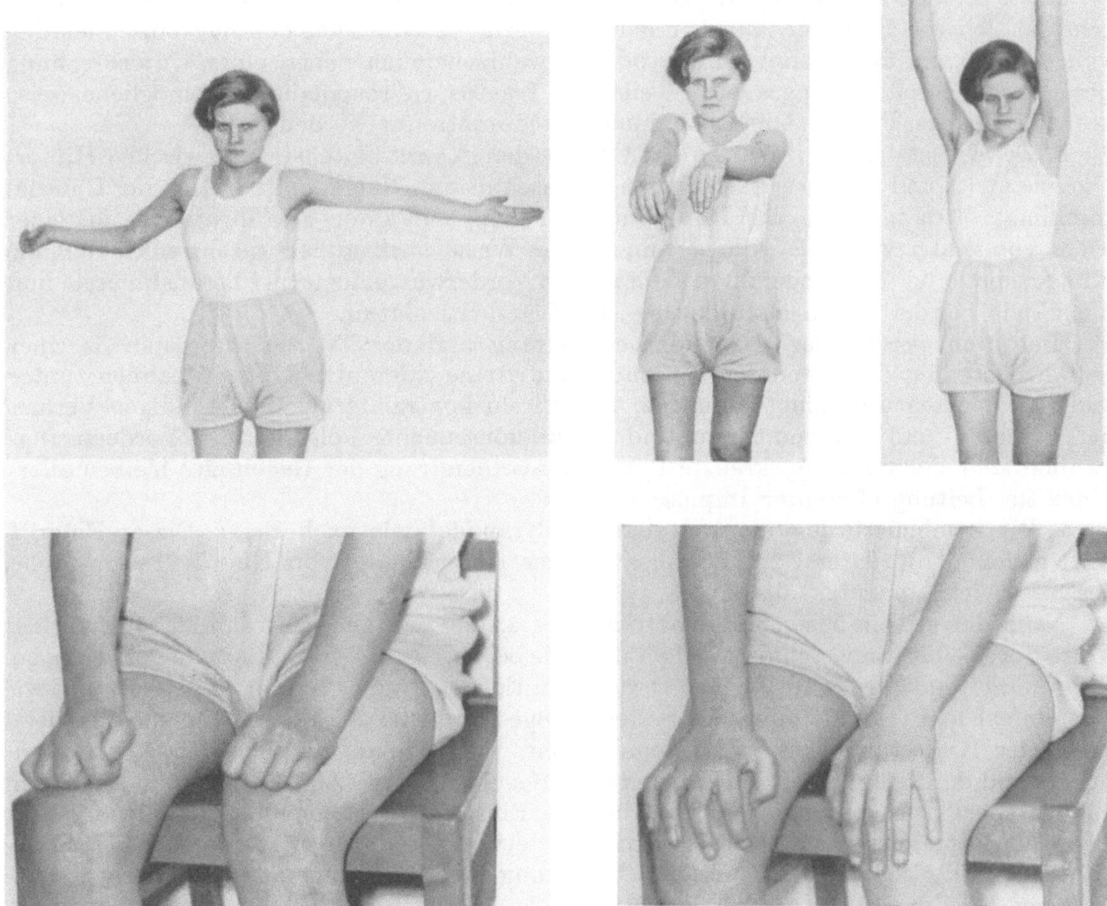

Abb. 37. Fall 3. Zustand $1^1/_2$ Jahre *nach* einer cervicalen kombinierten Pyramido-Extrapyramidotomie rechts. Die Hyperkinese ist beseitigt; mit den distalen Extremitätenabschnitten sind nur Massenbewegungen möglich.

Oberflächen- und Tiefensensibilität beiderseits nicht gestört. — *Psychisch* ist eine Änderung in der geistigen Leistungsschwäche, wie zu erwarten, nicht eingetreten. Das Kind hat die Schule nicht mehr besucht. Der Versuch einer Schulausbildung und Berufsvorbereitung in einer entsprechenden Anstalt wird ins Auge gefaßt (Abb. 37).

## Die Technik der cervicalen Pyramidotomien.

Die Durchschneidung des Pyramidenseitenstranges wird ebenfalls gleichseitig zur Lokalisation der Hyperkinese vorgenommen, gewöhnlich in Höhe des 2. oder 3. Cervicalsegmentes. Wegen der nachfolgenden Hemiparese erlaubt sich der Eingriff in der Regel nur bei einseitigen Bewegungsstörungen.

**1. Die laterale Pyramidotomie nach Putnam.** Nach der routinemäßigen Laminektomie des 2. und 3. Halswirbels wird die Dura in Längsrichtung eröffnet. Durch Fassen der 2. oder 3. Hinterwurzel wird das Mark unter leichtem Zug an der Wurzel fixiert und das auf 4 mm Klingenlänge eingestellte Chordotom wird nun unmittelbar lateral von der Eintrittsstelle der Hinterwurzel ins Mark eingestochen und bis zur gewünschten Tiefe von 4 mm eingeführt, wobei der Winkel zwischen Chordotomschaft und der Senkrechten etwa $10^0$ betragen soll. Anschließend wird die Klinge nach außen geschwenkt, bis die Klingenspitze am Lig. denticulatum herauskommt (s. Abb. 28 und 40).

An absteigenden Bahnen ist hiermit meist nur der Pyramidenseitenstrang unterbrochen worden.

**2. Die laterale Pyramidotomie nach Oliver.** a) Die erste Modifikation Olivers unterscheidet sich von Putnams Vorgehen lediglich darin, daß die Tiefe der Markeinschneidung von 4 auf 5 mm ausgedehnt wird, wodurch wahrscheinlich neben einer Unterbrechung des Pyramidenseitenstranges auch Teile des Tractus rubrospinalis und möglicherweise sogar Teile des Tractus spinothalamicus mit durchtrennt werden.

b) Bei der letzten Modifikation hat Oliver den ganzen Seitenstrang zwischen Hinterwurzeleintritt und Vorderwurzelaustritt durchschnitten. Nach dem Einstich der Chordotomklinge etwa in Höhe des Hinterwurzeleintritts und ihrer Einführung bis zu einer Tiefe von 5 mm wird die Klinge nun in der Weise nach außen geschwenkt, daß die Klingenspitze in der ungefähren Höhe des Vorderwurzelaustritts herauskommt und nicht, wie bei der ersten Modifikation, am Lig. denticulatum.

Hierdurch werden der Pyramidenseitenstrang und der Tractus rubrospinalis einer Seite vollständig durchtrennt, aber auch eine Reihe afferenter Leitungsbahnen, unter anderen der Tractus spinothalamicus, so daß ein kontralateraler vollständiger Verlust der Schmerz- und Temperaturempfindung die konsequente Folge ist. Die Vorderstrangbahnen und der noch ungekreuzte Pyramidenvorderstrang der Gegenseite bleiben allerdings zur Leitung efferenter Impulse erhalten.

**3. Die kombinierte laterale und ventrale Pyramidotomie nach Ebin.** Dieser Eingriff wird gleichfalls ipsilateral zur Lokalisation der Hyperkinese, von Ebin selbst in Höhe des 5. Cervicalsegmentes, ausgeführt.

Nach der gewöhnlichen Laminektomie des 4. und 5. Halswirbels und Eröffnung der Dura durch einen Längsschnitt wird ähnlich wie bei Putnams Pyramidotomie vorgegangen. Die Chordotomklinge wird für eine etwa 8 mm tief reichende Incision eingestellt und wie zur einfachen Pyramidotomie des Seitenstranges unmittelbar lateral von der Eintrittsstelle der Hinterwurzel ins Mark eingestochen. Der Winkel zwischen dem Chordotomschaft und der Senkrechten soll dabei etwas offener sein, etwa $20^0$ anstatt $10^0$. Nach dem bis zu einer Tiefe von etwa 8 mm reichenden Einstich in der genannten Richtung wird der Chordotomschaft nach vorn geschwenkt, etwa bis zur Ansatzstelle des Lig. denticulatum, und gleichzeitig mit dieser Schwenkung wird die Klinge aus dem Mark herausgezogen (s. Abb. 29).

Mit diesem Vorgehen kommt es zu einer Teilschädigung des gegenseitigen, noch ungekreuzten Pyramidenvorderstranges und zu einer praktisch kompletten Durchtrennung des gleichseitigen gekreuzten Pyramidenseitenstranges.

**4. Die kombinierte Pyramido-Extrapyramidotomie des Verfassers.** Auch diese Operation wird auf der Seite der Hyperkinese, am vorteilhaftesten in Höhe des 1. oder 2. Cervicalsegmentes, ausgeführt.

Laminektomie des 1. und 2. Halswirbels. Auf *der* Seite, auf welcher die Markeinschneidung erfolgen soll, werden die Wirbelbögen möglichst weit nach lateral reseziert, um sich später die Darstellung der Seitenfläche des Markes zu erleichtern. Die Dura wird aus dem gleichen Grunde nicht median, sondern paramedian — auf der Seite der Markincision — der Länge nach eröffnet und seitlich leicht eingekerbt. Die mit Haltefäden versehene Dura wird mit Pean-Klemmen belastet und dadurch angespannt. Vor dem Einstich wird die Klingenlänge des Traktotoms auf 9 mm eingestellt, was durch einen auf dem Traktotomschaft beweglichen Schieber, welcher durch die mit Raster versehene Millimetermarkierung des Schaftes arretiert wird, leicht zu bewerkstelligen ist (s. Abb. 40). Die Klinge des so eingestellten Traktotoms wird nun, unter leichter Fixierung des Markes an der 1. oder 2. Hinterwurzel, an einer Stelle ins Mark eingestochen, welche unmittelbar lateral vom Eintritt der Hinterwurzel, wenige Millimeter oberhalb der 2. oder unterhalb der 1. Hinterwurzel, gelegen ist. Die Klinge des Traktotoms wird dann behutsam in transversaler Richtung bis zum gegenseitigen Vorderstrang eingeführt, wobei die Klingenspitze auf einen Punkt zielt, welcher etwa in der Mitte zwischen Fissura mediana anterior und Vorderwurzelaustritt der Gegenseite gelegen ist (Pfeil 1 der Abb. 38). Wenn eine

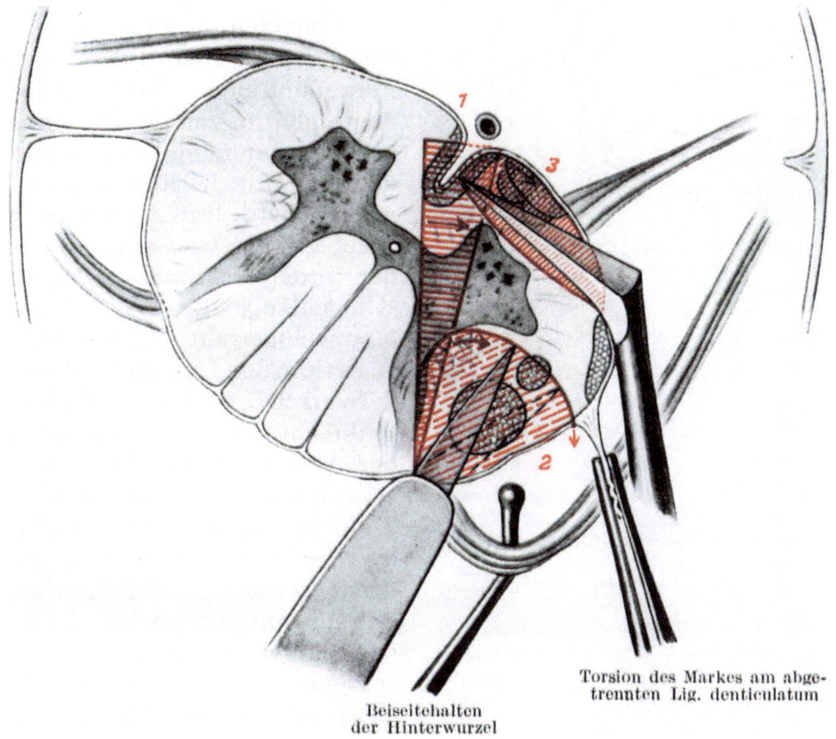


Abb. 38. Die cervicale kombinierte Pyramido-Extrapyramidotomie (halbschematisch). *1* Durchschneidung des kontralateralen Pyramidenvorderstranges; *2* Durchschneidung des homolateralen Pyramidenseitenstranges; *3* homolaterale Extrapyramidotomie (s. Text).

Tiefe von etwa 8—9 mm erreicht ist, wird der Schaft um wenige Grad hin und her geschwenkt. Die Einstichstelle ins Mark, am Hinterwurzeleintritt, bildet dabei den Drehpunkt für die leichten Schwenkungen. Hier ist besonders darauf zu achten, daß auf der Gegenseite die Pia mater nicht perforiert wird, wegen der Gefahr einer Verletzung der A. spinalis anterior, deren vollständiger Ausfall ja ein Zugrundegehen der infraläsionellen Vorderhornsäulen mit nachfolgender schlaffer Tetraplegie bedeuten würde. — Im allgemeinen wird man bei der 9 mm-Einstellung die Gegenseite nicht ganz erreichen. Sollte man sie dennoch erreichen, so ist bei behutsamer Klingenführung die Pia mater der Gegenseite am deutlich erhöhten Gewebswiderstand zu erkennen. Man wird in diesem Falle die Klinge um 1 mm zurückziehen, ohne die Pia und noch weniger die außerhalb und weiter medial gelegene A. spinalis anterior zu verletzen. — Nachdem die leichten Schwenkungen mit dem Traktotom ausgeführt worden sind, wird es herausgezogen. Der Schieber wird nun auf eine Klingenlänge von 5 mm eingestellt. Dann wird an der gleichen Stelle des Markes die Traktotomklinge nochmals zur lateralen Pyramidotomie, in gleicher Richtung wie vorher, aber nur bis zur 5 mm-Tiefenmarkierung, eingestochen. Anschließend wird die Klinge scharf nach außen geschwenkt, bis die Klingenspitze in

Höhe der Leiste des Lig. denticulatum an der Seitenfläche das Mark wieder verläßt (Pfeil 2 der Abb. 38). Auf diese Weise ist die dorsale Hälfte des Seitenstranges, d. h. der Pyramidenseitenstrang, total und der Tractus rubrospinalis subtotal, unterbrochen worden. Das Mark sollte während der Durchführung dieser beiden Schnitte in seiner Lage möglichst nicht verändert werden, um eine Verzerrung des Markquerschnittes mit Veränderung der Topographie der langen Rückenmarksbahnen zu vermeiden. — Die 3. Markincision entspricht ganz der Putnamschen Extrapyramidotomie. Hierzu wird das Lig. denticulatum von der Durainnenfläche abgetrennt, und, indem das Mark am Lig. denticulatum leicht um seine Längsachse gedreht wird, bringt man sich die seitliche Fläche des Markes und die Austrittsstelle der vorderen Wurzel zur Darstellung. Die Klingenlänge des Traktotoms bleibt auf 5 mm eingestellt. In der Mitte zwischen Insertion des Lig. denticulatum und Vorderwurzelaustritt wird die Klinge nahezu senkrecht ins Mark eingestochen (Pfeil 3 der Abb. 38) und in Richtung auf die Fissura mediana anterior eingeführt. Ist eine Tiefe von 5 mm erreicht, dann werden die *vor* der ventralen Klingenschneide gelegenen extrapyramidalmotorischen Bahnen durchtrennt, indem der Traktotomschaft nach hinten geschwenkt wird unter gleichzeitigem Herausziehen der Klinge. Bei entsprechend sorgfältiger Handhabung kann man hierbei den etwas derberen elastischen Widerstand der Pia mater von innen spüren und gewissermaßen als Führung für die Klinge benutzen (Abb. 39 und 40).

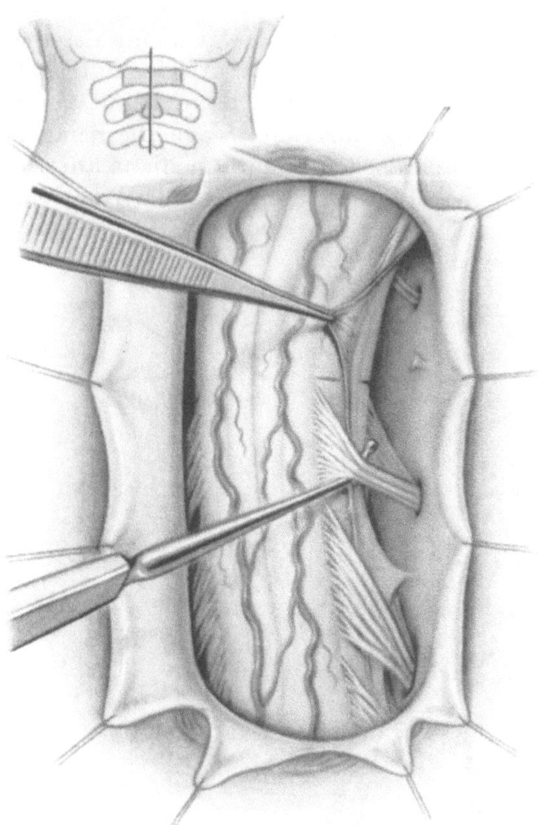

Abb. 39. Die cervicale kombinierte Pyramido-Extrapyramidotomie. (Operationsskizze mit eingezeichneten Markeinschnitten dorsal und ventral von der Leiste des Lig. denticulatum).

Bei Beachtung der erforderlichen Sorgfalt werden sich unangenehme Komplikationen vermeiden lassen. Es empfiehlt sich, nach Beendigung der Operation bei männlichen Patienten eine suprapubische Fistel anzulegen, welche über ein Zweiwegesystem mit einem Irrigator (der am Bett

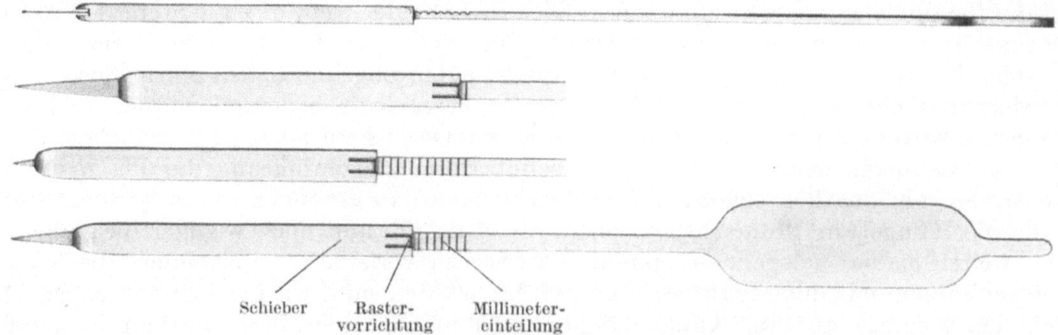


Abb. 40. Das für die cervicalen Markeinschneidungen verwendete Traktotom mit doppelschneidiger Klinge. Mit Hilfe eines Schiebers und einer Rastervorrichtung mit Millimetereinteilung ist die Klinge auf die gewünschte Länge einzustellen.

angebracht ist) und mit einem Urinsammelglas (das unter dem Bett steht) verbunden wird. Mit dieser Spülvorrichtung kann der Operierte schon am Tage nach der Operation selbständig stundenweise eine Blasenspülung vornehmen, wodurch bei Eintreten einer vorübergehenden Blasenlähmung die Gefahr einer aufsteigenden Harninfektion vermindert wird. Die Blasenlähmung klingt in der 2. bis 3. Woche p. op. ab.

Mit der kombinierten Hinterseiten-Vorderstrangdurchschneidung werden an absteigenden Bahnen homolateral der Pyramidenseitenstrang total, der Tractus rubrospinalis subtotal und die extrapyramidal-motorischen Bahnen (Tractus vestibulospinalis, reticulospinalis, tectospinalis) ebenfalls total unterbrochen. Auf der Gegenseite wird wahrscheinlich gerade eine partielle Schädigung des ungekreuzten Pyramidenvorderstranges erreicht.

## 3. Epikrise zu den cervicospinalen Eingriffen.

Alle Operationen am Halsmark werden homolateral zur Lokalisation der Hyperkinese ausgeführt, ohne Unterschied, ob sie an den pyramidalen oder extrapyramidalen Leitungswegen angreifen.

1. Außer bei der Extrapyramidotomie nach PUTNAM werden in irgendeiner Form die Pyramidenbahnen geschädigt, da sonst in den meisten Fällen kein Dauerresultat zu erzielen ist.

2. Nur die Extrapyramidotomie nach PUTNAM kann mit gutem Gewissen doppelseitig ausgeführt werden, da sie kein Defizit in der willkürlichen motorischen Funktion hinterläßt.

3. Je mehr efferente Bahnen einer Markhälfte aber durchtrennt werden, desto sicherere, günstigere und dauerhaftere Resultate lassen sich erreichen, wenn auch ein Ansteigen der permanenten, postoperativen, spastisch-paretischen Symptome damit parallel geht.

4. Aus diesem Grunde sind die *halbseitigen Syndrome* stets für die operative Behandlung zu bevorzugen, selbst wenn bzw. gerade wenn die Hyperkinese einen extremen Grad erreicht hat und sehr quälend ist.

Zur Behandlung der *Athétose double* ist der doppelseitigen Vorderstrangdurchschneidung (bilaterale Extrapyramidotomie nach PUTNAM) der Vorzug zu geben. Wenn mit diesem Eingriff auch keine Beseitigung der unwillkürlichen Bewegungen zu erreichen ist, so vermag sie doch in etwa der Hälfte der Fälle zu einer dauerhaften Besserung der Bewegungsstörung zu führen, ohne daß gleichzeitig eine Beeinträchtigung der Willkürmotorik erfolgt. Günstigere Resultate läßt die Extrapyramidotomie anscheinend im Kindes- und Jugendlichenalter erzielen. Ohne Wirkung blieb der Eingriff bei den pyramidalen paraspastischen Formen der LITTLEschen Krankheit, bei der Torsionsdystonie und beim PARKINSON-Tremor.

Zur Behandlung des PARKINSON-*Tremors* müssen die pyramidalen Leitungswege möglichst vollständig unterbrochen werden, weshalb sich für die Anwendung der cervicalen Operationsmethoden eigentlich nur der *Hemi*parkinsonismus eignet. Die Ergebnisse scheinen besser zu sein, wenn auch der Tractus rubrospinalis durchtrennt wird. Die totale Seitenstrangdurchschneidung nach OLIVER verspricht daher die sichersten und dauerhaftesten Resultate zu geben, wodurch allerdings auch das Ausmaß der postoperativen Hemiparese zunimmt. Bei leichteren Tremorformen kann allerdings schon die einfache laterale Pyramidotomie nach PUTNAMs Originalmethode ausreichen, welche wegen der guten Rückbildung der willkürlichen motorischen Funktion unter Umständen auch einmal doppelseitig ausgeführt werden kann. Die Symptome der Akinese und der Rigidität werden durch die lateralen Pyramidotomien praktisch nicht beeinflußt, weshalb der Schütteltremor das hervorstechende Merkmal der Erkrankung sein muß.

Zur Behandlung *extrem schwerer halbseitiger Hyperkinesen* (Hemichoreoathetosen, einseitige Torsionsdystonien) empfiehlt sich die radikale, aber mit großer Sicherheit erfolgreiche kombinierte Pyramido-Extrapyramidotomie des Verfassers. Die hiermit erreichte nahezu vollständige Unterbrechung *aller* Efferenzen einer Seite bietet die sicherste Garantie gegen die sonst sehr häufigen „Rezidive" gerade der schweren Bewegungsstörungen.

*Vorteile der cervicospinalen Methoden.* Die Anatomie des Halsmarkes und die Topographie der Bahnensysteme erlauben ein sehr exaktes chirurgisches Vorgehen, welches sich insbesondere durch eine große Treffsicherheit in der selektiven Ausschaltung bestimmter Bahnen — auch in der Hand verschiedener Operateure — auszeichnet. Die technische Durchführung der Eingriffe ist relativ einfach und die Operationsbelastung gering.

Schwere einseitige Bewegungsstörungen sind sicher und vollständig zu beseitigen. Bestimmte Formen von doppelseitigen Bewegungsstörungen (Athétose double) können durch eine in einer Sitzung ausführbare Operation (bilaterale Extrapyramidotomie) zwar nicht beseitigt, aber doch gebessert werden.

*Nachteile der cervicospinalen Methoden.* Nur die einseitigen Bewegungsstörungen können wirklich wirkungsvoll beeinflußt werden, da der Erfolg im wesentlichen auf Kosten pyramidaler Lähmungen erkauft wird.

Die *Mortalität* der cervicalen Eingriffe liegt nach der allgemeinen Erfahrung unter 10% (PUTNAM 0%, OLIVER 9%, EBIN 7,6%, TÖNNIS-SCHÜRMANN 6%).

*Anhangsweise* müssen gerade wegen ihres vollständigen Versagens einige Eingriffe genannt werden, zu deren Durchführung vermutlich zeitbedingte medizinische Auffassungen, um nicht zu sagen „Moderichtungen", Anlaß gegeben haben. — DELMAS-MARSALET und VAN BOGAERT (1934) versuchten, durch eine *chirurgische Zerstörung des Nucleus dentatus* die Erscheinungen eines postencephalitischen Parkinsonismus zu beeinflussen. Aber, obschon danach die Starre tatsächlich in einem gewissen Grade gelindert worden sein soll, ist der Tremor nach diesem Eingriff verschlimmert gewesen (was übrigens die tierexperimentellen Beobachtungen FULTONS und seiner Schule bestätigt — 1932). Unglücklicherweise ist aber das klinische Bild dieses Falles durch eine Thrombose der A. cerebellaris superior kompliziert worden und der postoperative Verlauf konnte nicht länger beobachtet werden, da der Patient 10 Tage nach der Operation starb.

Im Hinblick auf die bekannte Tatsache, daß Emotionen den PARKINSON-Tremor zumindest vorübergehend verstärken, ist die *präfrontale Lobotomie* versucht worden. Der Zustand solcher Patienten wurde jedoch durch diese Maßnahme nicht geändert, wenn auch von RAO und MOREA (1949) in einem Falle das augenblickliche Sistieren des Tremors und eine Verminderung der Starre mitgeteilt wurde. Daß die präfrontale Lobotomie zur Behandlung des Torticollis ergebnislos ausgeführt worden ist, wird in dem entsprechenden Abschnitt noch erwähnt werden (WOHLFAHRT und FORSOCK, GIRARD, BORDET und DÉVIC).

In der Hoffnung auf eine möglicherweise erfolgende Verbesserung der Hirndurchblutung versuchten GARDNER und WILLIAMS (1949) und RIESSNER (1951) durch eine *bilaterale cervicale Sympathektomie* einen günstigen Einfluß auf die Erscheinungen des Parkinsonismus auszuüben. Der praktische Wert dieser Eingriffe ist jedoch, wie nicht anders zu erwarten, gleich Null gewesen.

## IV. Der Torticollis spasticus.

Die Besprechung der operativen Behandlung des spastischen Schiefhalses soll in einem besonderen Abschnitt erfolgen, weil sich allein für dieses Krankheitsbild inzwischen eine Art Standardoperation herausgehoben hat. Das ist nicht schwer zu verstehen, wenn man bedenkt, daß die pathologische Tonusveränderung des Schiefhalses wie bei sonst keiner anderen striären Erkrankung auf eine eng umschriebene Muskelgruppe beschränkt bleibt. Hierdurch ist konsequenterweise die möglichst vollständige Unterbrechung der efferenten Erregungszuflüsse insofern erleichtert, als ja bereits eine segmentale periphere Denervierung zum Ziele führen muß. Deshalb haben sich die sehr frühen Versuche peripherer Nervendurchschneidungen und Nervenwurzelresektionen bei extrapyramidalen Hyperkinesen und Dystonien auch nur beim Torticollis bewähren können, während sie zur Behandlung anderer Bewegungs- und Tonusstörungen extrapyramidaler Herkunft versagt haben und deswegen bald wieder aufgegeben wurden.

Die Eingriffe an den cervicalen Nervenwurzeln haben beim Torticollis schnell an Bedeutung gewonnen, so daß schließlich die ganz alten Verfahren der Muskel- und Muskelsehnendurchtrennungen ganz verdrängt wurden und ihnen heute nur noch ein historisches Interesse entgegengebracht wird.

Die *Myotomie* der beim spastischen Schiefhals beteiligten Halsmuskeln wurde wohl zuerst von einem deutschen Militärchirurgen, ISAAC MINNIUS (1641), angewandt. Er versuchte, den Torticollis mit einer einfachen Durchtrennung des Kopfnickermuskels zu bessern. Gegen Ende des vorigen Jahrhunderts wurde dieser Gedanke erneut von KOCHER, MIKULICZ (1895) und DE QUERVAIN (1896) aufgegriffen. MIKULICZ empfahl die Excision der unteren $^2/_3$ des M. sternocleidomastoideus ohne den N. accessorius zu schädigen; DE QUERVAIN führte 2 Incisionen aus, mit der ersten durchtrennte er den M. sternocleido und mit der zweiten die Muskeln des suboccipitalen Dreiecks. — Auch die *Tenotomie* des M. sternocleido, welche von DUPUYTREN (1912) empfohlen wurde, wird heute kaum noch angewandt, es sei denn im Säuglingsalter. — Es ist erstaunlich, daß die ersten Schritte zu einer Denervation der am Krampf beteiligten Muskeln bereits vor einem Jahrhundert getan wurden. Die erste *Durchschneidung peripherer Nerven* beim Schiefhals wurde von BUJALSKI (1834) mitgeteilt, welcher die isolierte Resektion des N. accessorius am Hals angab. Anderen Quellenangaben zufolge soll ROMBERG im Jahre 1853 auf die Möglichkeit einer Durchschneidung der Äste des spinalen N. accessorius in einem Falle von Torticollis hingewiesen haben und sei DE MORGAN (1867) der erste gewesen, welcher diesen Nerven durchschnitten hat, um die Spasmen zu bessern. Im Jahre 1890 hat COLLIER den spinalen N. accessorius mit einem Silberdraht abgeklemmt. Aussichtsreicher wurden die Resultate durch das Vorgehen von KEEN (1891), welcher mit seiner neuen Methode die *extradurale Wurzeldurchschneidung* begründet hat. Er führte eine an der hinteren Mittellinie beginnende und 2 cm unterhalb des Ohrläppchens endende, etwa 7—8 cm lange, horizontale Incision aus, mit welcher die daruntergelegenen Muskeln und die hinteren Äste der ersten 3 Halsnervenwurzeln, an der Stelle ihres Austrittes aus den Wirbeln, auf der krampfenden Seite durchtrennt wurden. Mit diesem Verfahren haben die vorerwähnten Myotomien, Tenotomien und Neurotomien bereits nicht mehr konkurrieren können. Später wurde von FINNEY und HUGHSON (1925) KEENS Operation auch doppelseitig ausgeführt und mit einer beidseitigen Durchschneidung des N. accessorius am Hals kombiniert. Kurze Zeit darauf schloß COLEMAN (1927) noch die 4. hintere Cervicalwurzel in die Resektion ein, wodurch die Ergebnisse weiter verbessert worden seien.

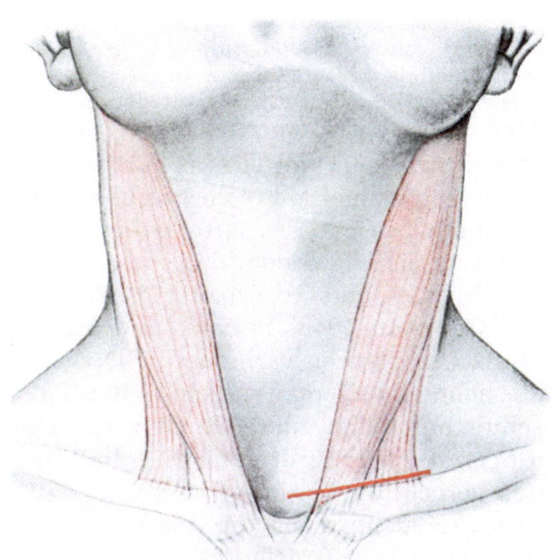

Abb. 41. Die Tenotomie des M. strenocleidomastoideus nach DUPUYTREN.

Die entscheidende Wendung in der chirurgischen Behandlung des Torticollis spasticus brachte aber das Jahr 1915, als TAYLOR die *intraspinale Durchschneidung der hinteren Wurzeln* der ersten 4 Halsnerven in Verbindung mit einer Durchtrennung des spinalen N. accessorius für den spastischen Schiefhals angab. TAYLOR war zu diesem Vorgehen durch die Erfolge mit der FOERSTERschen Operation (hintere Rhizotomie — 1908) angeregt worden, welcher ja als Grundgedanke eine quantitative Verminderung der peripheren afferenten Reize zur Besserung der Spasmen zugrunde lag. Der nächste sehr wesentliche Schritt in der chirurgischen Behandlung des spastischen Schiefhalses ist nach dem amerikanischen Schrifttum in CUSHINGs Fall getan worden, welcher von McKENZIE (1924) mitgeteilt wurde. Hier sind neben den sensiblen auch die *motorischen* Wurzeln des 1., 2. und 3. Cervicalsegmentes intradural durchschnitten und gleichzeitig der spinale N. accessorius durchtrennt worden.

In Wirklichkeit aber hat ohne Zweifel FOERSTER (1920) als erster die Durchschneidung der ersten 3—4 cervicalen Hinterwurzeln mit einer Durchschneidung auch der *motorischen* Wurzeln und der intraspinalen Fasern des N. accessorius kombiniert. Damit hat FOERSTER den Grundstein zu einer in ihren wesentlichen Teilen noch heute allgemein gültigen Standardtechnik in der chirurgischen Behandlung des spastischen Schiefhalses gelegt. DANDY (1930) hat zu FOERSTERs Operation zusätzlich den N. accessorius am Hals durchtrennt und, nach seiner letzten Mitteilung, hat er bei späteren Operationen die Hinterwurzeln bewußt geschont. Diese letzte Modifikation, die doppelseitige intradurale Durchschneidung der ersten 3 motorischen cervicalen Wurzeln und der intraduralen Accessoriuswurzeln mit einer später erfolgenden Durchtrennung des peripheren Astes vom N. accessorius am Eintritt in den Kopfnickermuskel, hat als die FOERSTER-DANDY*sche Operation* Eingang in die Neurochirurgie gefunden und darf auch heute noch als die wirksamste Behandlungsmethode des organischen spastischen Schiefhalses gelten. Die Ergebnisse in der chirurgischen Behandlung dieses Krankheitsbildes konnten bis jetzt durch kein anderes Verfahren überzeugend verbessert werden, obschon manche Versuche hierzu unternommen wurden.

In den 40er Jahren wurden vereinzelt auch beim spastischen Schiefhals *Operationen am Zentralnervensystem* versucht. So hat KLEMME (1940—1942) in seiner Serie von Cortectomien eine Besserung der Symptome beim Torticollis mitgeteilt, die aber, wie KLEMMES Angaben überhaupt, berechtigte Zweifel aufkommen lassen. DAVID und Mitarbeiter (1952) sahen in einem ihrer Fälle, in denen zum Torsionsspasmus des Armes ein spastischer Torticollis hinzukam, nach Entfernung der Area 4 und 6 den Schiefhals verschwinden, aber bereits nach $4^1/_2$ Monaten in vollem Umfang wiederkehren! MEYERS (1942) hat mit seiner subcorticalen Durchschneidung der pallidofugalen Verbindungen in einem Falle von Torticollis gleichfalls einen Mißerfolg buchen müssen. Die Versuche, im letzten Jahrzehnt auch mit der präfrontalen Lobotomie auf die Erscheinungen des spastischen Schiefhalses einzuwirken, müssen ebenfalls als ergebnislos angesehen werden (WOHLFAHRT und FORSOCK, GIRARD, BORDET und DÉVIC). Die Wirkungslosigkeit der in 3 Fällen bei diesem Krankheitsbild vom Verfasser versuchten cervicalen Extrapyramidotomie ist bereits im vorangehenden Abschnitt mitgeteilt worden.

Im Krankengut von TÖNNIS hat sich in 52 Fällen die Operation nach FOERSTER-DANDY in ihrer Originalmethode sehr gut bewährt. Die Zahl der Mitteilungen über gute und ausgezeichnete sowie dauerhafte Behandlungsergebnisse mit dieser Technik ist inzwischen so umfangreich geworden, daß nicht alle Autoren genannt werden können (OLIVECRONA 1931, PUTNAM und Mitarbeiter 1949, LAZORTHES und ANDUZE 1949, DAVID, HÉCAEN und TALAIRACH 1948, POPPEN und MARTINEZ-NIOCHET 1951 u. v. a.).

Einzelne Autoren variieren die Operation, indem sie die Resektion nach caudal durch Einbeziehung weiterer Wurzeln in den Fällen erweitern, in denen auch proximale Rumpfabschnitte beteiligt sind. So ist schon DOWMAN (1931) sehr dafür eingetreten, daß man den operativen Eingriff dem Einzelfall anpassen müsse, um den individuellen Besonderheiten gerecht zu werden. Das heißt, daß es gegebenenfalls erforderlich ist, den Eingriff soweit auszudehnen, bis die Ausschaltung der nervösen Innervation fast aller am Krampf beteiligten Muskeln gelungen ist. So sehr einleuchtend diese Empfehlungen scheinen, so wird man sich doch vor von vornherein allzu sehr ausgedehnten Wurzelresektionen scheuen, um der für den Patienten (und für den Operateur!) unangenehmen Situation zu entgehen, daß hernach der Kopf abgestützt werden muß, weil er selbständig nicht mehr aufrecht gehalten werden kann. Darüber hinaus haben der 4., 5. und 6. Cervicalnerv auch andere Muskeln mit wichtigen Funktionen zu versorgen, so daß sie besser erhalten bleiben (z. B. der N. phrenicus, welcher aus dem 4. Cervicalnerven hervorgeht und die Schlundmuskeln, welche den Schluckakt besorgen). In nicht ganz befriedigenden Ergebnissen nach der FOERSTER-DANDYschen Operation muß zunächst exakt analysiert werden, welche Muskelgruppen für das Weiterbestehen des Krampfes verantwortlich zu machen sind und welchem Segment sie innervatorisch angehören. Dann ist in einer zweiten Operationssitzung durch die selektive Ausschaltung der entsprechenden motorischen Wurzeln unter Umständen doch noch ein befriedigendes Resultat zu erreichen. In der Regel wird man aber, wie wir gesehen haben, in diesen Fällen mit einfacheren Maßnahmen zum Ziele kommen. Das ist durch eine von SCHALTENBRAND (1938) zur Denervierung der noch an einem Krampf beteiligten Muskeln mitgeteilte konservative Maßnahme zu erreichen: eine mehrmals anzuwendende systematische Infiltration der gesamten Halsmuskulatur, auch der tiefen Muskelgruppen (!) mit ausgiebigen Mengen einer 0,5%igen Novocainlösung (bis zu 100 $cm^3$ und mehr). Hierdurch wird nach SCHALTENBRAND eine „länger dauernde, lokalisierte, neurale Atrophie und Deafferenzierung“ der betroffenen Halsmuskeln erreicht. Später kann unter Umständen durch Zusatz von kleinen Dosen absoluten Alkohols eine Dauerschädigung der neuromuskulären Endapparate herbeigeführt werden, was sich uns aber bisher nicht als unbedingt notwendig erwiesen hat. In der Nachbehandlung hat sich uns dieses Vorgehen jedenfalls als vorteilhaft und aussichtsreich zur Beeinflussung von Reststörungen erwiesen.

*Die Technik der* FOERSTER-DANDY*schen Schiefhalsoperation.* Dieser Eingriff wird grundsätzlich doppelseitig ausgeführt. Von einem hinteren Mittelschnitt aus werden die Bögen des 1.—3. Halswirbels entfernt und ein kleines Stück der Hinterhauptsschuppe reseziert, gerade soviel, daß das Hinterhauptsloch erweitert ist. Die Dura wird längs

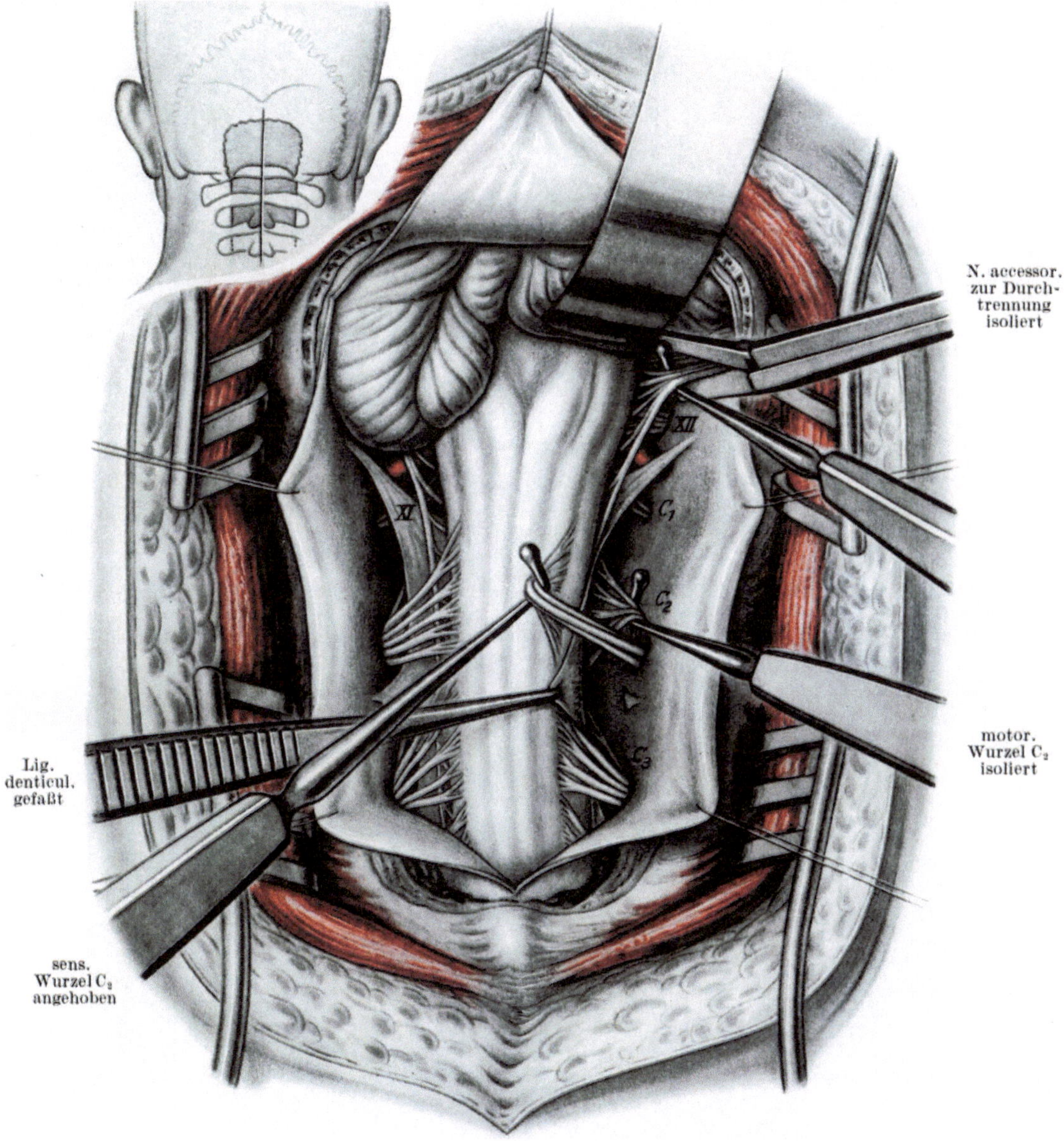


Abb. 42. Die FOERSTER-DANDYsche Schiefhalsoperation, die doppelseitige, intradurale Durchschneidung der drei ersten motorischen Wurzeln und der Wurzeln des N. accessorius (Operationsskizze).

eröffnet und kranial durch Y-förmige, seitliche Incisionen gespalten. Auf einem stumpfen Nervenhäkchen wird beiderseits die Wurzel des N. accessorius angehoben und nach Aufsetzen eines Silberclip durchtrennt. In der gleichen Weise werden nach Ablösen des Lig. denticulatum auf beiden Seiten nacheinander die 1.—3. vordere Wurzel auf dem Häkchen angehoben und zwischen 2 Clips durchtrennt. Die Dura wird durch eine fortlaufende Naht dicht geschlossen (s. Abb. 42). — Nach Beendigung der Operation wird ein SCHANZscher Watteverband angelegt und, wenn der Patient ins Bett gelegt worden ist, wird der Kopf zwischen zwei seitlich unter das Kissen geschobene Sandsäcke gelagert. — Etwa 1 Woche nach dem intraduralen Eingriff wird auf beiden Seiten der N. accessorius peripher durchschnitten und zwar an der Stelle seines Eintritts in den Kopfnickermuskel. Hierzu geht man von einem kleinen Schnitt entlang des Vorderrandes vom

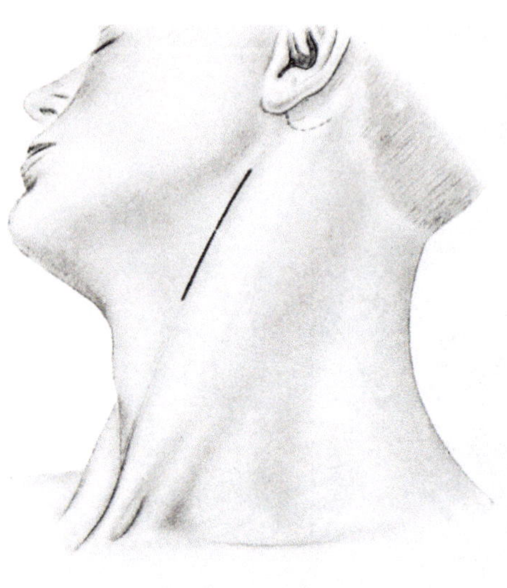

a

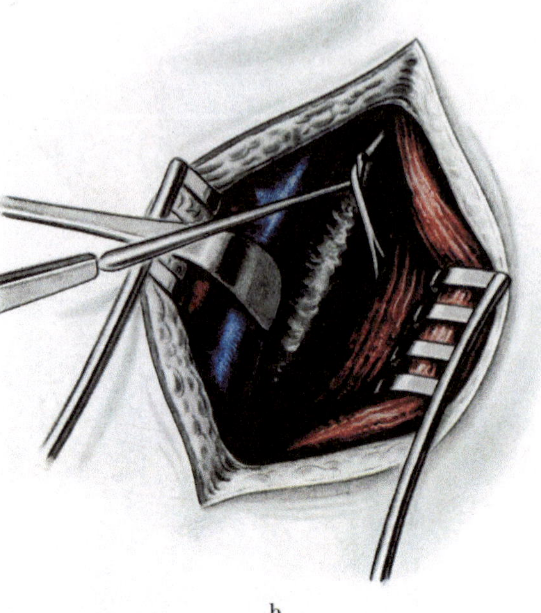

b

Abb. 43a u. b. Durchschneidung des den M. sternocleidomastoideus versorgenden Astes vom N. accessorius. a Schnittführung am Vorderrand des Kopfnickermuskels; b Operationsskizze, der Nerv, welcher lateral von den Halsgefäßen verläuft und an der Medialseite in den Muskel tritt, ist angehoben.

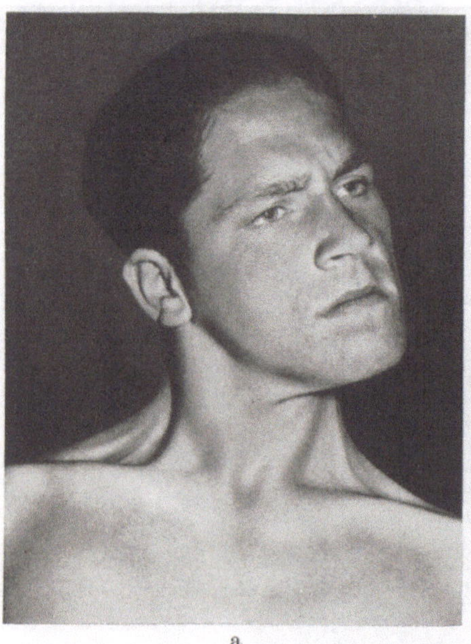

a

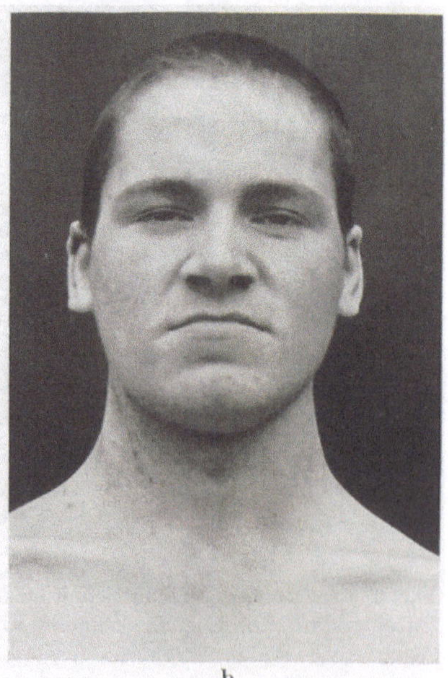

b

Abb. 44a u. b. Torticollis spasticus eines 17jährigen *vor* und *nach* der Foerster-Dandyschen Operation.

M. sternocleidomastoideus aus, hält den Muskel mit einem Haken nach lateral und sucht an der Medialseite des Muskels, zwischen oberem und mittlerem Drittel, den Nerven auf. Dieser wird dann nicht nur durchtrennt, sondern auch ein Stück reseziert, um eine Regeneration zu verhindern (s. Abb. 43). — Den Schanzschen Watteverband sollte man grundsätzlich 2—3 Wochen belassen, da dieser eine vorübergehende Nackenschwäche gut überwinden hilft. Im Anschluß sind ausgiebige heilgymnastische Übungen von großem Wert. Die Patienten müssen eine normale Kopfhaltung und -bewegungen neu erlernen, da ja die Kraft und Bewegungsfähigkeit der am Krampf beteiligt gewesenen Muskeln durch eine weitgehende Unterbrechung ihrer nervösen Innervation herabgesetzt wurde.

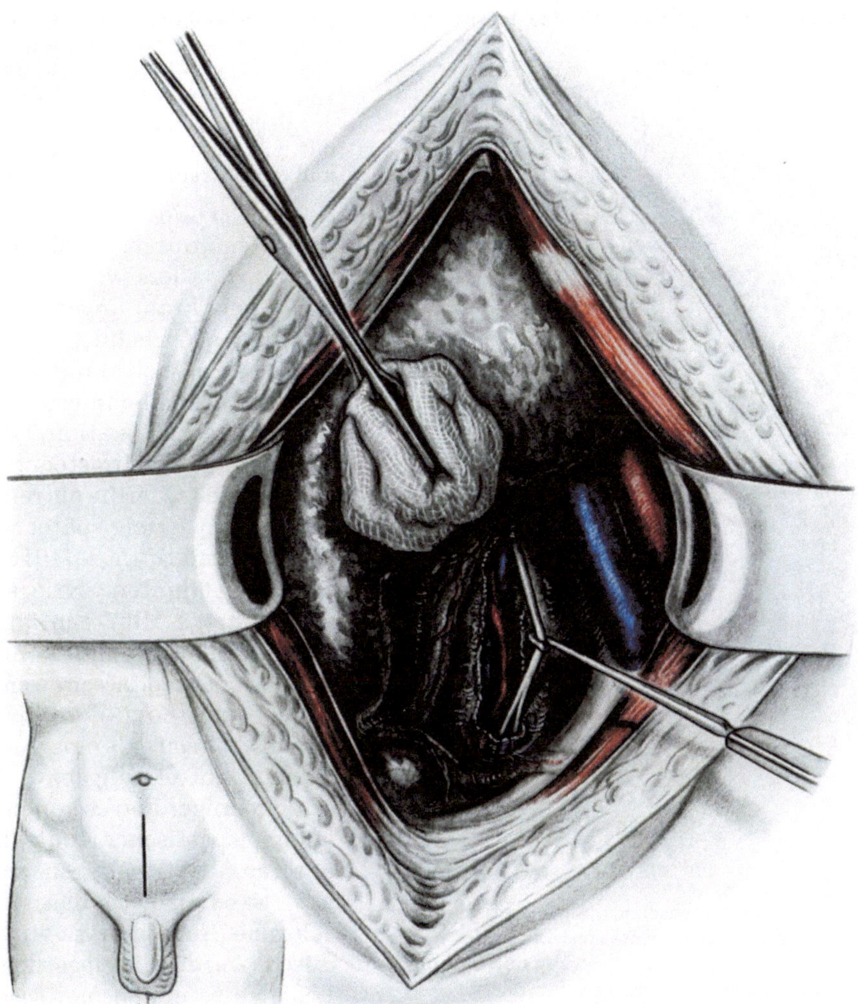

**Abb. 45.** Die Seligsche Operation, Durchschneidung des N. obturatorius beim Adduktionsspasmus der unteren Gliedmaßen. Der Peritonealsack ist stumpf abgeschoben und der medial von den Iliacalgefäßen auf der Beckenfascie liegende N. obturatorius ist angehoben.

## Anhang: Die schweren spastischen Zustände.

Störungen dieser Art haben mit dem engeren Thema der extrapyramidalen Hyperkinesen eigentlich nichts mehr zu tun. Trotzdem muß ihnen im Rahmen einer Besprechung der Chirurgie der Hirn- und Rückenmarksbahnen, welche sich insbesondere mit den pathologischen Zuständen des motorischen Systems befaßt, ein kurzes Wort gewidmet werden. Unser Interesse soll hier vor allem den *hochgradigen paraspastischen Lähmungen der unteren Gliedmaßen mit quälenden Kontrakturen* gelten, wie sie sich im Verlauf bestimmter degenerativer Systemerkrankungen einstellen (Encephalomyelitis disseminata, spastische Spinalparalyse, funikuläre Myelosen; aber auch beim pyramidalen Little oder nach spinalen Meningitiden).

Die peripheren Eingriffe an den Muskeln und Sehnen, wie sie noch heute von den Orthopäden zur Beseitigung der Schrumpfungsfolgen durch die Kontrakturen ausgeführt werden, sollen unberücksichtigt bleiben. Ebensowenig scheint es angebracht, an dieser Stelle auf die Neurotomien (STOFFEL) und die Radikotomien (MUNRO, FOERSTER) näher einzugehen. Beim *Adduktionsspasmus* der Oberschenkel in den paraplegischen Fällen der LITTLEschen Krankheit wird der Vorteil der Durchschneidung des N. obturatorius von verschiedenen Autoren hervorgehoben (SELIGsche Operation). Die Freilegung des Nerven geschieht extraperitoneal von einem Rectusaußenrandschnitt aus. Bei doppelseitiger Durchtrennung kann man einen tiefreichenden Mittelschnitt am Unterbauch benutzen. Der Peritonealsack wird stumpf von der lateralen Bauchwand abgeschoben, bis die Iliacalgefäße freigelegt sind. Unterhalb der medial von der Arterie verlaufenden V. iliaca externa verläuft der N. obturatorius, welcher auf der Beckenfascie gut zu sehen ist. Er wird mit einem stumpfen Häkchen angehoben und durchtrennt (Abb. 45).

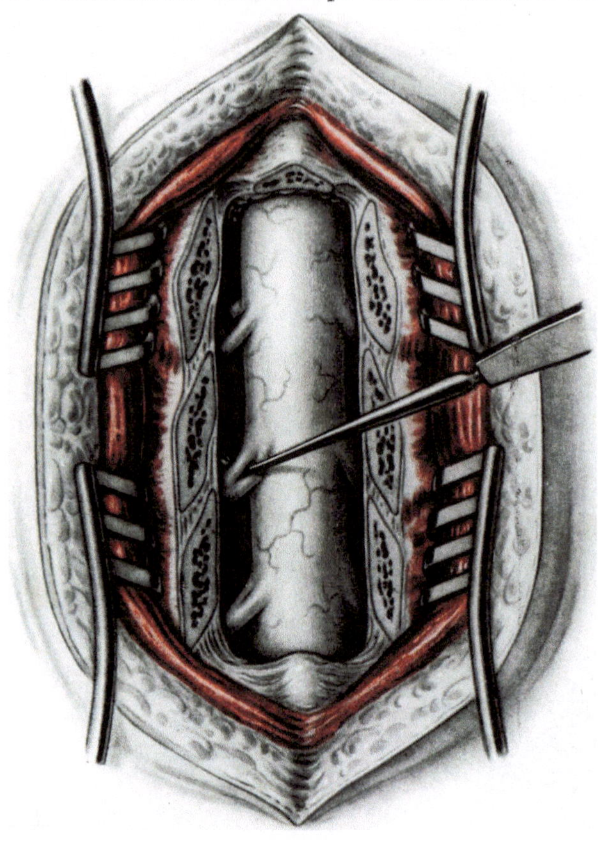

Abb. 46. Die extradurale Durchschneidung motorischer Wurzeln bei spastischen Zuständen. Operationsskizze; der motorische Anteil der oberen Wurzel links ist bereits durchschnitten, der darunter gelegene wird gerade isoliert.

Die *Myelotomia transversa*, eine totale Querdurchschneidung des Markes, wurde zuerst von CUSHING (1910) bei einer Frau angewandt, welche infolge von Wirbelmetastasen an einer kompletten Querschnittslähmung mit unerträglichen Schmerzen litt. Unter der gleichen Indikation, nämlich zur Bekämpfung heftigster Schmerzen, wurde die Querdurchtrennung des Markes mit Erfolg später von FEDOR KRAUSE und SULTAN (1916) bei querschnittsgelähmten Kriegsverletzten ausgeführt. Mit Einführung der Schmerzchordotomie konnte dieser Weg wieder verlassen werden. Nun ist es aber SORGO (1952), welcher meines Wissens als einziger die quere Markdurchtrennung bzw. die Exstirpation einiger Marksegmente zur Behebung spastischer Kontrakturen der unteren Extremitäten ausgeführt hat. Er exstirpierte das infraläsionell gelegene Lumbalmark in toto. Dadurch wurde die spastikerzeugende Läsion des ersten motorischen Neurons artefiziell in eine solche des zweiten (peripheren) motorischen Neurons abgeändert. Die Folge war eine schlaffe Lähmung der unteren Gliedmaßen, allerdings auch mit allen den bekannten unangenehmen, neurovegetativen Ausfallserscheinungen, welche die Prognose so sehr trüben. Der Eingriff hat sich wohl nicht durchsetzen können.

Die **Myelotomia longitudinalis,** eine Spaltung des Markes durch einen Längsschnitt in der Mittellinie (Sagittalebene), wurde von PUTNAM (1934) zur Durchschneidung der in der Commissur kreuzenden Schmerzfasern durchgeführt. PUTNAM hat diese „commissurale Chordotomie“ nur cervical — von $C_4$—$D_3$ — ausgeführt, um damit die wegen der Nähe der Phrenicuszentren gefahrvoller erscheinende cervicale Vorderseitenstrangchordotomie zu ersetzen. Dieser zur Bekämpfung von Schmerzen im Gebiet proximaler Rumpfabschnitte angewandte Eingriff wurde durch die medulläre und mesencephale Chordotomie überflüssig. Der Gedanke einer über mehrere Segmente ausgedehnten Längsspaltung des Markes wurde aber von BISCHOF (1951) für die Behandlung *para-*

*plegischer Kontrakturen* wieder aufgegriffen. Man hielt sich an FOERSTERs Auffassung der Notwendigkeit einer Unterbrechung des peripheren Reflexbogens zur Abschwächung der afferenten Muskeldehnungsreflexe. Es hatte sich aber gezeigt, daß FOERSTERs Hinterwurzeldurchschneidung zur Bekämpfung der spastischen Kontrakturen mit häufigen Rezidiven belastet war. Außerdem führte der Eingriff zu ausgedehnten Sensibilitätsausfällen. Die Wiederkehr der spastischen Tonuserhöhung nach der hinteren Rhizotomie führt BISCHOF darauf zurück, daß die intramedullären Schaltneuronen (die Strangzellen oder indirekten Kollateralen KÖLLIKERs) den anfänglichen Tonusverlust nach der Hinterwurzeldurchschneidung kompensieren können.

„Bei den indirekten Kollateralen handelt es sich um die Zwischenschaltung eines anderen Neurons, das nichts anderes als eine Strangzelle ist, die im Grau des Rückenmarkes liegt. Die Neuriten

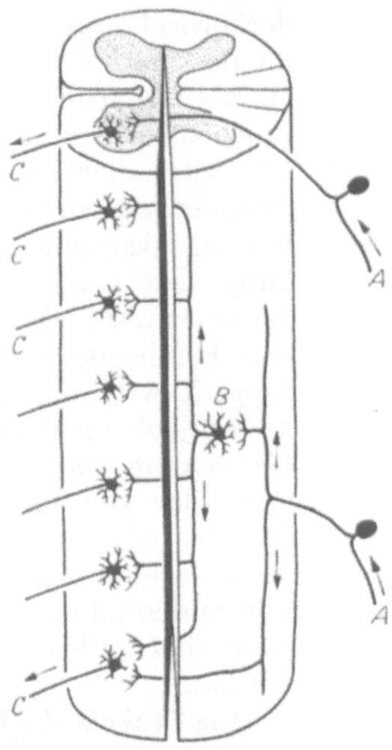


Abb. 47. Schematische Darstellung der intramedullären Schaltneurone (die Strangzellen oder indirekte Kollateralen KÖLLIKERs) mit Einzeichnung der Längsincision in der Frontalebene. *A* Zwei sensible Neurone; *B* eine Strangzelle; *C* zahlreiche motorische Neurone.

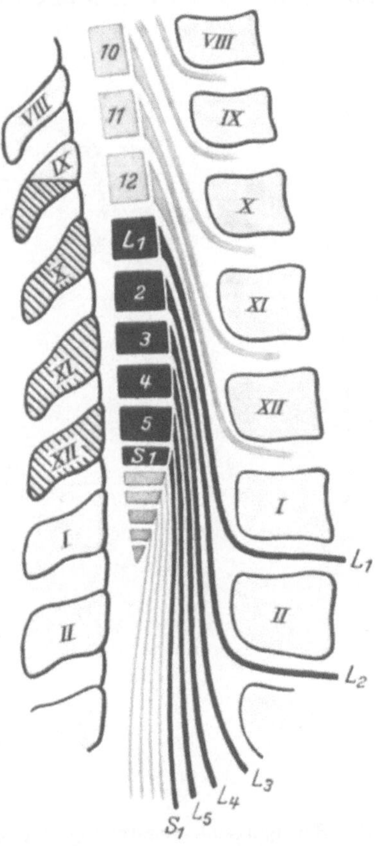


Abb. 48. Schematische Darstellung der Ausdehnung der Laminektomie und der Markincision bei der lateralen longitudinalen Myelotomie nach BISCHOF. Die schraffiert gezeichneten Dornfortsätze und Wirbelbögen werden reseziert. Die Ausdehnung der Längsincision reicht über die schwarz gezeichneten Rückenmarkssegmente.

teilen sich in auf- und absteigende Längsfasern. Von beiden gehen Kollateralen und je eine Endfaser (terminale Kollaterale) aus, welche die Erregungen auf die motorischen Vorderhornzellen übertragen, Die Reflexzelle selbst wird erregt durch eine Kollaterale der sensiblen Längsfaser" (KÖLLIKER). Im Hinterhorn, in welchem die peripheren afferenten Reize des entsprechenden Segmentes ankommen, trennen sich die Wege der afferenten Erregungen. Ein Teil fließt dem segmentalen Vorderhorn zu, ein Teil gelangt nach zentral zum Thalamus, dem Sammelbecken afferenter Zuflüsse, zum Kleinhirn und anderen subcorticalen Strukturen. Die Kollateralen KÖLLIKERs können wohl als das anatomische Substrat des segmentalen physiologischen Tonus der Muskulatur angesehen werden; sie verbinden das Hinter- und das Vorderhorn gewissermaßen zu einer physiologischen Funktionseinheit. Anscheinend kann sich der Reiz eines peripheren Hautbezirkes über das segmentale Hinterhorn durch die Vermittlung der Strangzellen auf die Vorderhörner der ganzen Extremität ausbreiten. Das heißt, daß jede Meldung von der Peripherie, welche in das Hinterhorn gelangt, nicht nur dortselbst, sondern auch in den benachbarten Segmenten eine Zustandsänderung hervorruft (Abb. 47).

BISCHOF vermutete, daß die longitudinale Rückenmarksspaltung mit Unterbrechung der kollateralen Hinter-Vorderhornverbindung den Tonus der entsprechenden Gliedmaßenmuskulatur dauerhaft herabsetzen müsse, da hierdurch der periphere Reflexbogen in seiner tonisierenden Funktion ausgeschaltet wird. Bei diesem Vorgehen ist nicht zuletzt ein großer Vorteil auch darin zu sehen, daß keine motorischen und sensiblen Bahnen geschädigt werden. Im Gegenteil, BISCHOF nimmt sogar an, daß die noch funktionierenden supranucleären Pyramidenanteile durch die Ausschaltung der pathologischen Einflüsse auf den Muskeltonus eventuell aktiviert werden können.

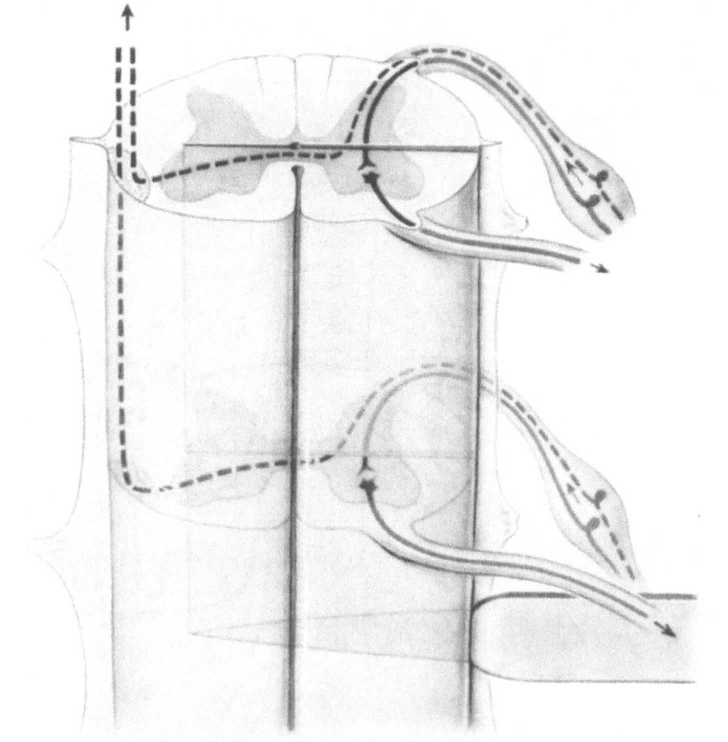

Tractus spinothalamicus

Abb. 49. Schematische Darstellung der lateralen longitudinalen Myelotomie zur Unterbrechung der Hinter-Vorderhornverbindung.

Zu wenig berücksichtigt ist meines Erachtens, daß mit der *lateralen* longitudinalen Myelotomie auch die Endstrecke des 1. motorischen Neurons der Pyramidenbahnfasern zum Vorderhornzellapparat — zumindest auf der Seite des Markeinschnittes — unterbrochen wird. Das bedeutet eine zusätzliche Verminderung der motorischen Innervation, also eine Verstärkung der bereits vorhandenen Parese. Die zukünftige Erfahrung mit diesem Eingriff wird daher lehren müssen, ob nicht doch der *hinteren* medianen Myelotomie der Vorzug zu geben ist, da mit dieser sicher keine Verbindungen von den Pyramidenbahnen zu den Vorderhornzellen zerstört werden.

*Die Technik der lateralen longitudinalen Myelotomie.* Die Längsspaltung des Rückenmarkes wird in der Frontalebene in Höhe der lumbalen Intumeszenz ausgeführt. Für diesen Eingriff eignen sich nur die schweren paraplegischen Kontrakturen der Beine.

Die Laminektomie wird vom 10. bis einschließlich 12. Brustwirbel durchgeführt (Abb. 48). Die nach caudal überragende Spitze des Dornes vom 9. Brustwirbel kann zur besseren Übersicht mitentfernt werden, während der Bogen stehen bleibt. Eine Erleichterung für die spätere Markincision ist die möglichst radikale Resektion der Bögen nach lateral. Nach Eröffnung der Dura durch einen Längsschnitt bleibt es der persönlichen Erfahrung des Operateurs überlassen, welcher Zugang zur Durchschneidung der Hinter-Vorderhornverbindung gewählt wird, d. h., ob der senkrechte Längsschnitt ins Mark von dorsal oder von lateral her geführt wird. Wir haben uns, wie BISCHOF, für die laterale Schnittführung entschieden. Das ist die Längsspaltung des Markes in der Frontalebene (Abb. 49). Hierzu wird zunächst die am weitesten proximal gelegene Zacke des Lig. denticulatum gefaßt und von der Dura abgetrennt. Durch behutsamen Zug an der abgelösten Zacke vom Lig. denticulatum wird das Mark leicht gedreht. Unmittelbar vor dem Lig. denticulatum wird das Traktotom, dessen Klingenlänge mit dem Schieber auf 7 mm eingestellt ist, in einem rechten Winkel ins Mark eingestochen. Durch Beiseiteschieben der nächsttiefergelegenen Hinterwurzel kann der Schnitt in der Frontalebene über $1—1^1/_2$ Segment ausgeführt werden. Nun wird die nächste Zacke des Lig. denticulatum gefaßt, abgetrennt und leicht angezogen. Die Hinterwurzel wird nach oben beiseitegehalten und der Schnitt kann nun wieder $1—1^1/_2$ Segment weiter nach caudal geführt werden. Schrittweise wird

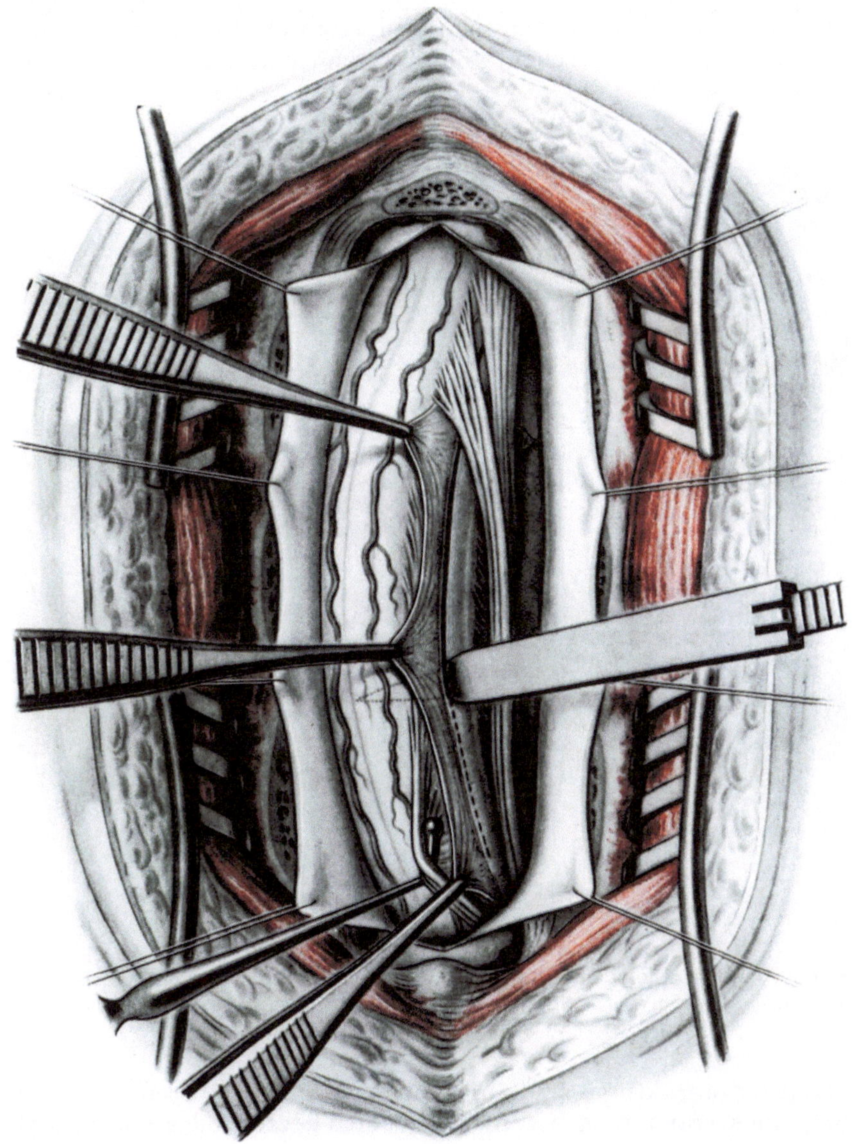

Abb. 50. Die laterale longitudinale Myelotomie in Höhe der lumbalen Intumeszenz. Operationsskizze; die senkrechte Längsincision des Markes erfolgt in der Frontalebene in Höhe der Leiste des Lig. denticulatum und reicht gewöhnlich vom 1. Lumbal- bis 1. Sacralsegment. Das Mark wird am abgetrennten Lig. denticulatum etwas gedreht, die Hinterwurzeln werden beiseite gehalten (s. Text).

in dieser Form der Schnitt nach caudal geführt, bis die vollständige Längsspaltung des Markes von $L_1$—$S_1$ erreicht ist, ohne daß eine Hinterwurzel geopfert werden muß. Das sacrale parasympathische Zentrum, welches bei $S_2$ und $S_3$ gelegen ist, wird bewußt geschont, während eine Schädigung der lumbalen vegetativen Versorgung der Blase nicht ganz zu umgehen ist (sympathisches Reflexzentrum der Blase $D_{12}$—$L_2$). Es genügt, den Eingriff auf einer Seite durchzuführen, da bei einer Tiefe von 6—7 mm auch die Hinter-

Vorderhornverbindung der anderen Seite unterbrochen wird. Bei der Schnittführung ist besonders darauf zu achten, daß die Traktotomklinge wirklich in der Mitte des Markes, etwa in Höhe des Zentralkanals, zu liegen kommt. Nur dann ist es möglich, eine Läsion der Vorderhorn- oder Hinterhornzellen zu vermeiden, welche ja möglichst erhalten bleiben sollen (Abb. 50).

Die *Wirkung der lateralen longitudinalen Myelotomie* tritt sofort ein. Vom Augenblick der Durchschneidung an sind die Spasmen und Krämpfe in den Muskeln, welche den durchtrennten Segmenten entsprechen, völlig verschwunden. Es besteht eine muskuläre

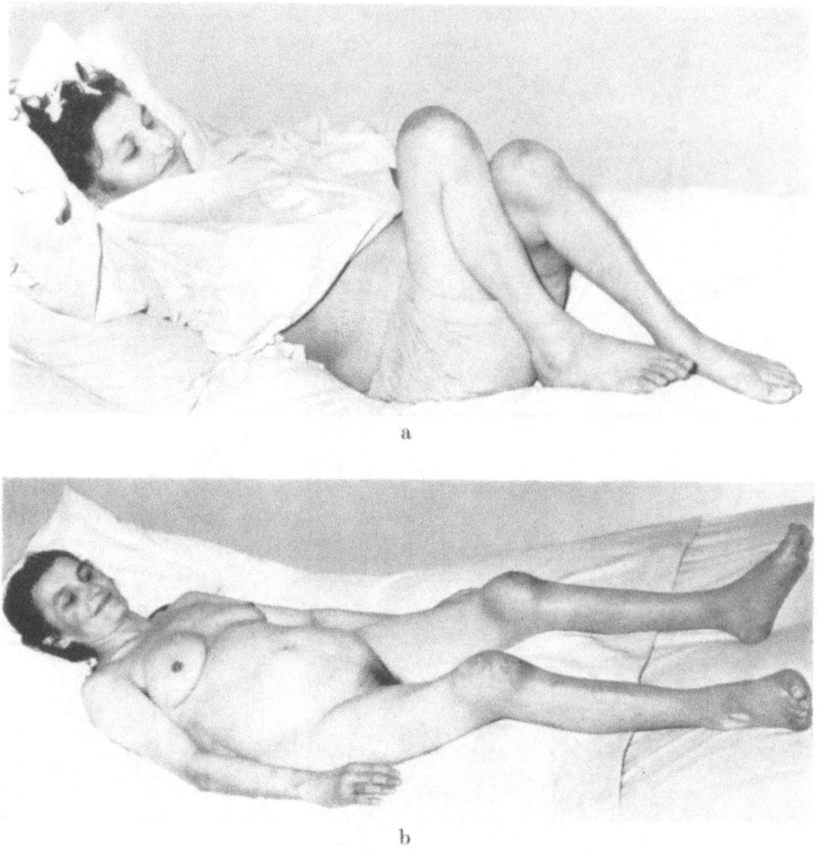

a

b

Abb. 51. Spätstadium einer multilokulären Systemerkrankung (M. S.) mit schweren spastischen Kontrakturen beider Beine bei einer 35jährigen Patientin *vor* (a) und *nach* (b) einer lateralen longitudinalen Myelotomie von $L_1$ bis $S_1$.

Hypotonie und die Kontrakturen sind aufgehoben, wenn nicht bereits tendinöse und artikuläre Schrumpfungsveränderungen vorliegen. Fehlen letztere oder sind sie geringfügig, so können wieder schwache aktive Bewegungen ausgeführt werden, die vorher unmöglich waren. Die Sehnenreflexe können p. op. fehlen, desgleichen Pyramidenzeichen (Abb. 51). Wenn vor dem Eingriff auch ein sensibler Querschnitt bestand, dann sind später die Befunde der Sensibilität unverändert. Haben vorher aber keine oder nur leichte Sensibilitätsstörungen vorgelegen, so ist als Operationsfolge eine Herabsetzung der Schmerz- und Temperaturempfindung von $L_1$ an nach distal zu finden, welche einseitig stärker ausgeprägt sein kann. In unseren Fällen hat bereits vor der Operation eine Blasenentleerungsstörung vorgelegen (komplette Harnverhaltung), welche nachher unverändert weiter fortbestand. In der Nachbehandlung sind orthopädische Maßnahmen wie Quengeln, Myotomien, Tenotomien, Plastiken u. a. zur weiteren Verbesserung des endgültigen Operationsresultates von großem Wert.

## Zusammenfassende Besprechung.

Die Chirurgie der extrapyramidalen Hyperkinesen kann erst auf die Erfahrung eines halben Jahrhunderts zurückblicken. Sie befindet sich offensichtlich immer noch in einem Stadium des Versuchens und Probierens. Trotz alledem haben aber die Ergebnisse, insbesondere der letzten 2 Jahrzehnte, gezeigt, daß nach Anwendung bestimmter neurochirurgischer Eingriffe, wenngleich nicht immer eine Beseitigung, so doch eine Unterdrückung oder Linderung der hyperkinetischen Symptome erwartet werden darf.

Die Resultate der meisten neurochirurgischen Operationen, welche zur Besserung der unwillkürlichen Bewegungen empfohlen werden, erlauben aber erst dann ein kritisches Urteil über ihre Brauchbarkeit, wenn der Eingriff mindestens 1—2 Jahre zurückliegt. Es sind eben zu viele Faktoren, welche zu einer vorübergehenden Besserung führen können [wie z. B. allein die psychologische Erschütterung einer größeren chirurgischen Maßnahme bei einem Kranken mit einem chronischen Leiden; oder die Folgen einer Rand- bzw. Ödemwirkung oder eine Art von „Schlag in das System" (Zülch), „Zusammenbruch der Arbeitsgemeinschaft" (Foerster), „Katastrophenreaktion" (Goldstein), „Diaschisis" (v. Monakow)]. Darüber hinaus müssen auch in manchen Fällen die natürlichen Schwankungen des Leidens in der endgültigen Beurteilung des Erfolges einer chirurgischen Maßnahme berücksichtigt werden. Operierte Fälle, welche nur einige Monate nach der Operation verfolgt wurden, haben bedauerlicherweise schon zu manchen unberechtigten enthusiastischen Schlußfolgerungen Anlaß gegeben, welche nicht nur ungern, sondern auch nicht leicht zu berichtigen sind.

Nachdem in der Einleitung versucht wurde, ganz allgemeine Richtlinien für die Indikation zu einer Operation zusammenzustellen, sollen zum Schluß schlaglichtartig einige Punkte zur operativen Anzeigestellung genannt werden, welche speziell die Form der Bewegungsstörung betreffen, da der Erfolg des chirurgisch-therapeutischen Vorgehens weitgehend hiervon abhängt.

1. *Die hyperkinetisch-hypotonen Syndrome* (nichtrhythmische Bewegungen).
a) Die Choreoathetosen.
b) Der Hemiballismus.
c) Die Torsionsdystonie.
d) Der Torticollis spasticus.

2. *Die akinetisch-hypertonen Syndrome* (rhythmische Bewegungen).
a) Der Parkinson-Tremor.
b) Die Parkinson-Starre.

**1. Die hyperkinetisch-hypotonen Syndrome bzw. die nichtrhythmischen Dyskinesien** sind unter Umständen bereits durch Eingriffe am extrapyramidal-motorischen System in den verschiedenen Ebenen (cortical — subcortical — spinal) günstig zu beeinflussen.

a) Allein die Bewegungsstörung der ***Choreoathetosen*** ist durch Eingriffe, welche auf die *parapyramidalen* Projektionsfelder und -leitungswege der verschiedenen Ebenen beschränkt bleiben, zu bessern. Die günstigen Ergebnisse werden aber offensichtlich durch eine zusätzliche partielle Schädigung des Pyramidensystems in der Ebene des Eingriffs vermehrt.

*Cortical:* Subpiale Resektion oder Unterschneidung der Felder 8, 6 und der ventralen Teile des Feldes 4 (Bucy u. a.). = Eingriff vorwiegend an den parapyramidalen Projektionsfeldern der Rinde, daher postoperativ keine bleibendenParesen (möglicherweise aber transitorische Halbseitensymptome).

*Subcortical:* Der Nutzen herdförmiger Ausschaltungen im äußeren Segment des Globus pallidus und einer Unterbrechung der pallidofugalen Verbindungen muß sich erst noch herausstellen (Spiegel-Wycis, Guiot u. a.) = Eingriff im Bereich der subcorticalen Rücksteuerungskreise, daher postoperativ keine kontralateralen Paresen.

*Cervical:* Bilaterale Extrapyramidotomie bei der Athétose double (Putnam, Tönnis-Schürmann) = Eingriff an den im Vorderstrang absteigenden, mehrgliedrigen, extrapyramidalen Bahnen, daher postoperativ keine Paresesymptome.

Bei schweren choreoathetotischen Halbseitensyndromen besser die kombinierte Pyramido-Extrapyramidotomie (SCHÜRMANN) = Eingriff an den extrapyramidalen *und* pyramidalen Bahnen, daher postoperativ stets Hemiparese.

b) Beim seltenen ***Hemiballismus*** reicht die alleinige Schädigung extrapyramidaler Strukturen in den verschiedenen Ebenen offenbar nicht aus. Wegen der Einseitigkeit ist diese Bewegungsstörung aber mit einer großen Sicherheit durch ein radikaleres Vorgehen, d. h. durch Einbeziehung der Pyramidenbahn, zu beseitigen.

*Cortical:* Resektion des Feldes 4 (BUCY, ALPERS und JAEGER) = Eingriff an der pyramidalen motorischen Rinde, daher postoperativ stets Hemiparese.

Resektion der Felder 4 *und* 6 (MEYERS); als postoperative Folge ebenfalls eine Hemiparese.

„Lineare Rindenincision" zwischen Feld 4 und 4s (MEYERS und Mitarbeiter) = Eingriff (Längsincision) zwischen der motorischen Rinde und dem „Suppressor"-Streifen, postoperativ keine permanente Parese.

*Subcortical:* Laterale Pedunkulotomie (WALKER) = Eingriff an der Pyramidenbahn in Höhe der Hirnschenkel, daher postoperativ stets Hemiparesesymptome zu erwarten.

Der Nutzen von gezielten pallidären und subpallidären Ausschaltungen ist noch umstritten und unsicher (SPIEGEL-WYCIS) = Eingriff an den extrapyramidalen Rücksteuerungskreisen, daher postoperativ keine kontralateralen Paresesymptome zu erwarten.

*Cervical:* Die lateralen Pyramidotomien (PUTNAM, OLIVER) oder die kombinierte Pyramido-Extrapyramidotomie (SCHÜRMANN) = Eingriffe an den Pyramidenbahnen, daher postoperativ stets Hemiparesen zu erwarten.

c) Die ***Torsionsdystonie*** tritt glücklicherweise gleichfalls in der Regel halbseitig in Erscheinung, was ihre totale chirurgische Beseitigung erleichtert. Ohne eine ausgiebige Zerstörung im Gebiet des pyramidal-motorischen Systems ist meines Wissens bis heute kein dauerhafter Erfolg bei diesem Krankheitsbild erzielt worden.

*Cortical:* Exstirpation des Feldes 4 (BUCY, DAVID u. a.) = Eingriff an der motorischen Rinde, daher kontralaterale Parese als postoperative Folge.

*Subcortical:* Laterale Pedunkulotomie (WALKER, WERTHEIMER und MANSUY) = Eingriff an der Pyramidenbahn, daher postoperativ kontralaterale Hemiparese die Folge.

*Cervical:* Kombinierte Pyramido-Extrapyramidotomie (SCHÜRMANN) = Eingriff an den extrapyramidalen *und* pyramidalen Bahnen, daher postoperativ ipsilaterale Hemiparese die Folge.

d) Beim ***Torticollis spasticus*** darf heute die Operation nach FOERSTER-DANDY als die Methode der Wahl gelten. Alle anderen bisher versuchten Eingriffe am zentralen Nervensystem haben in diesen Fällen ausnahmslos enttäuscht.

2. Unter den **akinetisch-hypertonen Syndromen bzw. den rhythmischen Dyskinesien** muß eine besonders strenge Auswahl der chirurgisch beeinflußbaren Krankheitsbilder getroffen werden. Bis vor kurzem ist unter den mannigfaltigen Erscheinungen der PARKINSON-Syndrome nur der *Tremor* neurochirurgisch zu bessern gewesen. Neuerdings scheint auch auf das schwerwiegende Phänomen einer subcorticalen Muskeltonusstörung, auf die *Rigidität und Starre*, durch chirurgische Maßnahmen ein gewisser Einfluß ausgeübt werden zu können.

a) Der ***Tremor,*** darin stimmen die meisten Autoren überein, kann durch eine Unterbrechung der Pyramidenbahn in irgendeiner Höhe, d. h. irgendwo in ihrem Verlauf, gebessert oder sogar beseitigt werden. Allerdings sind postoperativ immer mehr oder weniger schwere Hemiparesen zu erwarten. Ohne ausgiebige Läsionen im Bereich des pyramidalen Systems ist diesem Symptom chirurgisch kaum beizukommen, wenn sich nicht auch in Zukunft die jüngsten Erfolge der Eingriffe an den subcorticalen Rücksteuerungskreisen bestätigen sollten (Pallidotomien und Ansotomien).

*Cortical:* Totale Entfernung der motorischen Rinde, Area 4 (BUCY u. a.) = Eingriff im Bereich des pyramidalen Systems, daher folgt postoperativ kontralateral eine Parese.

*Subcortical:* Ventrale Capsulotomie (BROWDER) = Eingriff an den corticopetalen parapyramidalen Verbindungen, aber auch partielle Pyramidenbahnläsion am Knie der inneren Kapsel, daher postoperativ transitorische, aber auch permanente Hemiparesen.

Pallidotomie und Unterbrechung der pallidofugalen Verbindungen (MEYERS, FÉNÉLON, GUIOT) und Ansotomie (SPIEGEL und WYCIS) = Eingriffe an den extrapyramidalen Rücksteuerungskreisen, daher postoperativ kein Defizit der willkürlichen motorischen Funktion.

Laterale Pedunkulotomie (WALKER) = Eingriff an der Pyramidenbahn, daher postoperative kontralaterale Hemiparese die Folge.

*Cervical:* Laterale Pyramidotomie (PUTNAM, OLIVER),

kombinierte laterale und ventrale Pyramidotomie (EBIN),

kombinierte Pyramido-Extrapyramidotomie (SCHÜRMANN) = Eingriffe an den Pyramidenbahnen, daher ipsilaterale spinalspastische Hemiparesen als Operationsfolge.

Da alle diese Eingriffe, mit Ausnahme der Pallidotomie und Ansotomie, zu postoperativen Lähmungen geringeren oder stärkeren Grades führen, eignet sich für ihre Anwendung nur der Hemiparkinsontremor.

b) Auf die ***Rigidität*** und ***Starre*** des PARKINSON-Syndroms konnte bisher durch keine chirurgische Maßnahme ein nachhaltiger Einfluß ausgeübt werden. Neuerdings wird dem Eingreifen an den extrapyramidalen Rücksteuerungsverbindungen in dieser Hinsicht eine bemerkenswert günstige Wirkung nachgesagt. Der Pallidotomie mit Unterbrechung der pallidofugalen Verbindungen (GUIOT) oder der Ligatur der A. chorioidalis anterior (COOPER), welche zu einer umschriebenen Malacie im Gebiet des inneren Pallidumgliedes, der intersegmentären pallidären und pallidofugalen Verbindungen führen soll, wird eine Besserung der Symptome der Muskelstarre nachgesagt.

*Cortical:* Kein Einfluß.

*Subcortical:* Pallidotomie (GUIOT),

Ligatur der A. chorioidea anterior (COOPER) = Eingriffe an den extrapyramidalen Rücksteuerungskreisen, daher keine postoperativen Paresen.

*Cervical:* Kein Einfluß.

Es ist kaum anzunehmen, daß ein Operateur mit allen Operationsmethoden vertraut ist. Trotzdem darf man von ihm erwarten, daß er vor der Durchführung irgendeines Eingriffes die Möglichkeiten und Chancen kritisch gegeneinander abzuwägen versteht. Da sich bislang für die Mehrzahl der unkontrollierten Bewegungen kein Standardverfahren herausgehoben hat, würde er mit Gewißheit bei unkritischer Wahl des operativen Vorgehens im Einzelfall große Enttäuschungen erleben und dadurch versucht sein, der operativen Behandlung der Hyperkinesen voreilig jede günstige Wirkung abzusprechen. Daß aber bei richtiger Indikationsstellung und sorgfältiger Auswahl der zur Operation geeigneten Patienten die Chirurgie der extrapyramidalen Bewegungsstörungen zu einem Segen für manchen chronisch leidenden und gequälten Kranken werden kann, wird nicht zu bestreiten sein.

Abschließend muß nochmals herausgestellt werden, daß die Chirurgie der extrapyramidalen Hyperkinesen bis jetzt noch keinen Standardeingriff hervorgebracht hat. Selbst in den Händen der erfahrensten Chirurgen lassen sich das Ergebnis und die Folgen eines Eingriffs nicht immer mit Sicherheit voraussagen. Nach dem augenblicklichen Stand der operativen Möglichkeiten ist bedauerlicherweise zuzugeben, daß in den glücklicheren Fällen nur *eine* Körperseite von der Hyperkinese betroffen ist, da nur solchen Kranken mit hinreichender Sicherheit durch die erhöhten Chancen eines radikaleren Vorgehens wirklich dauerhaft geholfen werden kann. Ganz gleich, in welcher Ebene und an welcher Struktur der Eingriff vollzogen wird, scheint ja neben der Wahl des richtigen Schädigungsortes auch die Menge der unterbrochenen Verbindungen bzw. die Anzahl der durchschnittenen Fasern oder die Größe des Läsionsherdes, d. h. ganz einfach das Quantum der zerstörten nervösen Elemente an der entsprechenden Stelle, eine nicht unmaßgebliche Rolle für den Erfolg zu spielen. Auf der anderen Seite wird

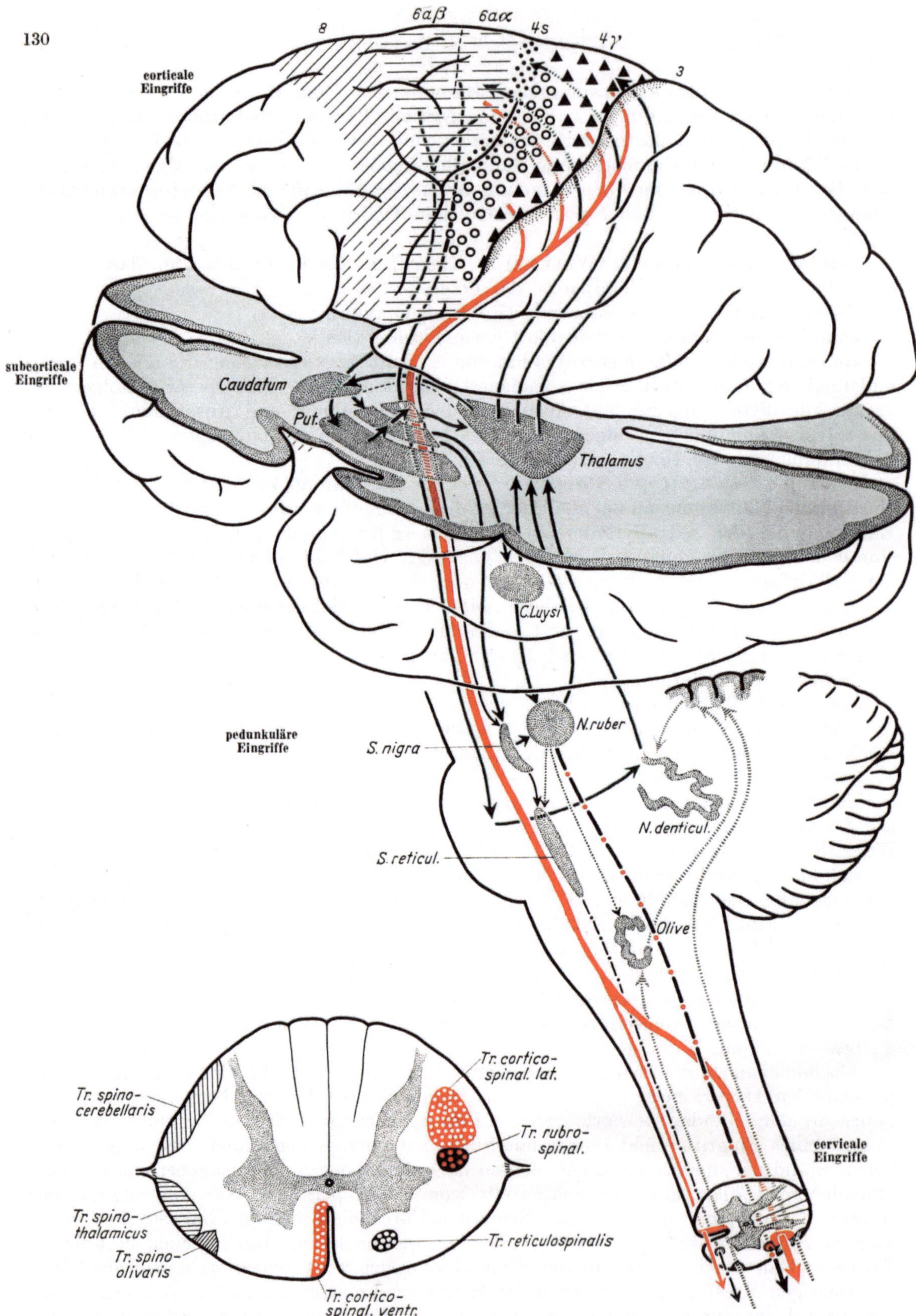


Abb. 52. Die verschiedenen Eingriffsorte in der chirurgischen Therapie der extrapyramidalen Motilitätsstörungen (schematisch).

aber durch ein gelegentlich erzieltes ausgezeichnetes Resultat die Hoffnung gestärkt, daß zukünftig doch noch eine Methode entwickelt werden kann, durch welche die unwillkürlichen Bewegungen vollständig und permanent zu beseitigen sein werden, ohne daß gleichzeitig eine Lähmung dafür in Kauf genommen werden muß. Bevor aber eine solch ideale Lösung erreicht werden kann, muß noch eine Reihe unbekannter Zusammenhänge in der Pathogenese und Pathophysiologie der unkontrollierten Bewegungen aufgeklärt werden.

## Literatur.


ABBIE, A. A.: The blood supply of the lateral geniculate body, with a note on the morphology of the choroidal arteries. J. of Anat. **67**, 491 (1933).
— The morphology of the forebrain arteries; with especial reference to the evaluation of the basal ganglia. J. of Anat. **68**, 433 (1934).
ADRIAN, E. D.: Double representation of the feet in the sensory cortex of the cat. J. of Physiol. **98**, 16 (1940).
ALAJOUANINE, T., J. LE BEAU et R. HOUDART: Résection corticale de la zone motrice (aires 4 et 6) dans un cas d'athétose localisée au bras gauche. Revue neur. **79**, 134 (1947).
— — — Résection corticale de la zone motrice (aires 4 et 6) dans un cas d'hémiparkinson gauche. Revue neur. **79**, 137 (1947).
ALEXANDER, L.: The vascular supply of the striopallidum. Proc. Assoc. Res. Nerv. a. Ment. Dis. **21**, 77 (1942).
ALPERS, B. J., and R. JAEGER: Hemiballism and its control by ablation of the motor cortex. Arch. of Neur. **64**, 285 (1950).
ANSCHÜTZ, O. O.: Hirnoperation bei Hemiathetose. Berl. klin. Wschr. **1910**, 1687.
ARING, C. D., and J.F. FULTON: Relation of the cerebrum to the cerebellum. II. Cerebellar tremor in the monkey and its absence after removal of the principal excitable areas of the cerebral cortex (areas 4 and 6a, upperpart). III. Accentuation of the cerebellar tremor following lesions of premotor cortex (Area 6a, upperpart). Arch. of Neur. **35**, 439 (1936).
BANNWARTH, A.: Die Erkrankungen des extrapyramidal-motorischen Systems. Fortschr. Neur. **10** 74 (1938).
BAUDOUIN, A., A. THÉVENARD et F. FÉNÉLON: Nouveaux cas de maladie de Parkinson opérés par interruption souspallidale et variations sur la technique personelle. Revue neur. **86**, 247 (1952).
BISCHOF, W.: Die longitudinale Myelotomie. Zbl. Neurochir. **11**, 79 (1951).
BONIN, G. v.: Architecture of the precentral motor cortex and some adjacent areas. In P. C. BUCY, The Precentral Motor Cortex, Bd. 2, S. 7. Urbana, Illinois: University of Ill. Press 1949.
—, and P. BAILEY: The Neocortex of Macaca Mulatta. Urbana, Illinois: University of Ill. Press **1947** (1645).
BRODMANN, K.: Vergleichende Lokalisationslehre der Großhirnrinde in ihren Prinzipien dargestellt auf Grund des Zellbaues. Leipzig: Johann Ambrosius Barth 1909. 324 S.
BROWDER, J.: Parkinsonism — Is it a Surgical Problem? N. Y. State J. Med. **47**, 2589 (1947).
— Section of the fibers of the anterior limb of the internal capsule in parkinsonism. Amer. J. Surg. **75**, 264 (1948).
BUCY, P. C.: Cortical exstirpation in the treatment of involuntary movements. Proc. Assoc. Res. Nerv. a. Ment. Dis. **21**, 551 (1942).
— The neural mechanisms of athetosis and tremor. J. of Neuropath. **1**, 224 (1942).
— Surgical relief of tremor at rest. Amer. Surg. **122**, 933 (1945).
— Cortical exstirpation in the treatment of involuntary movements. Amer. J. Surg. **75**, 257 (1947).
— The surgical treatment of abnormal involuntary movements. Surg. etc. **90**, 376 (1950).
—, and D. N. BUCHNANAN: Athetosis. Brain **55**, 479 (1932).
—, and T. J. CASE: Athetosis. II. Surgical treatment of unilateral athetosis. Arch. of Neur. **37**, 983 (1937).
— — Tremor. Physiological mechanism and abolition by surgical means. Arch. of Neur. **41**, 721 (1939).
BUJALSKI: Zit. nach ROMBERG.
CAMPBELL, A. W.: Histological Studies of the Localization of Cerebral Function. Cambridge: University Press **1905**. 360 S.
COBB, ST., J. L. POOL, J. SCARFF, R. S. SCHWAB, A. E. WALKER and J. C. WHITE: Section of "U"-Fibers of motor cortex in cases of paralysis agitans (Parkinson's disease). Arch. of Neur. **46**, 57 (1950.)
COLEMAN, C. C.: The treatment of spasmodic torticollis by intradural posterior root section and extracranial division of the spinal accessory. Virginia Med. Monthly **53**, 761 (1927).
COLLIER, M.: Spasmodic torticollis treated by nerve ligature. Lancet **1890**, 1354.
COOPER, I. S.: Ligation of the anterior choroidal artery for involuntary movements — parkinsonism. Psychiatr. Quart. **27**, 317 (1953).

— Persönliche Mitteilung 1954.

COOPER, I. S.: Surgical occlusion of the anterior choroidal artery in parkinsonism. Surg. etc. **99**, 207—219 (1954).

— Surgical alleviation of parkinsonism: Effects of occlusion of the anterior choroidal artery. J. Amer. Geriatr. Soc. **2** 691—718 (1954).

CUSHING, H.: Zit. nach H. PEIPER.

DANDY, W. E.: An operation for the treatment of spasmodic torticollis. Arch. Surg. **20**, 1021 (1930).

DAVID, M., et H. HÉCAEN: Traitement neurochirurgical des dyskinésies (mouvements choréoathétosiques, dystonies, tremblements). Semaine Hôp. **1946**, 209.

— — et B. COLOMB: Deux nouvelles observations des mouvements involontaires traités par excision corticale. Revue neur. **78**, 588 (1946).

— — et J. TALAIRACH: Résultats éloignés des cortectomies dans le traitement des dyskinésies. Revue neur. **80**, 53 (1948).

— — — Traitement chirurgical des dyskinésies. XVIIIe Réunion Neurologique Internationale, Paris, 7—8 Juillet. 1952.

DELMAS, J., et A. DELMAS: Voies et centres nerveux. Paris: Masson & Cie. **1949**. 194 S.

DELMAS-MARSALET, P., et L. VAN BOGAERT: Sur un cas de myoclonies rhythmiques continuées déterminées par un intervention chirurgicale sur le tronc cérébral. Revue Neur. **64**, 728 (1935).

DOWMAN, C. E.: Spasmodic torticollis. Surg. etc. **53**, 836 (1931).

DUPUYTREN, G.: Zit. nach FINNEY u. HUGHSON.

DUSSER DE BARENNE, J. G., H. W. GAROL and W. S. MCCULLOCH: Functional organization of sensory and adjacent cortex of the monkey. J. of Neurophysiol. **4**, 324 (1954).

— — — Physiological neuronography of the cortico-striatal connections. Proc. Assoc. Res. Nerv. a. Ment. Dis. **21**, 246 (1941).

EBIN, J.: Combined lateral and ventral pyramidotomy in treatment of paralysis agitans. Arch. of Neur. **62**, 24 (1949).

ECONOMO, C. v., u. G. N. KOSKINAS: Die Cytoarchitektonik der Hirnrinde des erwachsenen Menschen. Wien u. Berlin: Springer 1925. 810 S.

FÉNÉLON, F.: Essais de traitement neurochirurgical du syndrome parkinsonien par intervention directe sur les voies extrapyramidales immédiatement sousstriopallidales (aux lenticulaire). Revue neur. **83**, 437 (1950).

—, et F. THIÉBAUT: Résultats du traitement neurochirurgical d'une rigidité parkinsonien par intervention striopallidale unilatérale. Revue neur. **83**, 280 (1950).

FERRIER, D.: The functions of the brain. London: Smith, Elder & Co. 1876. 323 S.

FINNEY, J. M. T., and W. HUGHSON: Spasmodic torticollis. Ann. Surg. **81**, 255 (1925).

FOERSTER, O.: Über eine neue operative Methode der Behandlung spastischer Lähmungen mittels Resektion hinterer Rückenmarkswurzeln. Z. orthop. Chir. **22**, 203 (1908).

— Vorderseitenstrangdurchschneidung im Rückenmark zur Beseitigung von Schmerzen. Berl. klin. Wschr. **1913**, 1499.

— Torticollis spasticus. Zbl. Chir. **47**, 1106 (1920).

— Zur Analyse und Pathophysiologie der striären Bewegungsstörungen. Z. Neur. **73**, 1 (1921).

— Über die Vorderseitenstrangdurchschneidung. 2. Jahresverslg der Ver.igg Südostdtsch. Psychiater und Neurologen 5./6. März 1927 in Breslau. Arch. f. Psychiatr. **1927**, 707.

— Schlaffe und spastische Lähmung. In BETHE-BERGMANNS Handbuch der normalen und pathologischen Physiologie. Berlin: Springer 1929.

FOERSTER, O., u. O. GAGEL: Die Vorderseitenstrangdurchschneidung beim Menschen. Z. Neur. **138**, 1 (1932).

FRAZIER, C. H.: Surgery of the Spinal Cord. New York: D. Appleton & Co. 1918. 668 S.

— Siehe SPILLER, FRAZIER u. VAN KAATHOVEN 1906.

FREEMAN, W., and J. W. WATTS: Psychosurgery. Springfield Ill.: Ch. C. Thomas 1942.

FULTON, J. F., E. G. T. LIDDELL and D. MCRIOCH: Relation of the cerebrum to the cerebellum. I. Cerebellar tremor in the cat and its absence after removal of the cerebral hemispheres. Arch. of Neur. **28**, 542 (1932).

GARDNER, W. J., and G. H. WILLIAMS jr.: Interruption of the sympathic nerve supply to the brain-effect on Parkinson's syndrome. Arch. of Neur. **61**, 413 (1949).

GIRARD, BORDET et DÉVIC: Zit. nach DAVID u. a.

GUILLAUME, J.: Conséquences physiopathologiques et thérapeutiques des interventions circonscrites sur l'écorce cérébrale rolandique. Congrès des médecins aliénistes et neurologistes de Frances, XLVIe session, Marseille, 49—77, 1948.

GUIOT, G., et S. BRION: Traitement des mouvements anormaux par la coagulation pallidale. Technique et résultats. Semaine Hôp. **28**, 49 (1952).

—, et S. FORJAZ: La tractotomie mesencéphalique par voie temporale. Revue neur. **79**, 733 (1947).

—, et J. PECKER: Traitement du tremblement parkinsonien par la pyramidotomie pédonculaire. Semaine Hôp. **25**, 2620 (1949).

— — Tractotomie mesencéphalique antérieure pour tremblement parkinsonien. Revue neur. **81**, 387 (1949).

HABERMANN, H.: Diagnose, Differentialdiagnose und Therapie der extrapyramidalen Erkrankungen. „Paracelsus". Arch. prakt. Med. **12**, 1 (1951).
HAMBY, W. B.: Discussion to the communication of J. BROWDER. "Parkinsonism — Is it a surgical problem?" N. Y. State J. Med. **47**, 2592 (1947).
HASSLER, R.: Extrapyramidal-motorische Syndrome und Erkrankungen. In MOHR u. STAEHELINS Handbuch der inneren Medizin, Bd. V/III Neurologie, S. 676—904. Berlin-Göttingen-Heidelberg: Springer 1953.
HESS, W. R.: Beiträge zur Physiologie des Hirnstammes. Leipzig: Georg Thieme 1930/31 u. 1938.
— Physiologische Aspekte der extrapyramidalen Motorik. Nervenarzt **15**, 457 (1942).
HINES, M.: The "motor" cortex. Bull. Johns Hopkins Hosp. **40**, 313 (1937).
HORSLEY, V.: The Linacre Lecture on the Function of the So-called Motor Area of the Brain. Brit. Med. J. **2**, 125 (1909).
—, and R. H. CLARKE: The structure and functions of the cerebellum examined by a new method. Brain **31**, 45 (1908).
JACOB, A.: Die extrapyramidalen Erkrankungen. Berlin: Springer 1923.
JERMUTOWICZ, W.: Un cas d'hémiballismus partiellement amélioré après intervention périphérique. Revue neur. **55**, 374 (1931).
KANKI, S., and T. BAN: Corticofugal connections of frontal lobe in man. Med. J. Osaka Univ. **3**, 201 (1952) (in engl. Sprache).
KEEN, W. W.: A new operation for spasmodic wry neck, namely division or exsection of the nerves supplying the superior rotator muscles of the head. Ann. Surg. **13**, 44 (1891).
KLEMME, R. M.: Surgical treatment of dystonia, paralysis agitans and athetosis. Arch. of Neur. **44**, 1926 (1940).
— Surgical treatment of dystonia with report of one hundred cases. Proc. Assoc. Res. Nerv. a. Ment. Dis. **21**, 596 (1942).
— The neural mechanism of paralysis agitans. Arch. of Neur. **50**, 367 (1943).
KOCHER, TH.: Zit. nach O. FOERSTER (Torticollis spasticus 1920).
KÖLLIKER, A.: Nervensystem des Menschen und der Tiere. In Handbuch der Gewebslehre des Menschen, 6. Aufl., Bd. II, S. 122. Leipzig: Wilhelm Engelmann 1890.
KRAUSE, F.: Zit. nach H. PEIPER, Die Chirurgie des Rückenmarks und seiner Häute. In KIRSCHNER-NORDMANN, Die Chirurgie, Bd. III, S. 881—996. Wien: Urban & Schwarzenberg 1948.
LASHLEY, K. S., and G. CLARK: The cytoarchitecture of the cerebral cortex of Ateles: a critical examination of architectonic studies. J. Comp. Neur. **85**, 223 (1946).
LAZORTHES, G., et H. ANDUZE: Torticolis et rétrocolis spasmodiques traités par l'opération de MCKENZIE-DANDY. Revue neur. **81**, 367 (1949).
LEKSELL, L.: A stereotaxic apparatus for intracerebral surgery. Acta chir. scand. (Stockh.) **99**, 229 (1949).
— Persönliche Mitteilung Sept. 1953.
LISI, L. DE, P. PERRIA e U. SACCHI: Contributi alla terapia chirurgia delle ipercinesia. I. Tremore parkinsoniano. Atti III Riunione Sezione Ligure-lombardo-piemontese della Soc. Ital. Neurol., 4—6 Giugno 1948. Minerva med. (Torino) **1948**.
— — — Contributi alla terapia chirurgica delle ipercinesia. II. Tremore post-apoplettico ed attività soppressoria corticale. Sistema nerv. (Milano) **1**, 1 (1949).
— — — Contributi alla terapia chirurgica delle ipercinesia. III. Atetosi doppia, tremore parkinsoniano ed attività soppressoria corticale. Sistema ner. (Milano) **1**, 6 (1949).
— — — Pathophysiologische Betrachtungen über die Neurochirurgie der Hyperkinesen. Zbl. Neurochir. **10**, 98 (1950).
MARTIN, J. P.: Hemichorea resulting from a local lesion of the brain. (The syndrome of the body of Luys.) Brain **50**, 637 (1927).
MASHANSKY, F. J.: Traitement chirurgical des mouvements involontaires des extrémités appliqué au parkinsonisme postencéphalitique. J. de Chir. **46**, 877 (1935).
MCKENZIE, K. G.: Intrameningeal division of the spinal accessory and roots of the upper cervical nerves for treatment of spasmodic torticollis. Surg. etc. **39**, 5 (1924).
METTLER, F. A.: Observations on the consequences of large subtotal lesions of the simian spinal cord. J. Comp. Neur. **81**, 3 (1944).
— H. W. ADES, E. LIPMAN and E. A. CULLER: The extrapyramidal system. An experimental demonstration of function. Arch. of Neur. **41**, 948 (1939).
MEYERS, R.: The modification of alternating tremors, rigidity and festination by surgery of the basal ganglia. The diseases of the basal ganglia. Proc. Assoc. Res. Nerv. a. Ment. Dis. **21**, 602 (1942).
— Surgical interruption of the pallidofugal fibers. Its effect on the syndrome of paralysis agitans and technical considerations in its application. N. Y. State J. Med. **42**, 317 (1942).
— The present status of surgical procedures directed against the extrapyramidal diseases. N. Y. State J. Med. **42**, 535 (1942).
— Surgical experiences in the therapy of certain "extra-pyramidal" diseases: a current evaluation. Acta psychiatr. (Københ.) **67**, 42 (1951).
— D. B. SWEENY and J. T. SCHWIDDE: Hemiballismus: aetiology and surgical treatment. J. Neurol., Neurosurg. a. Psychiatry **13**, 115 (1950).

Minnius, I.: Zit. nach Finney u. Hughson (spasmodic torticollis — 1925).
Mikulicz, J.: Über die Exstirpation des Kopfnickers beim muskulären Schiefhals, nebst Bemerkungen zur Pathologie dieses Leidens. Zbl. Chir. **22**, 1 (1895).
Money, R. A.: Discussion of paper by W. L. Reid. Studies on the tremor-rigidity syndrome. I. Surgical treatment of human subjects. Med. J. Austral. **2**, 532 (1948).
Morgan, C. de: A case in which severe spasmodic contraction of cervical muscles is produced by movement. Lancet **1867**, 128.
Naffziger, H. C.: Discussion of paper by P. C. Bucy and T. J. Case: Athetosis. II. Surgical treatment of unilateral athetosis. Arch. of Neur. **37**, 1017 (1937).
Nasaroff, N. N.: Über Alkoholinjektionen in die kortikale Hirnsubstanz bei Athetose. Zbl. Chir. **54**, 1478 (1927).
Niemeyer, P.: Tratamento cirurgico do tremor parkinsoniano, da atetose e outras hipercinesias (14 casos operados). Med. cir. farm. (Brasil.) **116**, 654 (1945).
Oldberg, E.: Discussion of paper by T. J. Putnam: Results of treatment of athetosis by section of extrapyramidal tracts in the spinal cord. Arch. of Neur. **39**, 272 (1938).
Olivecrona, H.: Der spastische Schiefhals und seine Behandlung. Arch. klin. Chir. **167** (1931).
Oliver, L. C.: Surgery in Parkinson's disease. Division of lateral pyramidal tract for tremor. Report on 48 operations. Lancet **1**, 910—913 (1949).
— The present position of surgery in the treatment of Parkinsonism, Practitioner **163**, 541 (1949).
— Surgery in Parkinson's disease: complete section of the lateral column of the spinal cord for tremor. Lancet **1**, 847—848 (1950).
Oppenheim, H.: Lehrbuch der Nervenkrankheiten. Berlin: S. Karger 1898.
Paillas, J. E., J. Boudouresques, J. Cain et J. Tamalet: Hémimyoclonies datant de 30 ans avec hémiplegie posttraumatique. Sédation après opération de Bucy. Revue neur. **70**. 139 (1947).
— — et J. Pellegrin: Trois observations de dyskinésies traitées par intervention sur le cortex (aires 4 et 6). Revue neur. **80**, 557 (1948).
Papez, J. W.: A summary of fiber connections of the basal ganglia. Proc. Assoc. Res. Nerv. a. Ment. Dis. **21**, 21 (1942).
Parkinson, J.: An essay on the shaking palsy. London: Sherwood, Neely & Jones 1817.
Payr, O. O.: Athetose. Münch. med. Wschr. **1921**, 1570.
Peiper, H.: Die Chirurgie des Rückenmarks und seiner Häute. In Kirschner-Nordmanns Handbuch, Die Chirurgie, Bd. III, S. 881—996. Wien: Urban & Schwarzenberg 1948.
Penfield, W., and T. Rasmussen: The cerebral cortex of man. A clinical study of localization of function, S. 248. London: Macmillan & Co. 1950.
Pollock, L. J., and L. Davis: Muscles tone in Parkinsonian states. Arch. of Neur. **23**, 303 (1930).
Poppen, J. L., and A. Martinez-Niochet: Spasmodic torticollis. Surg. Clin. N. Amer. **1951**, 883—890.
Puech, P., H. Fischgold, Th. Gibert et C. Dreyfus-Brisac: Absences, épilepsie bravias-jacksonienne droite et athétose brachiale droite. Résultats de l'excision corticale limitée. Revue neur. **81**, 760 (1949).
Putnam, T. J.: Treatment of athetosis and dystonia by section of extrapyramidal motor tracts. Arch. of Neur. **29**, 504—521 (1933).
— Myelotomia longitudinalis, a commissural cervical chordotomy for pain of the upper extremities, Arch. of Neur. **32**, 1189 (1934).
— Results of treatment of athetosis by section of extra-pyramidal tracts in the spinal cord. Arch. of Neur. **39**, 258 (1938).
— Relief from unilateral paralysis agitans by section of the pyramidal tract. Arch. of Neur. **40**, 1049 (1938).
— Paralysis agitans and athetosis: Manifestations and methods of treatment. Arch. of Neur. **43**, 170 (1940).
— Treatment of unilateral paralysis agitans by section of the lateral pyramidal tract. Arch of Neur. **44**, 950 (1940).
— The operative treatment of diseases characterized by involuntary movements (tremor, athetosis). Proc. Assoc. Res. Nerv. a. Ment. Dis. **21**, 666 (1941).
— The surgical treatment of the dyskinesias. Ann. Western Med. a. Surg. **1949**.
— The neurology and neurosurgery of cerebral palsies and related disorders. Nerv. Child. **8**, 170—176 (1949).
—, and E. Herz: Results of spinal pyramidotomy in the treatment of the Parkinsonian syndrome. Arch of Neur. **63**, 357 (1950).
— — and C. H. Glaser: Spasmodic torticollis, III. Surgical treatment. Arch of Neur. **61**, 227 (1949).
Puusepp, L.: Cordotomia posterior lateralis (fascic. Burdachi) on account of trembling and hypertonia of the muscles in the hand. To the physiology of the posterior columns in the human body. Fol. neuropath. eston. **10**, 62 (1930).
Quervain, F. de: Le traitement chirurgical du torticolis spasmodique d'après la méthode de Kocher. Semaine méd. **16**, 405 (1896).
Rao, L., and R. Morea: Suggestion de tratamiento de los sindromes parkinsonianos por la lobotomia prefrontal (nota previa). Semana méd. **56**, 133 (1949).

REID, W. L.: Studies on the tremor-rigidity syndrome. I. Surgical treatment of human subjects. Med. J. Austral. **2**, 481 (1948).
RIECHERT, T.: Persönliche Mitteilung 1953.
— R. HASSLER u. M. WOLFF: Methodik der gezielten Hirnoperation. Jahrestgg der Dtsch. Ges. Neurol. u. Dtsch. Ges. Neurochir. 25. bis 27. Sept. 1952 in Hamburg.
—, u. M. WOLFF: Über ein neues Zielgerät zur intracraniellen elektrischen Ableitung und Ausschaltung. Arch. f. Psychiatr. u. Z. Neur. **186**, 225 (1951).
RIESSNER, D.: Cervikale Sympathektomie beim PARKINSON-Syndrom. Kolloquium ehem. Mitarbeiter von TÖNNIS in Köln. Jan. 1952.
RIZZATTI, E., e G. MORENO: Cordotomia laterale posteriore nella cura delle ipertonie extrapiramidali postencefalitiche. Schizofrenie **5**, 117 (1936).
ROMBERG, M. H.: Lehrbuch der Nervenkrankheiten des Menschen, Bd. II, S. 53—56. Berlin: A. Duncker 1851.
— Zit. nach CURTIS MARSHALL in A. E. WALKER, A History of Neurological Surgery, S. 303. Baltimore: Williams & Wilkins Company 1951.
ROTHMANN, M., u. A. SCHÜLLER: Zit. nach O. FOERSTER, 1913, 1927.
— M.: Über die hohe Durchschneidung des Seitenstranges und Vorderstranges beim Affen. Verh. Berl. Physiol. Ges. 1902, S. 12—16 (Arch. Anat. usw.).
— Über die Ergebnisse der experimentellen Ausschaltung der motorischen Funktion und ihre Bedeutung für die Pathologie. Z. klin. Med. **48**, 10 (1903).
SACHS, E.: The subpial resection of the cortex in the treatment of Jacksonian epilepsy (HORSLEY-Operation) with observations on Area 4 and 6. Brain **58**, 492 (1935).
— Trans. Amer. Neur. Assoc. **68**, 80 (1942).
SCHALTENBRAND, G.: Klinik und Behandlung des Torticollis spasticus. Dtsch. Z. Nervenheilk. **145**, 36 (1938).
SCHÜLLER, A.: Über operative Durchtrennung der Rückenmarksstränge (Chordotomie). Wien. med. Wschr. **1910**, 2292.
SCHÜRMANN, K.: Die Durchschneidung der Pyramidenvorderstränge und benachbarter extrapyramidaler Bahnen bei spastischen Zuständen und unwillkürlichen Bewegungen. Zbl. Neurochir. **9**, 136 (1949). — Dtsch. Z. Nervenheilk. **163**, 27 (1949).
— Über das Spätergebnis der chirurgischen Behandlung extrapyramidaler Bewegungsstörungen und paraplegischer Zustände. (Bericht über 33 Fälle.) Dtsch. Z. Nervenheilk. **169**, 24 (1952). Nervenarzt **24**, 252 (1953).
— „Tractotomia postero-lateralis et ventralis“ oder „Kombinierte Hinterseiten-Vorderstrangdurchschneidung“. Ein neues Operationsverfahren bei halbseitigen extrapyramidalen Hyperkinesen. Jahrestagg Dtsch. Ges. Neurol. u. Dtsch. Ges. Neurochir. 25. bis 27. Sept. 1952 in Hamburg. Dtsch. Z. Nervenheilk. **170**, 61 (1953).
— Die extrapyramidalen Hyperkinesen. (Übersichtsreferat.) Zbl. Neurochir. **13**, 223 (1953).
— Offene chirurgische Eingriffe am Zentralnervensystem bei Bewegungsstörungen. Ref. Kongr. der Ges. Dtsch. Neurologen und Psychiater, 20. Sept. 1955 in Hamburg. Dtsch. Z. Nervenheilk. **175**, 191—204 (1956).
—, u. H. TELLENBACH: Ein extrapyramidales Anfallssyndrom und seine Behandlung. Mschr. Psychiatr. **1926**, 378 (1953).
SCOTT, M.: Cerebral and spinal operations in a case of severe postencephalitic tremors. Arch. of Neur. **51**, 168 (1944).
SELIG, H.: Intrapelvine extraperitoneale Resektion des Nervus obturatorius und anatomische Studien über die Topographie dieses Nerven. Arch klin. Chir. **103**, 994 (1914).
SJÖQVIST, O.: Surgery in Parkinsons's disease. Zbl. Neurochir. **14**, 16—21 (1954).
SORGO, W.: Die lumbosakrale Myelektomie zur Behandlung der paraplegischen Kontrakturen der Beine. Acta neurochir. (Wien) **2**, 240 (1952).
SPIEGEL, E. A.: Siehe auch H. T. WYCIS.
—, and H. T. WYCIS: Physiological and psychological results of thalamotomy. Proc. Roy. Soc. **42**, 84 (1949).
— — Thalamotomy recording in man with special reference to seizure discharges. Electroencephalogr. Clin. Neurophysiol. **2**, 23 (1950).
— — Pallidothalamotomy in chorea. Trans. Phil. Neurol. Soc. Arch. of Neur. **64**, 295 (1950).
— — Effect of thalamic and pallidal lesions upon involuntary movements in choreoathetosis. Trans. Amer. Neur. Assoc. **75**, 234 (1950).
— — Thalamotomy and Pallidotomy for treatment of Choreic movements. Acta neurochir. (Wien) **2**, 417 (1952).
— — Ansotomy in paralysis agitans. Arch of Neur. **71**, 598—614 (1954).
— — and J. W. BAIRD: Studies in Stereoencephalotomy. I. Topical relationships of subcortical structures to the posterior commissure. Confinia neur. (Basel) **12**, 121 (1952).
— — and H. FREED: Stereoencephalotomy, thalamotomy and related procedures. J. Amer. Med. Assoc. **148**, 446 (1952).

Spiegel, E. A., H. T. Wycis, H. Freed and A. J. Lee: Stereoencephalotomy. Proc. Soc. Exper. Biol. a. Med. **69**, 175 (1948).

— — M. Marks and A. J. Lee: Stereotaxic apparatus for operations on the human brain. Science (Lancaster, Pa.) **106**, 349 (1947).

Spiller, W.G., C. H. Frazier and J. J. A. van Kaathoven: Treatment of selected casas of cerebral, spinal and periperhal nerve palsies and athetosis by nerve transplantation. With the report of a case of athetosis benefited by operation. Amer. J. Med. Sci. **131**, 430 (1906).

—, and E. Martin: The treatment of persistent pain of organic origin in the lower part of the body by division of the anterolateral column of the spinal cord. J. Amer. Med. Assoc. **58**, 1489 (1912).

Stoffel, A.: Eine neue Operation zur Beseitigung der spastischen Lähmungen. Münch. med. Wschr. **1911**, 2493—2498.

— Zur Chirurgie der peripheren Nerven. 83. Verslg Dtsch. Naturforsch. u. Ärzte in Karlsruhe vom 24.—29. Sept. 1911.

Sultan, G.: Zit. nach H. Peiper, Die Chirurgie des Rückenmarks und seiner Häute. In Handbuch Kirschner-Nordmann, Die Chirurgie, Bd. III, S. 881—996. Wien: Urban & Schwarzenberg 1948.

Takebayashi, H.: "T-Tomy", a new technique in extrapyramidal surgery. Med. J. Osaka Univ. **2**, 517 (1951) (in engl. Sprache).

Talairach, J.: Persönliche Mitteilung 1953.

— J. de Ajuriaguerra et M. David: A propos des coagulations thérapeutiques sous-corticales. Étude topographique du système ventriculaire en fonction des noyaux gris centraux. Presse méd. **1950**, 697—701.

— — — Étude stéréotaxiques des structures encéphaliques profondes chez l'homme. Technique. — Intéret physiopathologique et thérapeutique. Presse méd. **1952**, 605.

— H. Hécaen, M. David, M, Monnier et J. de Ajuriaguerra: Recherches sur la coagulation thérapeutique des structures souscorticales chez l'homme. Revue neur. **81**, 4 (1949).

— J., J. E. Paillas et M. David: Dyskinésie de type hémiballique traitée par cortectomie frontale limitée puis par coagulation de l'anse lenticulaire et de la portion interne du globus pallidus. Amélioration importante depuis un an. Revue neur. **83**, 440 (1950).

Taylor, A. S.: Operation for relief of spasmodic torticollis. In A. B. Johnson, Operative Therapeusis; Bd. 1, S. XXXIV, 533, New York u. London: D. Appleton & Comp. 1915.

Thiébaut, F., E. Wolinetz et G. Guiot: Syndrome du noyau rouge avec tremblement du type de Benedict, traité par excision corticale. Revue neur. **78**, 612 (1946).

Tietze u. Foerster (1912): Zit. nach Foerster (Vorderseitenstrangdurchschneidung 1913).

Tönnis, W.: Die Chirurgie des Gehirns und seiner Häute. In Handbuch Kirschner-Nordmann, Die Chirurgie, Bd. III. Wien: Urban & Schwarzenberg 1948.

Tower, S. S.: Extrapyramidal action from the cat's cerebral cortex: motor and inhibitory. Brain **59**, 408 (1936).

Verbiest, H.: Neurosurgical experiences in the treatment of spasmodic torticollis, athetosis and parkinsonian tremor. Fol. psychiatr., néerl. **52**, 204 (1949).

Vogt, C., u. O. Vogt: Allgemeinere Ergebnisse unserer Hirnforschung. J. Psychol. u. Neurol. **25**, 221 (1919).

Walker, A. E.: Mesencephalic tractotomy. A method for the relief of unilateral intractable pain. Arch. Surg. **44**, 953 (1942).

— Cerebral pedunculotomy for the relief of involuntary movements: Hemiballismus. Acta psychiatr. (København.) **24**, 723—729 (1949).

— The surgical treatment of involuntary movements. Texas Rep. Biol. a. Med. **10**, 105 (1952).

— Persönliche Mitteilung 1954.

Wertheimer, P., et L. Mansuy: La pyramidotomie pédonculaire dans le traitement des dyskinésies. A propos de deux observations. Revue neur. **83**, 433 (1950).

Wilson, S. A. K.: Modern problems in neurology. Baltimore: William Wood & Co. 1940. 364 S.

Winslow, R., and I. J. Spear: Section of posterior spinal nerve roots for relief of gastric crises and athetoid and choreiform movements. J. Amer. Med. Assoc. **58**, 238 (1912).

Wohlfahrt u. Forsock: Zit. nach M. David u. a. (Traitement chirurgical des dyskinésies 1952).

Woolsey, C. N.: Patterns of sensory representation in the cerebral cortex. Federat. Proc. **6**, 437 (1947).

Wycis, H. T.: Siehe auch E. A. Spiegel u. a.

—, and E. A. Spiegel: Ansotomy in paralysis agitans. Confinia neur. (Basel), Sep.-Bd. **12**, 245 (1952).

— — The effect of thalamotomy and pallidotomy upon involuntary movements in chorea and athetosis. Zit. nach David, Hecaen, Talairach 1952.

Wyke, B.: Zit. nach Cobb, Pool, Scarff, Schwab, Walker u. White (Section of "U"-Fibers etc. 1950).

Zülch, K. J.: Diskussion zur Physiologie und Pathophysiologie der Motorik, Hyperkinesen usw. Freiburger Symposion. Heidelberg: Springer 1954. — Zbl. Neurochir. **14**, 48 (1954).

— Persönliche Mitteilung 1954.

# Psychosurgery.

By

EDUARD BUSCH.

With 13 figures.

## I. Development of modern psychosurgery.

The date of November 12, 1935 might with some reason be taken as the date of birth of modern psychosurgery. At this date EGAS MONIZ and PEDRO ALMEIDA LIMA were at last ready to perform their first intervention on the human frontal lobes in an attempt to relieve mental disease. It is true that psychosurgical procedures have been used previously, and even with effect. It has been assumed that operations, at least upon the skull, were carried out in prehistoric times in order to let out the devils who had changed formerly normal members of the tribe into shrieking maniacal demons, and the locations of some of these craniectomies make it probable that such operations were not in all instances carried out in traumatic disease. No certain knowledge has, however, come down to us, and the indication for what must have been a formidable surgical procedure may have been the demons of epilepsy or migraine—or the operations may have had quite different reasons. We know, however, that "trepanations" were carried out in the times of ROGER OF SALERNO, and SEVERINUS advised "trephinations" in melancholia and mania.

Subsequent to the spectacular rise of modern psychosurgery the work of a Swiss psychiatrist, BURCKHARDT, became known. BURCKHARDT described his operations in 1891 and seems to have performed the first ,,topectomies" in his six schizophrenics, mostly with auditory hallucinations. Several of his patients improved and became more amenable following excisions of variable amounts of temporal cortex carried out in several stages. BURCKHARDT's ideas met with no succes — they were forgotten and first unburied following the work of MONIZ.

The birth of psychosurgery is a good illustration of the usefulness of scientific collaboration and may convince even the most sceptical of the use of medical meetings. At the International Congress of Neurology in London 1935 BRICKNER communicated his detailed study of a patient of DANDY's with bilateral frontal lobectomy, and this report together with the experimental evidence of FULTON and JACOBSEN made fertile repercussions in the mind of EGAS MONIZ, who for several years had spent much thought on these problems. MONIZ brought to this study what may be called an "anatomical" mind—the preparations of RAMON Y CAJAL made him think of the felt of fibrils and their interspaced synapses, and the picture of psychical processes as currents moving in this network was always present in his mind. The fixed ideas of some psychotics, where the same train of thought is repeated again and again, made him think that the impulses in such brains were travelling repeatedly along the same pathways. "*To change these paths chosen by the impulses so as to modify the corresponding ideas and force thought into different channels*" was the purpose of his first operations. "*Being convinced of the importance of the prefrontal lobes in mental life, I chose this region*" and again "*by upsetting the existing adjustments and setting into movement other fibril-synapsis groups, I expected to be able to transform the psychic reactions and to relieve the patient thereby.*"

At the above mentioned date the first alcohol injection in the human frontal lobe was consequently carried out, and December 27, of the same year ALMEIDA LIMA performed the first „leucotomy" by means of the "leucotome".

In his paper "*How I came to perform prefrontal leucotomy*" from which the above quotations are taken, MONIZ quotes from his *Tentatives Operatoires: "We are certain that these experiments shall stir up keen discussions in the medical, psychiatric, psychological, social, philosophical and other fields*". The instant reactions to MONIZ's ideas were, however, only feeble. In Italy RIZATTI and in America MATTOS PIMENTA and FREEMAN and WATTS were among the few pioneers (1936). From Italy came the first technical modification when FIAMBERTI inaugurated the *transorbital* approach, either cutting part of the frontal lobe or injecting formalin—MARRIOTTI and SCIUTI later substituted the patients' own blood for formalin. ODY in 1936 tried unilateral frontal *lobectomy* and thought this operation preferable to the bilateral one of MONIZ.

Little interest was, however, shown by the medical profession as a whole. Most older neurosurgeons will from personal experience remember the feeble response which the report of FREEMAN elicited on the *International Congress of Neurology* in Copenhagen 1939. Even with the shadows of the coming war clouding the minds of the participants, one should have thought that reactions, positive or negative, would have been more vigorous. The responses, mostly adverse, were however of a singularly uninterested type. During the war work was going on in North and South America, while Europe was otherwise engaged, MONIZ and ALMEIDA meanwhile studiously and soberly continuing work in peaceful Portugal.

Even if interest quickened somewhat in different circles it might with some justice be said that the problem of psychosurgery was not seriously faced by the medical profession until the publication of the book *Psychosurgery* (1942) by FREEMAN and WATTS. The importance of the work done by these two pioneers lies not in the fact that they were among the first to take up psychosurgery, but in the singularly logical and purposeful way in which their work was performed. Dissatified with the technic of MONIZ they introduced a standard procedure called by them *lobotomy* which, even if imperfect, was a conspicuos advance towards more exact operations. While the psychosurgery of EGAS MONIZ may have its origin in theoretical considerations, it was still to a large extent purely empirical. Nobody knew if MONIZ's ideas of "breaking up patterns" were referable to anatomical and psychological facts. FREEMAN and WATTS not only examined their patients conscientiously, drawing conclusions from psychiatric and psychological studies, but they strove valiantly to correlate the effect of lobotomy with what was known of the anatomy of the frontal lobe, and they soon centred their attention on the *anterior thalamic radiation* directly connecting the frontal lobe and the thalamus. It happened that a number of workers in the thirties had occupied themselves in this field (METTLER, LE GROS CLARK a. o.) and especially had the experimental study of WALKER (1938) shown that the dorsomedial nucleus of the thalamus will degenerate if the frontal pole is excised, and that the thalamo-frontal pathway contains as well afferent as efferent fibres. As early as 1926 HERRICK suspected this and set up what he called "*a very attractive hypothesis, though it must be admitted, not adequately supported anatomically and physiologically*", namely that the "*thalamo-frontal connections provide for the addition within the prefrontal fields of affective impulses of thalamic origin*". FREEMAN and WATTS found in autopsies of lobotomized patients that the most outstanding change was a degeneration of the dorsomedial nucleus of the thalamus. Not only did FREEMAN and WATTS in their book try to link psychosurgical procedures with anatomical and physiological facts, but they also stressed the importance of section of the frontal lobe taking place in a special plane—which they rather surprisingly found to be represented by the coronal suture of the skull. They called this *the critical plane of section* and found that patients who had had their lobotomy anterior to this plane had insufficient relief from troublesome symptoms, but exhibiting no gross defects, while patients who had had their sections carried out posterior to this plane had serious complications—some dying with remarkable symptoms, while those who recovered exhibited a syndrome of inertia, disorientation and incontinence, which later changed into apathy and euphoric indifference. Operating under local anesthesia they found that they were able to sever about three-fourths of the white matter in the coronal plane (divided into four quadrants: right and left, upper and lower) until the fourth quadrant was cut, when sometimes within seconds, nervous tension would disappear, while the patient became confused and disorientated. They found that if these symptoms appeared during the operation they could feel fairly confident of a good result. In their book FREEMAN and WATTS also published a system of *postoperative treatment* and *training* and tried to define the field and the boundaries of these new surgical procedures. Even if other workers at the same time contributed much, and even if some conclusions later were found to be hasty and others doubtful, the work of FREEMAN and WATTS done with the heavy burden of daily routine added to patient exploration in a new field will always command respect. Their book is a conspicuous landmark in the history of psychosurgery.

Other neurosurgeons also modified the MONIZ-procedure, and as early as 1937 LYERLY performed the first "*open*" operation, sectioning the frontal lobes through a parasagittal craniotomy under direct vision using usual neurosurgical technic. The method has since been modified by several surgeons (POPPEN, SCARFF a. o.) and is widely used. Others tried to get a uniform plane of section in the "closed" lobotomy by elaborating special instruments and cranial localizers (LOVE, VIANNA a. o.), while some modified the MONIZ-leucotome (MCGREGOR and CRUMBIE, MCKENZIE a. o.). Many clung to simple instruments periosteal elevators, brain needles etc.

Even while interest was centred on *where* lobotomy most advantageously should be performed, the just as important question of *how much* should be cut was discussed. While enterprise at first was tempered by caution, succesful reoperations in previously incomplete lobotomies led to a feeling that as much as possible of the white matter should be sectioned. This led again to a realization of *the post-lobotomy syndrome*, which made it advisable to limit the section as much as possible consistent with effect on symptoms. In England CUNNINGHAM-DAX with RADLEY-SMITH used the MCGREGOR-CRUMBIE leucotome to perform "upper", "middle" and "lower" sections, while in other patients horizontal cuts were made. They concluded that there was some evidence that depressive patients were relieved by the lower section, aggressive patients by upper and paranoid schizophrenics by middle and horizontal cuts.

In 1945 HOFSTATTER a. o. reported on sectioning inferior quandrants only and reported as good results as those obtained in more extensive operations.

Some surgeons performed lobotomies in stages and this led to the introduction of *unilateral lobotomy*. Some patients improved following the first stage and in 1942 LYERLY stated that a complete unilateral lobotomy might be as effective as a partial bilateral one. Later on SCARFF and BUSCH reported favourably on unilateral lobotomy in the special field of otherwise intractable pain.

Work was now progressing in a number of places the world over, new ideas arose and old procedures were revived. ODY's early (1936) unilateral lobectomy was followed by the bilateral ones of PEYTON, NORAN and MILLER (1948) as a more exact and surgically satisfying procedure. Results, however, did not seem to warrant this extensive and time-consuming procedure when compared with the results obtained by more simple methods. The work of RYLANDER who meticulously examined patients following lobectomies performed in neurosurgical disease, corrected the previous assumption of lack of psychical defects following these operations. A wish for correlation of this mass of new evidence led to the publishing by *The Great Britain Board of Control* in 1947 of a material of 1000 lobotomized patients, showing a wide variation in technics and indications.

Another old technic revived was certainly simple and time-saving—if nothing else: The *transorbital lobotomy* of FIAMBERTI. A modification was presented (1948) by FREEMAN, who performed the operation in the coma following electro-shock. While complications were surprisingly low, effects seemed promising and personality defects rare, which made FREEMAN extend his indications considerably—not without opposition. FERNÁNDEZ-MORÁN also favoured this approach and reported results both from mechanical lobotomy and from injection of chemicals, among them novocaine. JONES and SHANKLIN found that the method might be of use in the group of patients which, irresponsive to shock-treatments, still presented no indication for major lobotomy.

In the hope of obtaining selective effect upon symptoms with the least possible defects, PENFIELD removed parts of frontal gyri (*gyrectomy*), but results were unconvincing. A more bold step in the same direction was taken in 1946, when the *Columbia-Greystone-Associates* took up the procedure to be known as *topectomy*. The whole project was admirably planned. Patients were studied and discussed by different and independent examiners and for the first time controls were used, closely matched with the patients undergoing surgery. The surgical procedure was excision of cortical tissue at symmetrical places in both frontal lobes, mostly in areas 9—10, but other operations were also used. Many useful points were gained from this study, and the operated patients showed a significantly higher percentage of improvement than the controls. Two years later the same group reported, that the attempt to find a correlation between the surgery done and the mental changes following had failed. Meanwhile the method of topectomy was taken up by several groups among whom LE BEAU reported considerable success as well in mental disease as in otherwise intractable pain. His excisions were mostly limited to areas 9—10. LE BEAU a. o. moreover reported that postoperative mental defects seemed considerably less than in the usual lobotomies. Another type of topectomy was introduced by CAIRNS and by LE BEAU, who excised the *gyrus cinguli* and found some effect in psychoneuroses and in pain, none in severe psychoses. The procedure was exact and surgically attractive and it was concluded that it might be of use in a restricted group of patients.

The method of topectomy made an appeal to most neurosurgeons, combining usual neurosurgical principles with as much exactitude as one can expect in this difficult field. The draw-back was the extensive cortical scars resulting. Still, this method would surely have had greater popularity, if SCOVILLE had not about the same time published his *selective cortical undercutting*. This method of bloodlessly undermining definitely localized areas of cortex, preserving its blood-supply, made its appeal to several workers. In his original operations SCOVILLE selected three different technics: Undercutting of *the lateral convexity* (mostly areas 9—10), of *the orbital surface* and of *the medial and cingulate areas*, and he hoped to be able to draw conclusions as to which procedure should be most appropriate in dealing with different symptoms. Results for the three different procedures have, however, up to now scarcely been significantly different—nor was any certain difference seen between the results of SCOVILLE's three procedures and the series of BUSCH, who undercut the medial surface and the medial half of the orbital surface. However, both series were too small to give certainty, and the important question of quantitative or qualitative effect of psychosurgery was still open.

As noted above several workers had centred their interest on the orbitomedial part of the frontal lobe and recently GRANTHAM, following air-studies, coagulated white matter just medial to the anterior horn by a diathermy-electrode introduced through a burr hole. He reported promising results in otherwise intractable pain and later in mental disease.

*Pool* of the *Columbia-Greystone* project tried *ligation of parasagittal veins* without effect, but introduced the method of thermo-coagulation of DUSSER DE BARENNE in this field as it previously had been used in focal epilepsy.

While interest so far had been focused on the frontal lobe, SPIEGEL and WYCIS turned to the other end of the thalamo-frontal system. Using an ingenious modification of the stereo-taxic HORSLEY-CLARKE apparatus they were able to make small and surprisingly exact lesions in the nuclei of the thalamus. During operation they were able to take electroencephalographic tracings from various subcortical nuclei, and as experience was gained the method seemed promising. It was shown that effect in mental disease was roughly parallel to that shown by frontal lobotomy. The method was taken up in several countries, among them France (TALAIRACH, and associates), Sweden (LEKSELL) and Germany (RIECHERT, KÖPKE a. o.), but its value in clinical routine is still to be proved.

*Temporal* (OBRADOR, PIMENTA a. o.), *parietal* (PIMENTA) and *occipital* (TORKILDSEN) lobotomies were tried, but without conclusive evidence. It seemed, however, that *temporal* lobotomy might be of help in special cases (see p. 163). The conclusion of TORKILDSEN in one case of *occipital* lobotomy (in a blind patient) was that no effect could be expected from this procedure, bur even this seems unwarranted as the patient was deteriorated. In a patient with auditory hallucinations FREEMAN excised the *amygdaloid nucleus* with some success.

Much useful evidence has been gathered by various teams, among them the *Boston* group, headed by GREENBLATT, ARNOT and SOLOMON, the above mentioned *Columbia-Greystone Project*, YAHN, PIMENTA and their associates, and several British groups. On an international basis correlation was sought through the *First International Conference on Psychosurgery* in Lisbon 1948 held under the auspices of EGAS MONIZ and planned by FREEMAN. Since then much work has been done, but, as might be expected, the problems of psychosurgery were found to be hydras—new problems arose from every one solved.

At the moment of writing there is no doubt that psychosurgery in one form or another is the only hope of numerous afflicted human beings. On the other hand it must always be recognized that these operations after all are destructive brain lesions, and it is to be hoped that they in the time to come will be supplanted by other, more adequate and less destructive, methods of treatment. Some promising beginning has been made by the introduction of drugs of the chlorpromazine and Rauwolfia groups. Psychosurgery, however, still retains the role in treatment which it in our opinion always has had—the *ultimum refugium* in otherwise intractable mental disease.

## II. Anatomical and physiological considerations.

Our knowledge of the inner anatomy of the human frontal lobe is still meagre. In the late thirties several workers interested themselves in these problems, mainly by doing degeneration studies in animals, but while valuable knowledge was gained by these means, it was of course evident, that conclusions drawn from such material must be irrelevant as to the human frontal lobe. In the human brain the frontal lobe goes posteriorly as far back as the Rolandic and the Sylvian fissures, the part lying rostral to the motor area being by MONIZ called the "prefrontal" area. The division of the frontal lobe into upper, middle and inferior gyri is of little practical use. More importance is to be attached to the cytoarchitectural divisions furnished by the pioneer work of BRODMANN, the VOGT's, ECONOMO a. o. Still, considerable uncertainty exists. Roughly the frontal lobe may be divided into an *agranular* portion (mainly motor, BRODMANN's areas 4—6), while area 8 and part of area 9 also are agranular together with the most posterior parts of the orbital surface. The rest of the frontal lobe is mainly *granular*.

*Afferent connections*, of the "prefrontal" areas arise in the nuclei of the thalamus (fig. 1) and from the painstaking studies of especially McLARDY it seems that in man as in animals (WALKER) a close *point-to-point relationship* exists between thalamic nuclei and definite parts of the frontal lobe. It seems that, grossly, the lateral part of the dorsomedial nucleus projects to the lateral convexity of the frontal lobe, while the medial part projects to the medial part and to the orbital surface. The anterior nucleus of the thalamus would a. o. seem to project to the cingulate gyrus. From the hypothalamus projections seem to go especially to the orbital surface.

*Efferent connections* (fig. 2) go from the frontal lobe to the thalamus—"a two-way-track" thus being established, even if the efferent pathways are considerably smaller in number than the afferent. Direct connections seem to go to the hypothalamus, indirect by way of the dorsomedial nucleus.

Even if the anatomical studies thus have given us a rude charting of the connections of the human frontal lobe with other parts of the brain, more, and more important, knowledge has been gained by physiological methods, especially by the "psychobiological" school started by THORNDIKE, FRANZ, LASHLEY a. o., who studied the behaviour of animals following excisions of differents parts of the brain. While the earlier workers were able to gain some evidence of connection between discriminating habits and various parts of the brain, the tendency later swung to the concept of "equipotentiality" of the cortex and a certain sense of frustration was felt as to the possibility of connecting form and function until the growing evidence of definite point-to-point relationship between cortical areas and various subcortical nuclei again gave some hope of finding definite patterns. The work done by FULTON and his associates has gone far in establishing such evidence and with the arrival of psychosurgery a great need and an unique chance came of correlating conclusions drawn from animal experiments and the human brain. In this field, also, pioneer work was done by FREEMAN and WATTS, who noted degeneration of the dorsomedial nucleus of the thalamus in lobotomized patients, and the work has been carried on by others, especially by MEYER and his coworkers GLEES a. o. The undoubtedly best and most informative surveys of these problems are at the moment of writing FULTON's book *Frontal Lobotomy and Affective Behaviour* (1951) and the work of MEYER and BECK (1954) to which the reader is referred. Here only a brief summary shall be given with strict reference to psychosurgical problems.

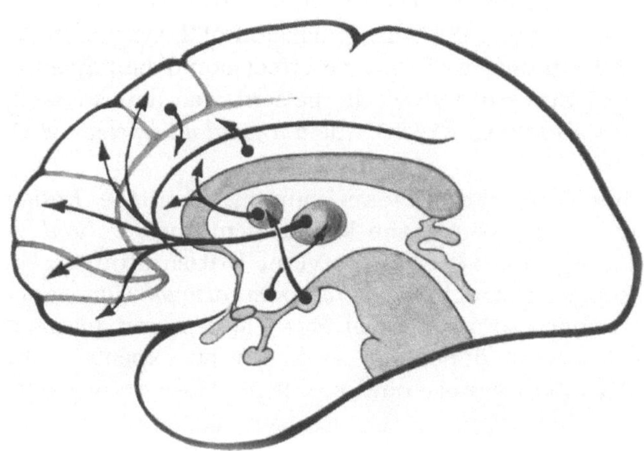

Fig. 1. Afferent connections of the human frontal lobe. After LE GROS CLARK.

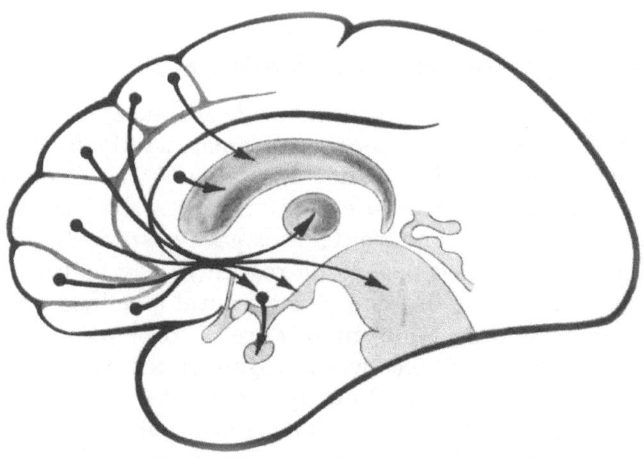

Fig. 2. Efferent connections of the human frontal lobe. After LE GROS CLARK.

Cytoarchitecturally the cortex is divided in three main divisions:

1. *Archipallium* (archicortex, allocortex) including the primitive rhinencephalon—olfactory bulb, tubercle, uncus, septum, dentate gyrus and hippocampus. This cortex mainly consists of three layers.

2. *Mesopallium* (palaeocortex) is six-layered, but of transitional type, and includes the posterior part of the orbital surface, the anterior part of the insula, pyriform, anterior hippocampus, cingulate gyrus and subcallosal regions.

3. *Neopallium* (neocortex, ectopallium) with six layers, fully developed.

Physiological studies have now shown that the mesopallium operates through the *visceral brain*—i. e. the ascending tracts of visceral impulses go into the hypothalamus, dividing into two groups, those to the anterior thalamic nuclei projecting to the cingulate gyrus, those going into the dorsomedial nuclei projecting to the transitional cortex of the posterior part of the orbital surface, the insula and the anterior tip of the temporal lobe. MACLEAN concludes that the phylogenetically older regions have to do with *visceral* and *emotional* reactions, while *intellectual* functions are associated with the newest and most highly developed parts of the frontal lobes. Recent physiological research has shown that several "visceral" responses can be obtained by stimulation of just these "visceral" parts of the brain, and confirmatory evidence is to be had from strychninization experiments. It would thus seem that we now have some evidence for the theory of PAPEZ (1937) that "*the hypothalamus, the anterior thalamic nuclei, the gyrus cinguli, the hippocampus and interconnections constitute a harmonious mechanism which elaborate the functions of central emotion as well as participate in emotional expression*".

The importance of these conclusions for surgery intended to influence the affective behaviour of patients will be evident, and their further importance for the various theories of the action of lobotomy clear. This will be discussed later when dealing with the type of lobotomy to be preferred, but it should already in this place be clearly stated that the theory of "equipotentiality" of the frontal cortex does *not* seem to be supported by what scanty anatomical and physiological evidence we do possess.

## III. Different forms of lobotomy.

### 1. The leucotomy of EGAS MONIZ.

Even if the original method of EGAS MONIZ now is mainly of historical interest it is still used in some clinics and no technic of psychosurgery would be complete without describing it. MONIZ designed the *cerebral leucotome* — a canula 11 cm. long with an external diameter of 2 mm. Through an opening 5 mm. from the end a loop of steel could be pushed out and again withdrawn.

MONIZ' own words are respectfully reproduced from his Les Premieres Tentatives Operatoires dans le Traitement de Certaines Psychoses (1936): "*On fait deux trous de trépan d'un centimètre de largeur dans la région frontale, un de chaque coté, à trois centimètres de la ligne médiane fronto-occipitale et dans une autre ligne perpendiculaire à la premiere et qui passe à trois centimètres en avant du tragus. La projection de cette ligne sur le lobe frontal correspond à peu pres a la limite postérieure de ce que nous avons conventionellement apellé le lobe préfrontal, partie du cerveau sur laquelle on provoque les destructions.*

*La dure-mère, une fois coupée, et le cortex découvert pour éviter les vaisseaux, on l'incise et on y introduit le leucotome, avec l'anse rentrée, premièrement dans la direction antéro-interne a la profondeur de 4,5 centimètres. Ensuite, on fait sortir l'anse et on tourne le leucotome d'un tour et demi. On fait rentrer l'anse dans la canule, en tirant le fil de l'appareil. Après, on retire le leucotome d'un centimètre et demi (3,5 ou 3 centimètres de profondeur) et après avoir fait sortir l'anse, de nouveau on le tourne pour faire une seconde coupe. On fait ensuite rentrer l'anse du leucotome et on enlève celui-ci. On introduit de nouveau le leucotome par la même ouverture du cerveau, mais cette fois-ci dans le sens antéro-externe du centre ovale pour exécuter des sections semblables.*

*La même opération se fait dans le centre ovale de l'autre lobe préfrontal. Pour executer l'operation que nous avons faite au début de nos tentatives chirurgicales, par les injections de l'alcool, la technique est tout à fait semblable. Il ne faut que substituer le leucotome par une aiguille de la série de celles de "de Martel" pour la ponction ventriculaire. A chaque place nous avons injecté 0,2 centimètre cube d'alcool absolu. Nous avons fait trois types de distribution d'injections sclérosantes d'alcool. En angle, c'est-à-dire dans la position des coupes faites par le leucotome. En triangle, c'est-à-dire quatre injections aux endroits où nous faisons maintenant les 4 coupes (internes et externes) et encore deux autres injections faites en deux points perpendiculaires à la base du crâne, à 3 et à 4 centimètres de profondeur. Un total de 6 injections dans chaque lobe préfrontal. Finalement, nous avons fait une autre série d'injections, 6 en triangle et encore deux autres obliques dans le plan perpendiculaire qui passe par le point d'entrée de l'aiguille. A cette dernière alcoolisation nous avons donné le nom de barrière du lobe préfrontal.*

*Nous n'avons pas abandonné entièrement l'alcoolisation des centres ovales préfrontaux. Nous pratiquons toujours, comme première intervention, les coupes indiquées par le leucotome; mais dans le cas au cours desquels nous avons eu besoin de réopérer, nous faisons alors des injections d'alcool plus faciles à réaliser dans ces cas, à travers la peau, à la hauteur des trous de trépan."*

In this same communication MONIZ deplores the lack of precision of this method and thinks it probable that in time to come precision may be attained. Still, in the twenty cases of his communication 35% were considered clinically cured, 35% improved, while 10% were unchanged.

## 2. Prefrontal lobotomy of FREEMAN and WATTS.

### a) Original method.

The coronal sutures are marked on the shaven skin and small incisions made so that bilateral burr holes 1 cm. in diameter can be placed in the lower part of the suture at a point 6 cm. above the zygoma and on a line approximately 3 cm. behind the outer margin of the orbit (fig. 3). The burr holes are extended upwards and downwards by means of a rongeur, the dura opened and an avascular part of the cortex coagulated. Through a small cortical incision a brain canula is inserted in the direction of the contralateral burr hole passing anterior to the ventricle. In case the ventricle is tapped, the needle is withdrawn and reintroduced in a more anterior direction. The sphenoidal ridge is now located in the same way at a depth of 4—5 cm. from the cortex. It is stated that the distance from the cortex to the median plane at the point of operation usually will be 5,5—6 cm. By means of these three land-marks—the *sphenoidal ridge*, the *medial longitudinal fissure* and the *coronal suture* the desired plane is located and the lobotomy performed by means of a blunt dissector, a brain canula or a leucotome, which is inserted to a depth of approximately 5 cm., a hemostat being clamped to the instrument at a right angle. An assistant checks the plane and the section is carried out by a sweeping movement downwards until the floor of the anterior fossa is reached, when it is withdrawn gently in a lateral direction, thus completing the lower cut. The upper part of the frontal lobe is now cut in the same manner and the incision irrigated with saline. A few drops of lipiodol or other contrast medium is introduced in the cut and the incisions in dura, muscle, galea and skin closed. Roentgenograms are taken in both projections. In the bed the patient is placed in a semi-Fowler position, which is maintained for 72 hours and blood-pressure, pulse, respiration and temperature recorded in the usual way. Constant supervision in the first days is necessary as the patient may be confused and try to remove his dressing, which should be fixed firmly by means of taping or similar means. If the patient is drowsy he should be turned in his bed every few hours to avoid bed-sores and pulmonary complications. If there is vomiting, fluid (the first days restricted to 1000 cc. daily) should not be given by mouth. The patient is allowed outside his bed after 4—6 days.

**Comment.** With various modifications this operation was for several years the most frequently performed form of lobotomy—variations mainly being in form and size of the instrument selected for the cut. Realising that a straight instrument must leave out sections of white matter above and below, several curved instruments were used in the attempt of making as complete a section as possible. The operation is quick, but most neurosurgeons soon had misgivings. The greatest drawback is the difficulty of maintaining the chosen plane of section (FREEMAN and WATTS's "critical plane of section")

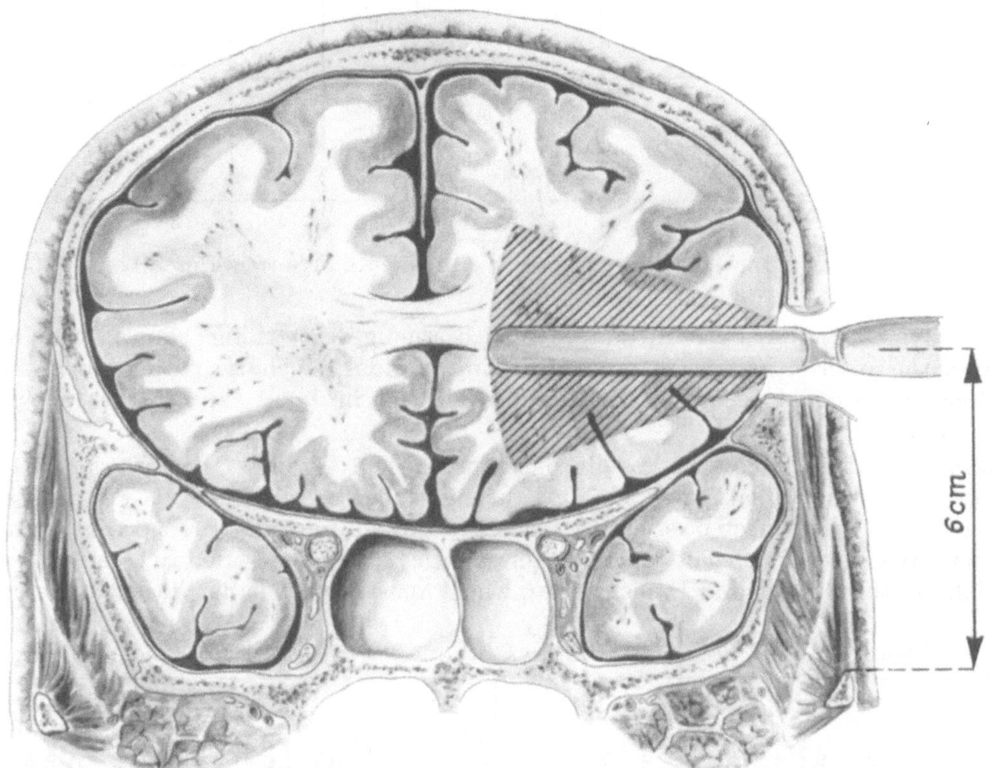


Fig. 3. Prefrontal lobotomy a. m. FREEMAN and WATTS. Original method.

Table 1. *Results of prefrontal lobotomy in schizophrenia.*
(From FREEMAN and WATTS, Psychosurgery, Springfield 1950.)

| Diagnosis | Number | Good % | Fair % | Poor % | Deaths operative % | Deaths later % |
|---|---|---|---|---|---|---|
| Catatonic . . | 128 | 39 | 35 | 20 | 2 | 4 |
| Hebephrenic . | 104 | 45 | 35 | 20 | — | — |
| Paranoid . . | 82 | 39 | 44 | 15 | — | 2 |
| Other . . . . | 14 | 22 | 36 | 36 | 6 | — |
| Total . . . . | 328 | 40 | 37 | 18 | 2 | 3 |

*Prefrontal lobotomy in schizophrenia.*
Present status of living patients — two to twelve years after operation.

| Diagnosis | Number | Employed % | Keeping house % | Home % | Institution % |
|---|---|---|---|---|---|
| Catatonic . . | 118 | 22 | 6 | 35 | 37 |
| Hebephrenic . | 103 | 15 | 11 | 37 | 37 |
| Paranoid . . | 80 | 18 | 9 | 42 | 31 |
| Other . . . . | 13 | 9 | 9 | 46 | 36 |
| Total . . . . | 314 | 21 | 8 | 38 | 33 |

and post-mortems all too frequently showed that the surgeon in spite of great care sectioned the frontal lobe in widely different planes in different patients. In some clinics

Table 2. *Results of prefrontal lobotomy 1949.*
(From FREEMAN and WATTS, Psychosurgery, Springfield 1950.)

| Diagnosis | No. | Good % | Fair % | Poor % | Deaths operative % | Deaths later[1] % |
|---|---|---|---|---|---|---|
| Schizophrenia . . . . . . . | 328 | 35 | 38 | 25 | 2 | 8 |
| Involutional psychoses . . . | 147 | 60 | 24 | 14 | 2 | 20 |
| Obsessive and psychoneuroses | 121 | 57 | 28 | 11 | 4 | 5 |
| Pain cases . . . . . . . . . | 21 | 43 | 38 | | 19 | 7 |
| Total . . . . . . . . . . . | 617 | 45 | 33 | 19 | 3 | 40 |

[1] Later deaths not included in tabulations. All patients were traced in 1949—1950.

preoperative air-studies were introduced, which among other things showed that a dilatation of the anterior horns was no rare finding in older psychotic patients and that no safe conclusions could be drawn from land-marks on the bony skull to the topography of the brain.

**Results.** Table 1 gives the results of FREEMAN and WATTS (Psychosurgery 1950) in schizophrenia, while table 2 gives the same authors' collected series (1949). For comparison is given (table 3) the collected series of PARTRIDGE and our personal series (table 4) with the FREEMAN-WATTS technic. The technic in these series may have varied to a certain extent, especially in the English and Danish series, where air-studies usually preceded operations.

Table 3. *Postoperative epilepsy.* After PARTRIDGE: Prefrontal leucotomy (1950).

| Cases still in hospital | | | | | | | | | | | | Cases discharged from hospital | | | | | | | | |
|---|---|---|---|---|---|---|---|---|---|---|---|---|---|---|---|---|---|---|---|---|
| Total | Deaths of operation | Delayed attributional deaths | Men Single occasion | Men Multiple attacks | Women Single occasion | Women Multiple attacks | Worse | Not improved | Conduct improved | Markedly improved | Improved to home level | Discharged against advice | Discharged though psychotic | Discharged psychotic relapsed | Discharged with psychotic traces | Discharged with psychotic traces and relapsed | Discharged recovered | Discharged recovered but relapsed | Recovered after relapse | Sustained recovery |
| *Incontestably schizophrenic cases* (without remissions). | | | | | | | | | | | | | | | | | | | | |
| 77 | 3 | 2 | 0/41 | 9/41 | 2/33 | 2/33 | 3 | 15 | 23 | 5 | 2 | 6 | 8<br>10 % | 1 | 7<br>9 % | 2 | 5<br>6.5 % | 1 | 0 | 6<br>7.8 % |
| *Preserved paranoid cases.* | | | | | | | | | | | | | | | | | | | | |
| 8 | 0 | 0 | 0 | 0 | 0 | 0 | 2 | 2 | 0 | 0 | 1 | 0 | 2<br>25 % | 0 | 0 | 0 | 1<br>12.5 % | 1 | 0 | 0 |
| *Schizophrenic cases with affective colouring* (without remissions). | | | | | | | | | | | | | | | | | | | | |
| 35 | 0 | 2 | 0/2 | 0/2 | 1/33 | 0/33 | 1 | 4 | 9 | 5 | 0 | 0 | 2<br>5.7 % | 1 | 4<br>11 % | 0 | 10<br>28.6 % | 1 | 1 | 9<br>25.7 % |
| *Recurrent schizophrenic cases* (with remissions). | | | | | | | | | | | | | | | | | | | | |
| 19 | 0 | 0 | 1/8 | 3/8 | 0/11 | 0/11 | 1 | 1 | 4 | 0 | 0 | 0 | 3<br>15.8 % | 0 | 1<br>5.3 % | 0 | 8<br>42 % | 4 | 3 | 4<br>21 % |
| *Other and non-classical schizophrenic cases* (without remissions). | | | | | | | | | | | | | | | | | | | | |
| 19 | 0 | 1 | 1/5 | 0/5 | 0/13 | 2/13 | 0 | 0 | 0 | 0 | 1 | 0 | 1<br>5.3 % | 0 | 4<br>21 % | 0 | 12<br>63 % | 0 | 0 | 12<br>63 % |

The technic seems to be abandoned in most psychosurgical centres—FREEMAN now mostly uses the transorbital technic, while more selective procedures have superseded this classical, but inexact procedure.

### b) Precision methods of FREEMAN and WATTS.

Later methods of lobotomy of FREEMAN and WATTS comprise three techniques: *Standard, radical* and *minimal.*

Table 4. *Results in 400 patients treated with lobotomy a. m.* FREEMAN-WATTS *(Copenhagen).* AC apparently cured; MI much improved; SI significantly improved; U unchanged; W worse; D deaths.

| | No. | AC | MI | SI | U | W | D |
|---|---|---|---|---|---|---|---|
| Schizophrenia | 322 | 2 | 9 | 122 | 182 | 1 | 6 |
| Manic depressive | 25 | 3 | 8 | 4 | 10 | 0 | 0 |
| Atypic. depressive psychosis | 4 | 0 | 1 | 2 | 1 | 0 | 0 |
| Involutional psychosis | 5 | 0 | 3 | 1 | 0 | 1 | 0 |
| Psychopathia | 24 | 0 | 3 | 12 | 8 | 0 | 1 |
| Psychogenic psychosis | 3 | 0 | 0 | 1 | 1 | 0 | 1 |
| Anankasmata (obsessive-compulsive reaction) | 16 | 4 | 0 | 4 | 7 | 0 | 1 |
| Epilepsy w. erethism. | 1 | 0 | 1 | 0 | 0 | 0 | 0 |
| Total | 400 | 9 | 25 | 146 | 209 | 2 | 9 |

The 9 deaths (D) are operative, making an operative mortality for the FREEMAN-WATTS-series of 2,25 %.

**Standard method.** As in the original technique the coronal suture and the midline are marked on the shaven skull (e.g. gentian violet), the position of the coronal suture in the midline being taken to be 13 cm. above the glabella in "normal" skulls, the lower end at a point 6 cm. above the zygoma and 3 cm. behind the lateral rim of the orbit. The 5 cm. long incisions are held open by means of retractors, burr holes, 1,5 cm. in diameter, made on both sides and enlarged upwards and downwards with a rongeur until they measure 2 cm. in the coronal line. The dura is incised, the cortex coagulated, and a canula, graduated in centimeters, made to pass from one burr hole to the other, the direction being controlled by a neurologist standing behind the patient and an applicator held against the contralateral burr hole. The diameter of the brain in this plane is now measured. Subsequently the sphenoidal ridge is located by introducing the canula in the coronal plane at an angle of 40° with the sagittal plane. The canula should strike the ridge at a depth of 4—5 cm.—if it goes deeper it will be in the middle fossa and must be reintroduced more anteriorly. The sphenoidal ridge is the most important guide to the *plane of section*, which will be somewhat (1—2 cms.) anterior to the marking of the coronal suture on the skin (the "13 cm. plane"); it is now marked on the skin and the lobotomy performed by means of the *precision leucotome* (fig. 4), this being inserted aimed at the contralateral burr hole. The section is carried out to a depth of half the brain diameter at this point *minus 1 cm.* in order to avoid the medial cortex and the anterior cerebral vessels. The instrument is now moved through an arc of 30—40°, the plane of section being controlled from above by the neurologist during the whole movement. Following this the cuts are irrigated with saline and deepened and extended by means of the *radial stab incisor*—a special instrument graduated in cms. The stab should pass into the corpus callosum and go to a depth nearly the full half of the brain diameter. Downwards the depth is controlled by feeling the resistance of the pia-arachnoid at a depth of 6—7 cms. One radial stab into the upper quadrant against the lower part of the falx completes the operation and the procedure is repeated on the other side. When the irrigating saline is clear lipiodol 0,5 $cm.^3$ is injected and the incisions closed as usual.

*Comment.* There is no doubt that this method is more precise than the original technique. FREEMAN and WATTS feel that they, using this technique, are able to perform a lobotomy within 2 mm. of a predetermined plane.

**Radical method.** In this procedure the plane of section may be 6—14 mm. *behind* the sphenoidal ridge, each millimeter being of importance for the later chances of readjustment of the patient.

As above the coronal suture and the midline is marked on the skin and a transverse incision made, 14 cm. long, above the suture. The pericranium is rougined away and the coronal and interparietal sutures identified. Burr holes, 1,5 cm. in diameter are made on each side 3,5 cm. lateral to the midline and enlarged with rongeurs until they measure 2 cm. in the coronal plane. The dura is incised, the cortex coagulated and incised. The sphenoidal ridge is located by means of the graduated canula being introduced in a plane posterior to the coronal suture, usually striking the ridge at a depth of 7—8 cm. The applicator held at the point 6 cm. above the zygoma and 3 cm. behind the rim of the orbit is now moved backwards to act as a guide to the cut, and it is stated that if the guide is moved 3 mm. posteriorly the knife will reach the base of the brain 10 mm. posteriorly to the ridge—if placed 4 mm. posteriorly the plane of lobotomy will be 12—13 mm. behind the ridge, and if moved only 2 mm. the plane will be 6 mm. posterior to the ridge. The method is stated to have a margin of error of 2 mm. When these measurements are

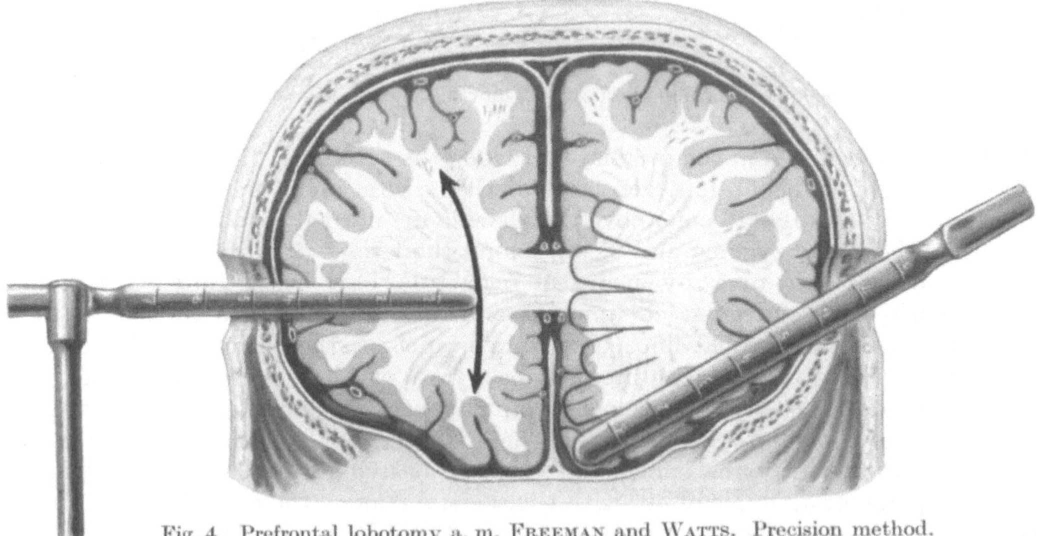

Fig. 4. Prefrontal lobotomy a. m. Freeman and Watts. Precision method.

made, the canula is reintroduced guided by the neurologist until it strikes the floor of the middle fossa at a depth of 1,5 cm. deeper than the anterior fossa. When the desired plane of section is marked the lobotomy is carried out by means of the precision leucotome, introduced to a depth of 6 cm., being swept through an arc of 30°—continously checked by the neurologist standing on the side. Medially the instrument is gently with-drawn without injuring the medial cortex. Following withdrawal, the leucotome is reintroduced and swept through 30° laterally again at a depth of 6 cm. After irrigation the fibres at the base of the frontal lobe are cut by radial stab incisions, the depth of the stabs varying between 7—8 cm., the pia-arachnoid being felt with the tip of the blunt instrument. The operation is completed by one stab against the falx and one laterally, after which the cuts are irrigated and the operation repeated on the other side. Lipiodol (0,5 cm.) is introduced and the wound closed.

*Comment.* Several neurosurgeons do not feel confident as to performing the cuts with the exactitude stated by Freeman and Watts and prefer to carry out „posterior" lobotomies under the guidance of the eye.

**Minimal operation.** This is the standard method (precision), but with the cuts into the upper quadrants omitted, stabs being made to the floor of the anterior fossa and one stab against the falx. Freeman and Watts mention another form of "minimal" operation—operating under local anesthesia they carry out the standard technique but stop when the patient becomes disorientated.

### c) Transorbital lobotomy.

Originally described by Fiamberti the technic of transorbital lobotomy has been perfected by Freeman, who for some reason performs the operation in the coma following electro-shock. For his first operations he used a common ice-pick, later a special leucotome, graduated in cm's and constructed of specially strong steel was constructed. Lifting the upper eyelid the instrument is placed against the vault of the orbit (fig. 5) keeping it parallel with the bony ridge of the nose and sligthly inclined to the midline. The instrument is said easily to penetrate the roof of the orbit in most cases, in others the bone is thickened and several taps with a hammer is necessary. When the 5 cm. mark is reached, the handle is pulled as far laterally as possible, severing the white matter at the base of the frontal lobe. The instrument is now returned halfway to the original position and driven to a depth of 7 cm. from the margin of the upper eyelid. A profile Roentgenogram is taken and the position checked. The instrument is now moved medially 15—20$^0$ and about 30$^0$ laterally, returned to the midline position and removed by a twisting movement. The operation is performed on the other side and the eyelids compressed in order to minimize bleeding.

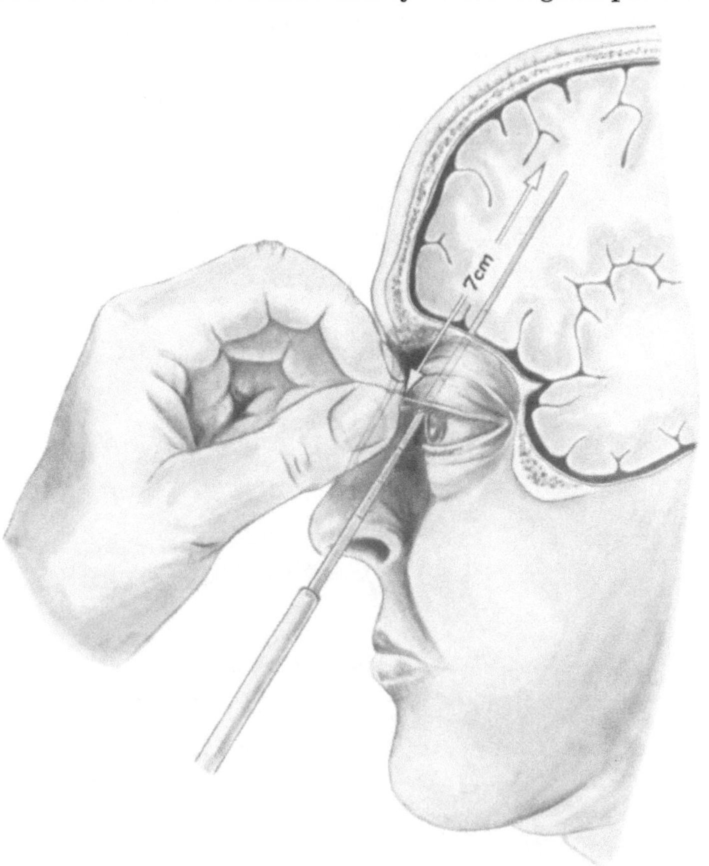


Fig. 5. Transorbital lobotomy a. m. FREEMAN.

FREEMAN thinks that this operation (*"sectioning fibres in the frontal lobe in the coronal plane corresponding with the bony ridge of the nose"*) as usually sufficient in patients with symptoms for less than one year and with less than six months hospitalization. Other patients demand in addition the "deep frontal cut": When the instrument has been moved laterally in an arc of 30$^0$ (see above) the handle is elevated strongly until it is nearly parallel with the orbital plate and then returned to the sagittal plane. By means of this movement the instrument should cut the thalamofrontal fibres in the neighbourhood of the caudate nucleus and some part of the orbital cortex should be undercut. FREEMAN has verified his sections in several postmortems and is satisfied with the procedure. Mortality has been singularly low and complications, mostly hemorrhage in the orbit, or escape of cerebrospinal fluid to the orbit, few. The patients are treated for some days with antibiotics and usually return home the day following the operation.

**Comment.** Most neurosurgeons would agree with WATTS, who feels that any procedure involving cutting of brain tissue is a major surgical operation and that disability constitutes the indication for lobotomy. In many clinics the patients listed by FREEMAN would not be considered candidates for any type of lobotomy. As to the technic itself, it seems to carry a remarkably low mortality and few complications. Still, if any lobotomy may be called a "blind" procedure, it is most certainly true of the transorbital variety.

## 3. Frontal lobotomy by the open method.

Originally introduced by LYERLY (1937) the open method has been used and modified by a number of neurosurgeons (POPPEN, SCARFF, BUSCH a. o.). The approach may be through a transverse incision just anterior to the coronal suture, through a midline incision 15 cm. long or perhaps best by two parasagittal incisions 4—5 cm. long extending forwards from the coronal suture on both sides 3—4 cm. from the midline. In any case access should be had to remove trephine buttons 2,5—3,5 cm. in diameter just

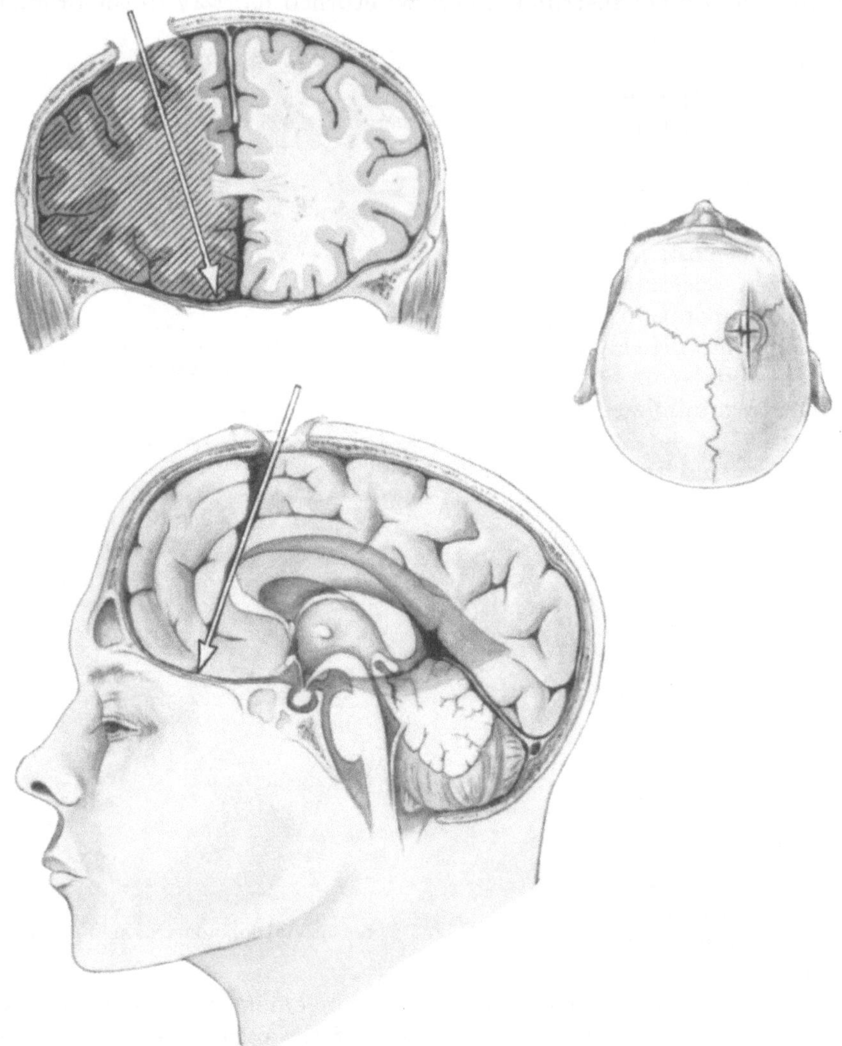

Fig. 6. Frontal lobotomy by open method (LYERLY).

anterior to the coronal suture, the posterior part of the buttons just touching the suture. When the buttons have been temporarily removed the dura is opened by a semicircular incision and the flap fixed by sutures. An avascular part of the cortex 1 cm. in diameter is removed without use of diathermy for microscopical study. Following hemostasis (diathermy) the sphenoid ridge is located by means of a graduated brain canula and the depth of the anterior fossa noted. The anterior horn is located by puncture and the lobotomy performed in the desired plane, usually just anterior to the sphenoid ridge. The anterior horn may be entered or it may frequently be depressed backwards by the spatula, the glia outside the ependyma usually being quite tough. The lobotomy may be performed by means of the suction canula with or without diathermy attachment, by a leucotome or other suitable instrument until the cortex on the orbital surface is reached. Medially the incision is carried as far as the cortex, care being taken not to injure the vessels from the anterior cerebral artery. Laterally the cut is made by a curved suction canula or a curved leucotome. When the lobotomy is felt to be as complete as desired (fig. 6) or is seen to have severed all white matter in the desired plane, the incision is washed out with saline, packed temporarily by jelfoam or spongostan with or without thrombine and the operation performed on the other side. When hemostasis is complete on both sides (control with lighted brain retractor and saline) the dura is closed with silk sutures, if necessary supplemented by a piece of jelfoam. The bone discs are replaced and the galea and skin sutured in the usual way. Dressings of adhesive straps have proved most effective in violent patients. Lipiodol or superoxide may be introduced in the cuts for visualization by Roentgen—superoxide being quite sufficient if the examination is carried out immediately following the operation.

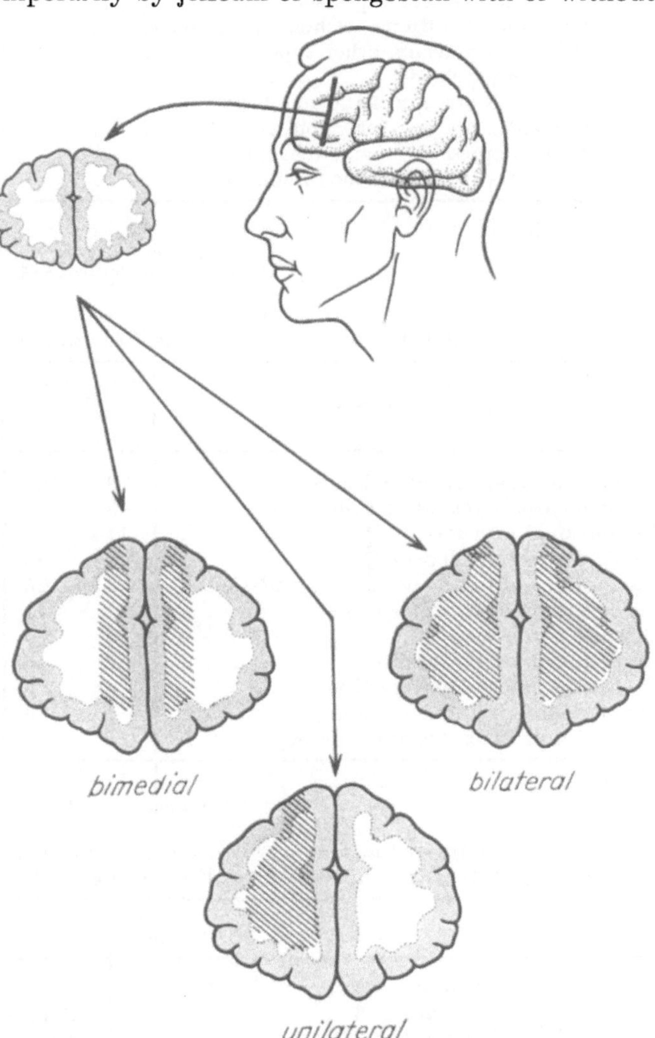


Fig. 7. Bimedial, bilateral and unilateral lobotomy a. m. Poppen. After Greenblatt and Solomon.

**Comment.** For the neurosurgeon this procedure has much to recommend it: The operation is performed under direct visual control; hemostasis can be had in the usual neurosurgical way; the vessels from the anterior cerebral artery are easily avoided in this approach; the operation is presumably somewhat more exact in localization than the "blind" lobotomies performed by means of skull measurements. Even so, brains differ and exactitude is not ideal and a preoperative encephalography always desirable. The operation can be made as partial or complete as desired—*Love* grades his operations (grade II a pyramid section with the apex at the burr hole leaving part of the white matter nedial and lateral to the pyramid intact, grade III as complete as possible), Busch and Poppen in suitable cases sectioning the white matter medial to the anterior horn only (fig. 7) [*bimedial lobotomy by open method*]. In a *total* lobotomy this approach is absolutely to be preferred—e.g. in patients previously lobotomized without or without satisfactory effect. As a disadvantage must be listed the necessity of parasagittal cortical incisions, the percentage of postoperative epilepsy being considerably larger than in lateral incisions (see p. 169). Attempts to carry out complete lobotomies by a lateral approach have, however, in our experience at least, proved unsatisfactory.

Table 5. *Results of open frontal lobotomy* (POPPEN) *as to mental status.* (After GREENBLATT, ARNOT, SOLOMON a. o.)

| Diagnostic category | No. | Good | Fair | Poor |
|---|---|---|---|---|
| Psychoneurosis, hypochondriasis . . . . . . | 3 | 3 | 0 | 0 |
| Psychoneurosis, obsessive-compulsive . . . . | 7 | 3 | 4 | 0 |
| Involutional psychosis . . . . . . . . . . | 12 | 11 | 0 | 1 |
| Manic-depressive, depressed . . . . . . . . | 15 | 8 | 5 | 2 |
| Paranoid conditions, without hallucination. . | 20 | 5 | 10 | 5 |
| Dementia praecox, other types . . . . . . . | 27 | 11 | 8 | 8 |
| Organic psychosis . . . . . . . . . . . . | 6 | 0 | 3 | 3 |
| Dementia praecox, katatonic type . . . . . | 35 | 2 | 13 | 20 |
| Dementia praecox, paranoid type . . . . . | 31 | 2 | 5 | 24 |
| Manic-depressive, manic (chronic) . . . . . | 5 | 1 | 0 | 4 |
| Dementia praecox, hebephrenic type . . . . | 18 | 1 | 1 | 16 |
| Totals. . . . . . . . . . . . . . . . . . | 179 | 47 | 49 | 83 |
| | 100 % | 26 % | 27 % | 47 % |

Observation time 1—4 years.

Table 6. *Results by diagnostic groups.* After GREENBLATT, ARNOT and SOLOMON (1950). Technic of POPPEN.

| Diagnostic category[1] | Good mental status | | Fair mental status | | Poor mental status | | Total | |
|---|---|---|---|---|---|---|---|---|
| | No. | % | No. | % | No. | % | No. | % |
| Psychoneurosis, hypochondriasis . . . . . | 3 | 100 | 0 | 0 | 0 | 0 | 3 | 100 |
| Psychoneurosis, obsessive-compulsive . . . | 3 | 43 | 4 | 57 | 0 | 0 | 7 | 100 |
| Involutional psychosis . . . . . . . . . | 11 | 92 | 0 | 0 | 1 | 8 | 12 | 100 |
| Manic-depressive, depressed . . . . . . . | 8 | 53 | 5 | 34 | 2 | 13 | 15 | 100 |
| Paranoid condition, without hallucinations . | 5 | 25 | 10 | 50 | 5 | 25 | 20 | 100 |
| Dementia praecox, other types . . . . . . | 11 | 41 | 8 | 29 | 8 | 30 | 27 | 100 |
| Organic psychosis . . . . . . . . . . . | 0 | 0 | 3 | 50 | 3 | 50 | 6 | 100 |
| Dementia praecox, katatonic type . . . . | 2 | 6 | 13 | 37 | 20 | 57 | 35 | 100 |
| Dementia praecox, paranoid type . . . . . | 2 | 6 | 5 | 16 | 24 | 78 | 31 | 100 |
| Manic-depressive, manic (chronic) . . . . | 1 | 20 | 0 | 0 | 4 | 80 | 5 | 100 |
| Dementia praecox, hebephrenic type . . . | 1 | 6 | 1 | 6 | 16 | 88 | 18 | 100 |
| Totals . . . . . . . . . . . . . . . . . . | 47 | 26 | 49 | 27 | 83 | 47 | 179 | 100 |

[1] Two cases unclassified.

Table 7. *Improved and unimproved groups according to diagnosis and type of operation.* After GREENBLATT and SOLOMON: Frontal lobes and schizophrenia (1953) compare fig. 6.

| | | Marked and moderate | Slight | Unimproved | | | Marked and moderate | Slight | Unimproved |
|---|---|---|---|---|---|---|---|---|---|
| Paranoid | Bimedial | 5 | 3 | 1 | Paranoid condition | Bimedial | 1 | | |
| | Bilateral | 6 | 4 | 4 | | Bilateral | 2 | | |
| | Unilateral | 7 | 1 | 2 | | Unilateral | | | 2 |
| | Total (33) | 18 (55 %) | 8 | 7 | | Total (5) | 3 (60 %) | | 2 |
| Catatonic | Bimedial | 5 | 1 | | Divolutional psychosis | Bimedial | 2 | | 1 |
| | Bilateral | 1 | 6 | 3 | | Bilateral | | | |
| | Unilateral | 1 | 3 | 2 | | Unilateral | 3 | | 4 |
| | Total (22) | 7 (32 %) | 10 | 5 | | Total (10) | 5 (50 %) | | 5 |
| Hebephrenic | Bimedial | 3 | 2 | 3 | Organic | Bimedial | | 2 | |
| | Bilateral | 5 | 1 | | | Bilateral | | 1 | |
| | Unilateral | | 5 | 5 | | Unilateral | | 1 | |
| | Total (24) | 8 (33 %) | 8 | 8 | | Total (4) | | 4 | |
| D. p. simplex | Bimedial | | | | Psychoneurosis | Bimedial | 1 | | |
| | Bilateral | | | 1 | | Bilateral | 1 | | |
| | Unilateral | | | 1 | | Unilateral | 1 | 2 | |
| | Total (2) | | | 2 | | Total (5) | 3 (60 %) | 2 | |
| D. p. other types | Bimedial | 3 | | 1 | Psychosis with psychopathic personality | Bimedial | 1 | | |
| | Bilateral | 2 | 1 | 1 | | Bilateral | | | |
| | Unilateral | | 1 | | | Unilateral | | 1 | |
| | Total (9) | 5 (56 %) | 2 | 2 | | Total (2) | 1 (50 %) | 1 | |

The open method is the most frequently used method in *unilateral* lobotomy (e.g. SCARFF).

**Results.** To illustrate results the series of the Boston group (technic of POPPEN) is shown in tables 5 and 6 (1950), while table 7 shows results also in partial lobotomies performed by the same approach (1953).

## 4. Coagulation lobotomy a. m. GRANTHAM.

Originally devised as a partial lobotomy for the relief of pain GRANTHAM's coagulation lobotomy has also been used in mental disease.

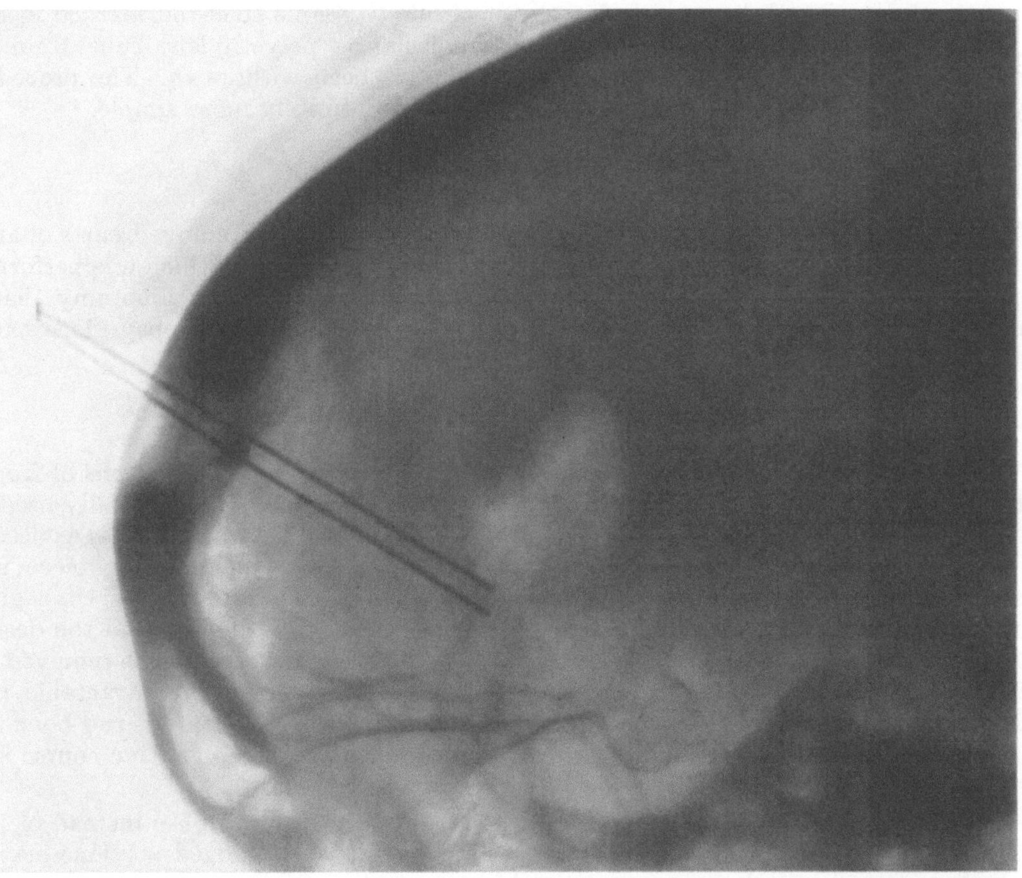

Fig. 8. Coagulation a. m. GRANTHAM. The electrodes are sheathed by thin polyethylene tubes.

Through one transverse coronal or through two parasagittal skin incisions burr holes are made 1,5—2 cm. from the midline, 6—8 cm. above the glabella. The burr holes may vary in diameter—we have found 2,5—3 cm. to be the most convenient size. When the dura has been opened, care being taken not to tear any vein the anterior horn is located by a ventricular needle and 8—10 cc of fluid is replaced with air or oxygen. A ventricular needle is passed to the floor of the anterior fossa about 1 cm. anterior to the tip of the anterior horn and the distance (usually 7—8 cm. measured. If the lesion—as done by GRANTHAM—is to be made 1 cm. anterior to the frontal horn and in the medial lower quadrant of the frontal lobe, electrodes isolated except for 1 cm. of their tips are introduced in both frontal lobes to a depth of 2 cm. short of the floor of the anterior fossa and their location checked by antero-posterior and lateral Roentgen exposures. If at the desired locations the coagulation is carried out by means of the DAVIS-BOVIE apparatus, where a power setting of 20 on the coagulation device applied to the unisolated extracranial part of the electrode is said to produce a cylindrical lesion approximately 12 mm.

in length and 8 mm. in dimater. The power setting is checked by grasping a bit of periosteum in a fine tooth bayonet forceps and applying the current, when there should be charring of the tissue in 3 seconds. When the coagulation has been carried through, the electrode is withdrawn 1 cm., and the current again applied in this new location, if a larger lesions is desire (fig. 8).

**Comment.** This procedure has much to recommend it: It is reasonably exact, there is no large cortical scar and the procedure may easily be repeated in an adjacent zone, if no effect is noted after the first attempt. It may of course be used in any other part of the frontal lobe—BUSCH has used it 1 cm. behind and medial to the tip of the anterior horn, thinking this region more likely to give results in mental disease. In order to be able to mark the site of the coagulation the electrode (a simple steel rod marked in cm., 0,6 mm. in diameter) is introduced through an isolating polyethylene tube 1 mm. in diameter and lipiodol injected when the electrode has been withdrawn. The procedure may not be as exact as the stereotaxic method, but is infinitely more simple.

## 5. Cortical excisions.

In the early forties PENFIELD for the purpose of psychosurgery removed parts of areas 6—8 symmetrically in both frontal lobes. This *prefrontal gyrectomy*, which was performed subpially, was, however, stated to give about the same results as lobotomy, had a more complicated technic and a higher incidence of postoperative epilepsy. Is seems to have been discontinued for the purposes of psychosurgery.

### a) Topectomy.

The name topectomy has become current for the selective partial ablations of frontal cortex which were introduced by POOL, HEATH and WEBER 1949 and especially used by POOL and LE BEAU: Through a usual craniotomy parts of the frontal cortex is excised in one or two stages. Two bone-flaps are hinged temporally or one midline piece may be removed temporarily giving access to the medial parts of both frontal lobes, the sagittal sinus lying in the middle of the field. The dura is opened on both sides and the desired parts of the frontal lobes removed by resection. POOL in his first operations removed the main parts of areas 9—10, while LE BEAU in benign psychoses or in intractable pain excises smaller amounts. After complete hemostasis the dura is sutured, the bone-flap or -flaps replaced and the galea and skin sutured. Immediate postoperative course is in most cases uneventful and sphincteric disturbances infrequent.

**Comment.** The idea of removing known portions of the frontal lobes instead of performing blind lobotomies will appeal to most neurosurgeons. Removed portions may be weighed, measured by volume and examined histologically. While the theory of topectomy is perfect, execution is more difficult, as orientation as to just where BRODMANN's or other topographical fields are situated in different brains is only possible with considerable uncertainty. Moreover, it will frequently be necessary to clip or coagulate vessels going beyond the fields actually excised, thus compromising the brain outside the chosen fields. Another drawback is the extensive meningocerebral scars resulting and the fear of a high percentage of postoperative epilepsy has subsequently been realised. Later modifications have to a certain extent neutralized these disadvantages: Instead of excision LE BEAU removes the chosen portions of cortex subpially by means of suction ("*decortication*"), while POOL employs *electrocoagulation* or *thermocoagulation*. Especially the latter technic, employed previously by DUSSER DE BARENNE in neurophysiology, seems to have much to recommend it, even if the temperature used by POOL (100° Celsius for as long as 10 secs.) seems excessive. Still, the work done by POOL in rationalizing the technic of lobotomy deserves the highest praise and prefrontal topectomy would undoubtedly have enjoyed a wider application if about the same time other, more satisfying, technics had not arisen.

## b) Cingulectomy.

It is especially the work done by SMITH, WARD and MCCULLOCH and of GLEES and collaborators which has drawn interest to the cingulate gyrus. It seemed certain that this area was of importance for autonomous function and the psychical responses noted in monkeys following ablation of the cingular area made the application of the facts noted in psychosurgery reasonable. The field was first explored by LE BEAU and CAIRNS who had somewhat similar experiences.

The cingular region may be reached bilaterally by a unilateral bone flap (left or right) tangential to the sagittal sinus. LE BEAU places his flap from 2 cm. in front of the coronal suture to 3 cm. above the orbital ridge. Following opening of the dura one frontal lobe is retracted from the falx, usually necessitating the coagulation of some parasagittal veins. The mesial parts of the frontal lobes are separated down to the corpus callosum, when the cingular gyrus is brought in view. The anterior part of the gyrus is now resected (CAIRNS) on both sides, or removed by aspiration (LE BEAU): Following the piercing of the pia in two or more places a fine suction tube is passed through these holes and the cortex aspirated avoiding the vessels passing up towards the convexity (fig. 9). Bleeding usually is slight and may be checked completely by temporary application of gelfoam with or without thrombine. LE BEAU actually leaves narrow bands of gelfoam soaked in lipiodol in the cavities for later verification by Roentgen. Moreover, he varies his "decortication" which usually is 3 cm. long and 1,5 cm. high by including parts of area 25 below the genu corporis callosi 2 cm. more ventrally, or by removing parts of areas 32, 2 cm. in front of the genu or area 12, near the orbital level.

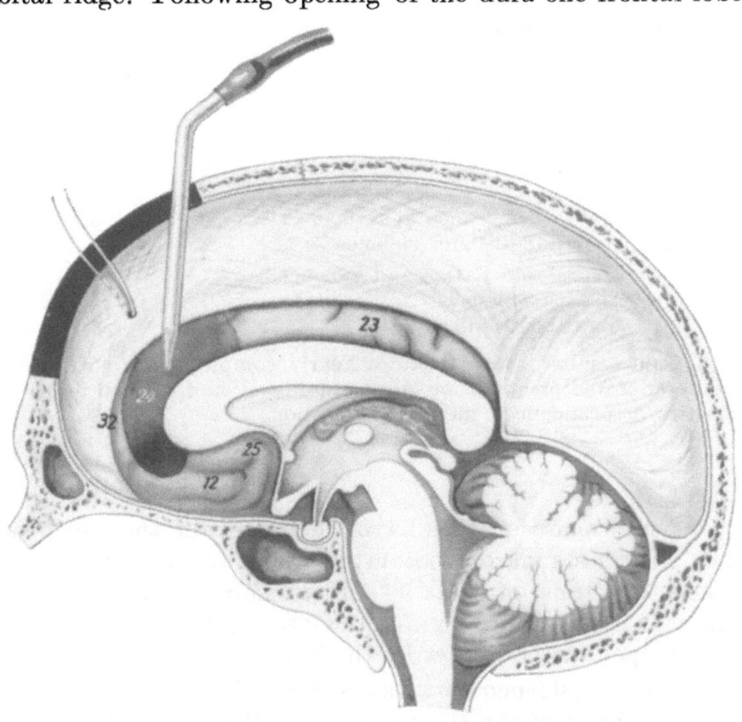

Fig. 9. Cingulectomy a. m. LE BEAU.

**Comment.** The operation performed by CAIRNS (see WHITTY et al.) and some of the operations of LE BEAU are typical agranular resections, presumably interfering with thalamo-cingular fibres coming from the anterior nucleus and not from the dorso-medial nucleus, which seems connected with the granular cortex. The operation compromises a considerably smaller area than SCOVILLE's undercutting of the medial surface which includes the cingular cortex. Results are said to be satisfactory in more benign psychoses and psychoneurotics (CAIRNS) and in intractable pain (LE BEAU), but to be insufficient in schizophrenia (table 8).

Belonging to this field is also the *cingulate cortex isolation* of LIVINGSTON, which procedure, however, presumably involves an uncertain amount of granular cortex: Using a transcortical aproach similar to the LYERLY-POPPEN procedure the parasagittal gray matter is denuded of subjacent white matter in a strip extending 2 cm. anterior to the tip of the frontal horn and posteriorly to a distance of 4 cm. along the roof of the lateral ventricle. LIVINGSTON undoubtedly is right in maintaining that this operation effectively isolates the cortex of the anterior cingulate gyrus, but other regions are also compromised. Good results are reported, but the technic seems to be less exact if less time-consuming than the technic of LE BEAU.

Table 8. *Clinical results of anterior cingulectomy.* (After LE BEAU.)

| Diagnosis | No. | Good results | Follow-up (years) |
|---|---|---|---|
| I. Depressive states | | | |
| a) with anxiety or pain | 5 | 0 | |
| b) with obsessive neurosis | 4 | 3 | 3, 1, $^3/_4$. |
| II. Excited states | | | |
| a) with hysteria | 3 | 2 | 3, 2. |
| b) w. psychopathic disorders | 3 | 0 | |
| III. Psychoses with violence | | | |
| a) dementia epileptica | 2 | 1 | $1^1/_2$. |
| b) schizophrenic syndrome | 2 | 2 | 5, 3. |
| IV. Epilepsy | | | |
| a) subnormal mental state | 5 | 3 | 4, $3^1/_2$, 2. |
| b) irritability and violence | 9 | 7 | $5^1/_2$, 4, $3^1/_2$, $3^1/_2$, $2^1/_2$, 1, $^1/_2$. |
| V. Mental retardation and violence | | | |
| a) with epilepsy | 7 | 5 | 3, 2, $1^1/_2$, $1^1/_2$, $^1/_2$. |
| b) without epilepsy | 4 | 3 | $3^1/_2$, $^3/_4$, $^1/_2$. |

"Good results" = complete or nearly complete cure with useful activity in patients with a not too deteriorated preoperative intellectual level, and marked improvement with at least some activity in cases of pronounced mental retardation.

## 6. Anterior lobotomies.

Several neurosurgeons have tried to evade the psychical defects following the FREEMAN-WATTS standard lobotomy by placing the cut more anteriorly in the frontal lobe. When topectomy of areas 9—10 had showed some effects one of the most active neurosurgeons in this field, WYLIE MCKISSOCK, introduced *rostral leucotomy*, at first performed by the open method, later by the blind method.

**Open rostral leucotomy** was performed through a transverse incision about 10 cm. long 1 cm. in front of the coronal suture. Bone discs 3—4 cm. in diameter were removed in the angle of the coronal and the sagittal sutures on both sides, small dural flaps turned medially and transverse incisions, 1—2 cm. in length made through the cortex with suction diathermy. The white matter was now divided by gentle suction forwards aiming slightly behind the point where the posterior surface of the frontal bone meets the roof of the orbit. Medially the division was carried to the cortex, laterally the division should extend for a distance of 2—3 cm. Hemostasis usually is easy. The dural flaps were sutured, the bone discs replaced and the insision closed in the usual manner.

*Comment.* This operation virtually is an undercutting of areas 9—10. It has the advantages of the undercutting procedure (see later) and supposedly is more exact than the topectomy performed by POOL as there is no danger of closing larger vessels. As results were disappointing in severe psychoses the procedure seems to have been discarded by MCKISSOCK in favour of

**Blind rostral leucotomy.** Incisions 3 cm. long are made 2 cm. to each side of the sagittal plane with the posterior limits at the coronal sutures (see later). The dura is opened just enough to allow a usual brain needle to be inserted in a forwards direction until its point strikes the roof of the orbit at the junction of its anterior and middle thirds. Following this the needle is withdrawn 1 cm. and the section made by "rotating the butt of the needle laterally, bringing the point nearer to the midline, and progressively withdrawing the needle as the butt is rotated steadily more laterally, a line parallel to the midline being cut in this way. The needle is then reinserted in the original line, and the butt rotated medially while the needle is again steadily withdrawn. A section is thus made about 2 cm. wide extending from 2 cm. in front of the coronal sutures forwards and downwards and ending just above the orbital roof about 2 cm. behind the frontal pole." Later McKISSOCK (personal communication) has modified the procedure "by making the burr holes further forwards and directing the needle backwards towards the posterior part of the orbital roof in order to divide the fibres in the medial, inferior and posterior quadrants."

*Comment.* The rostral leucotomy is not, as is the case with other partial lobotomies, intended for use in severe psychoses, but was planned for patients with "severe tension, agitation, hypochondriasis, obsessional states, anxiety neuroses, agitated depressions and

Table 9. *Comparison of results of prefrontal and open rostral leucotomy.* (After McKISSOCK.)

| Operation | No. | Greatly improved | Moderately improved | Slightly improved | No information | Worse |
|---|---|---|---|---|---|---|
| FREEMAN-WATTS . . . . | 21 | 10 | 4 | 3 | 4 | 0 |
| Open rostral leucotomy . | 28 | 1 | 10 | 11 | 6 | 0 |

The two series was as similar as possible. While results were better in the FREEMAN-WATTS-series personality change, postoperative confusion and incontinence were rare in the rostral procedures.

*Results of 100 rostral leucotomies.* (After McKISSOCK.)

| Operation | No. | Greatly improved | Moderately improved | Slighthly improved | No improvement | Died | No information |
|---|---|---|---|---|---|---|---|
| Open . . | 63 | 9 | 13 | 17 | 9 | 2 | 13 |
| Blind . . | 37 | 10 | 10 | 7 | 7 | 0 | 3 |

The results of blind rostral leucotomy lie between those of the blind FREEMAN-WATTS procedure and those of open rostral leucotomy. The effect in suitably selected cases seems adequate.

the like." The small cortical incision should mean a lower percentage of postoperative epilepsy than in operations involving larger parasagittal cortical incisions. Disadvantages will be the same as in other "blind" lobotomies—the danger of venous bleeding with subsequent hematoma or venous thrombosis and, not least, uncertainty of which part and how large a part of the white matter has been sectioned. It can easily be done in any mental hospital by a travelling neurosurgical team in the manner favoured in England. *Results* are shown in table 9.

## 7. Selective cortical undercutting.

### a) SCOVILLE's methods.

A definite step forward was made in 1947, when SCOVILLE published his technic of selective cortical undercutting of the frontal lobes. The aim of this operation is to isolate certain desired areas of the frontal cortex while preserving the blood-supply of the isolated parts and of the neighbouring areas so frequently compromised by cortical excisions. The plane of section is made at the relatively avascular zone between the gray and the white matter.

Through a trephine hole 3,5 cm. in diameter the dura is opened and the cortex incised in an avascular place for a distance of ca. 1 cm. Through this incision a fine suction canula with or without diathermy attachment is introduced in the white matter and the line of cleavage started, care being taken to move just under the cortex. Special brain spatulas (SCOVILLE) may be used (fig. 10). Bleeding is minimal and the cavity is usually dry if packed by spongostan with or without thrombine while the other side is being done. Arterial bleeding may occur, if the cortex is reached in a sulcus, which infrequently may happen especially on the medial side of the frontal lobe. The extent of the undercutting may be marked by fine wire loops of stainless steel (SCOVILLE), by clips, lipiodol or peroxide while tantalum dust is to be avoided (BAILEY, O., F. D. INGRAHAM, P. S. WEADON, A. F. SUSEN 1952). When hemostasis is complete the dura is sutured, the bone discs replaced and the skin incisions closed in the usual way.

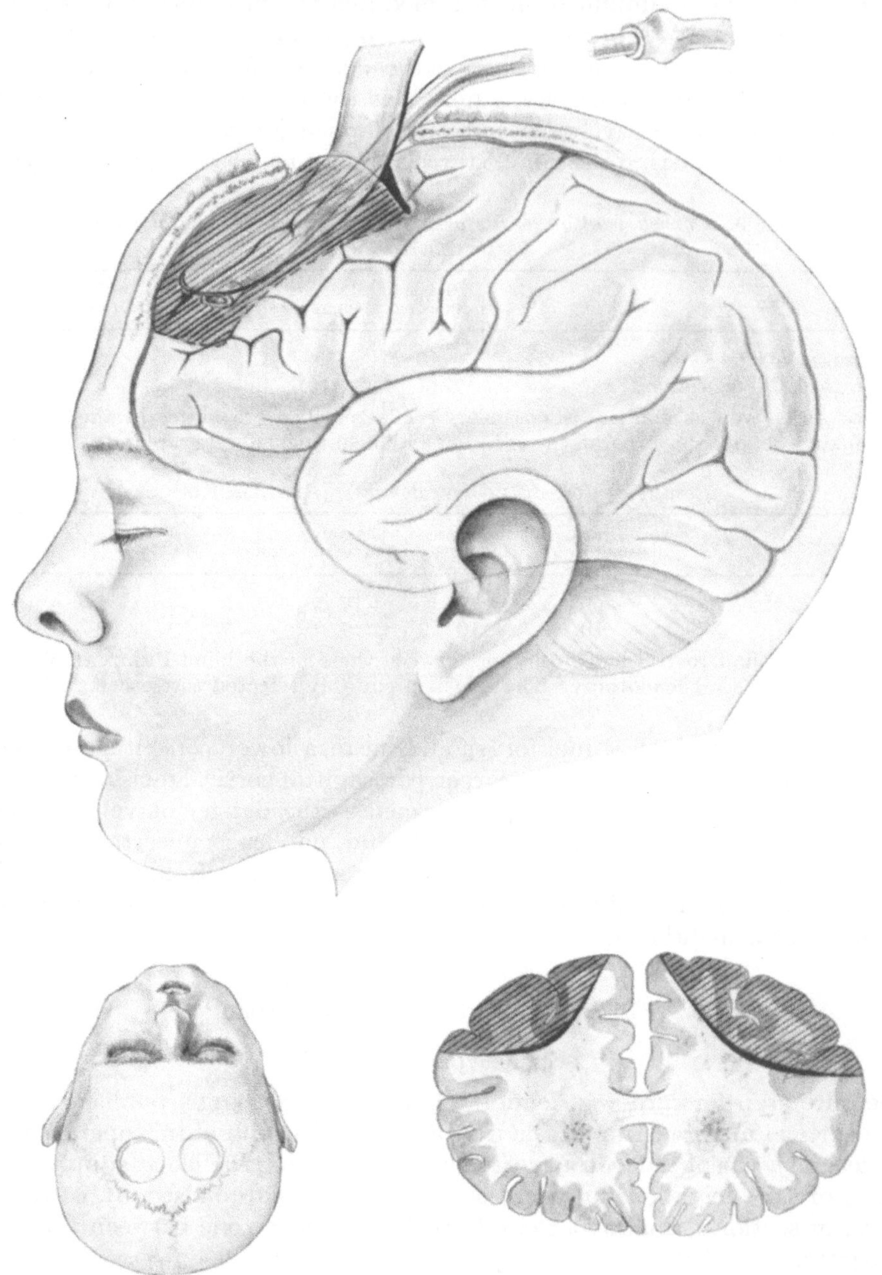

Fig. 10. Undercutting of superior surface a. m. SCOVILLE.

The undercutting procedure may be carried out in any desired location. SCOVILLE has performed his undercuttings in three different locations:

1. *Undercutting of superior surface*. This undercutting originally included some part of the medial surface, but is now limited to a rectangle measuring 7,5 cm. posterior to the frontal pole and 4 cm. lateral to the medial edge (fig. 10).

2. *Undercutting of the orbital surface.* The trephine hole is here placed low down in the frontal region, just not interfering with the frontal sinus and the orbital surfaces undercut in toto back to the temporal lobe laterally and the chiasmatic cistern medially (fig. 11).

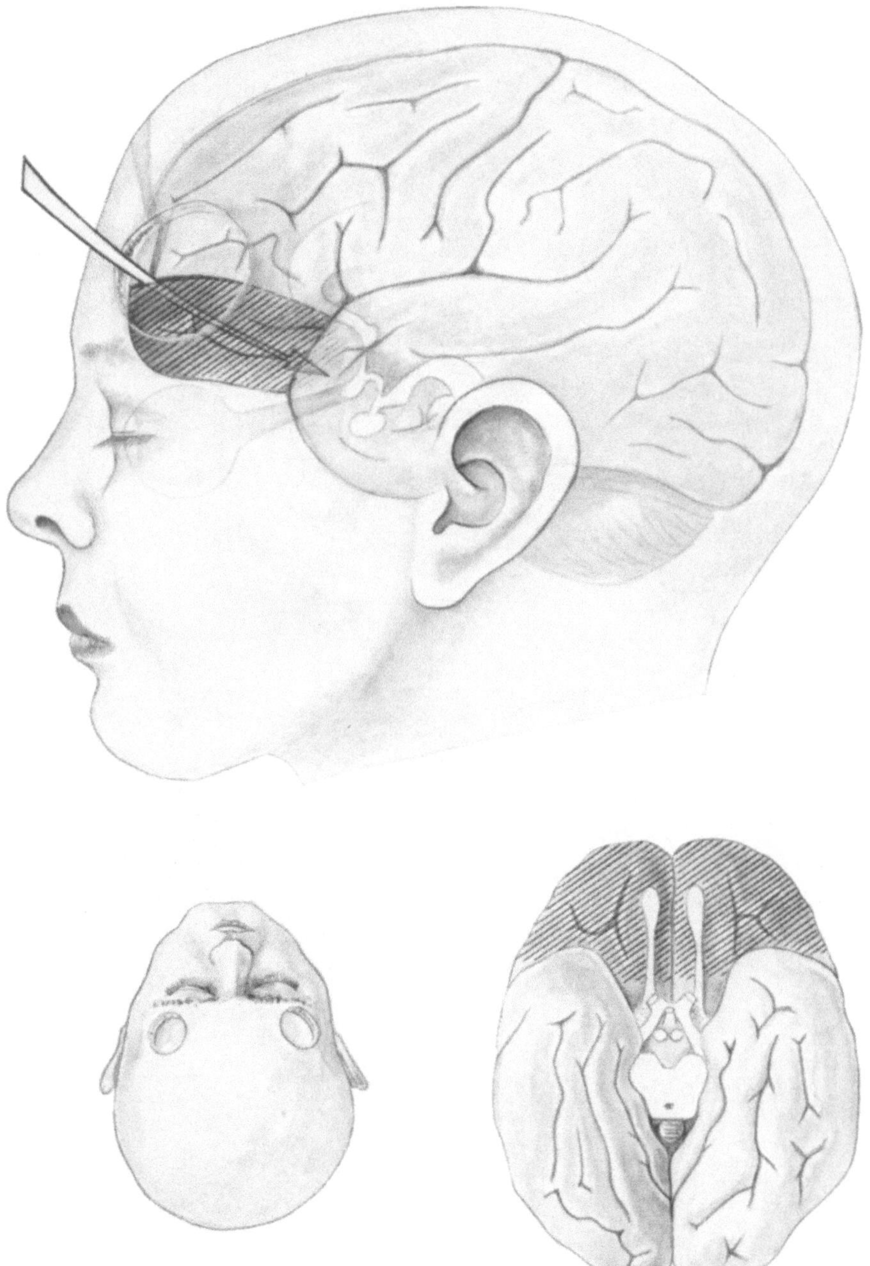

Fig. 11. Undercutting of orbital surface a. m. SCOVILLE.

3. *Undercutting of medial surface* including the anterior cingulate gyrus both above and below the corpus callosum. The trephine hole is here placed on either side of the midline halfway between the glabella and the coronal suture (fig. 12).

In all three types of undercutting SCOVILLE carries the peripheral limits of the cut superficially through the cortex to the pia-arachnoid by means of a spatula in order to make the isolation complete.

The surface undercut in these three types of operation is about the same, averaging 50—60 cm², the most extensive being the superior surface operation. For comparison it

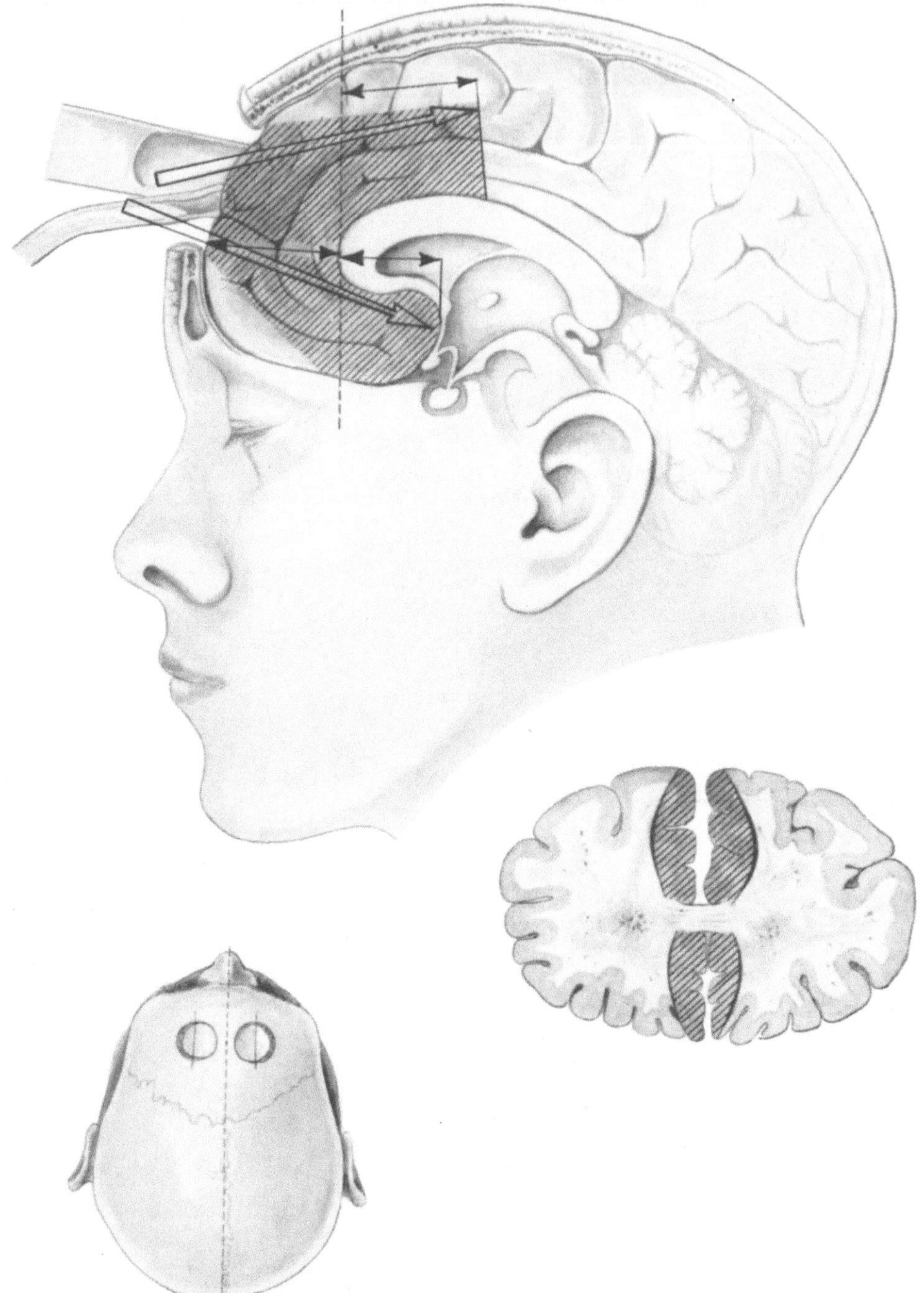

Fig. 12. Undercutting of medial surface a. m. SCOVILLE.

may be estimated that the usual FREEMAN-WATTS lobotomy isolates some 160 cm² of frontal cortex.

**Comment.** The undercutting procedure seems to be at least exact enough to warrant the expression "selective", when compared with the various other lobotomy procedures. The technic seems morover as atraumatic as possible in open operations and bleeding is reduced to a minimum. Interference with other cortical areas via vascular occlusion is extremely rare.

**Results.** SCOVILLE's results with his three procedures are listed in table 10, which, moreover, shows results in other operations. No certain difference was found between the three procedures in SCOVILLE's first publication. This, however, does not mean that no difference is to be found in suitable materials. Several neurosurgeons, who have worked in this field are inclined to think that while undercutting of the superior (lateral) surface of the convexity gives greater intellectual deficit, effects on affective symptoms in mental

Table 10A. *Classification of patients undergoing 7 types of temporal and frontal lobes operation.*

| Operations | Total cases | Avg. age (years) | Sex | Diagnostic category | | Duration illness (years) | Average follow-up (mos.) |
|---|---|---|---|---|---|---|---|
| | | | | Temporal lobe operations | | | |
| Uncotomy | 5 | 31 | F 5 | Schizophrenia | | 8 | 13 |
| | | | M 0 | Hebephrenic | 2 | | |
| | | | | Catatonic | 2 | | |
| | | | | Paranoid | 1 | | |
| Medial temporal lobotomy | 8 | 35 | F 5 | Schizophrenia | | 12 | 6 |
| | | | M 0 | Hebephrenic | 3 | | |
| | | | | Catatonic | 1 | | |
| | | | | Paranoid | 2 | | |
| | | | | Unclass. | 1 | | |
| | | | | Psych. w. epilepsy | 1 | | |
| | | | | Combined frontal and temporal operations | | | |
| Orbito-temporal lobotomy | 6 | 32 | F 6 | Schizophrenia | | 14 | 5 |
| | | | M 0 | Hebephrenic | 2 | | |
| | | | | Catatonic | 2 | | |
| | | | | Unclass. | 1 | | |
| | | | | Psych. w. epilepsy | 1 | | |
| | | | | Frontal lobe operations. | | | |
| Superior surface undercutting | 15 | 42 | F 7 | Schizophrenia | | 13 | 19 |
| | | | M 8 | Hebephrenic | 4 | | |
| | | | | Catatonic | 5 | | |
| | | | | Paranoid | 4 | | |
| | | | | Involutional | 2 | | |
| Orbital surface undercutting | 15 | 40 | F 9 | Schizophrenia | | 9 | 8 |
| | | | M 6 | Hebephrenic | 4 | | |
| | | | | Catatonic | 7 | | |
| | | | | Paranoid | 2 | | |
| | | | | Involutional | 2 | | |
| Medial and cingulate surface undercutting | 15 | 36 | F 10 | Schizophrenia | | 11 | 23 |
| | | | M 5 | Hebephrenic | 4 | | |
| | | | | Catatonic | 5 | | |
| | | | | Paranoid | 4 | | |
| | | | | Unclass. | 1 | | |
| | | | | Psych. w. epilepsy | 1 | | |
| Standard lobotomy | 15 | 38 | F 12 | Schizophrenia | | 9 | 4 |
| | | | M 3 | Hebephrenic | 4 | | |
| | | | | Catatonic | 2 | | |
| | | | | Paranoid | 3 | | |
| | | | | Unclass. | 1 | | |
| | | | | Psych. w. epilepsy | 1 | | |
| | | | | Psych. w. M. D. | 3 | | |
| | | | | Involutional | 1 | | |

Table 10B. *Psychiatric results of 3 types of medial temporal lobotomy compared with 3 types of fractional and 1 of complete frontal lobotomies.*

(From SCOVILLE, W. B., R. H. DUNSMORE, W. T. LIBERSON and A. PEPE in *Psychiatric Treatment* (Assoc. Res. Nerv. and Ment. Dis. **31**, 362.)

| Types of operation | No. of cases | No. of patients showing significant improvement | Degree of improvement (based on a maximum of 100) |
|---|---|---|---|
| Temporal lobe operations. | | | |
| Uncotomy . . . . . . . . . . | 4[1] | 0 (0%) | 6 |
| Medial temporal lobotomy . . . | 7[1] | 1 (14%) | 16 |
| Combined frontal and temporal operations | | | |
| Orbito-temporal lobotomy . . . | 6 | 5 (83%) | 50 |
| Frontal lobe operations. | | | |
| Superior surface undercutting . | 15 | 7 (47%) | 47 |
| Orbital surface undercutting . . | 15 | 7 (47%) | 32 |
| Medial and cingulate surface undercutting . . . . . . . . | 15 | 8 (53%) | 36 |
| Standard lobotomy . . . . . . | 15 | 7 (47%) | 35 |

[1] 1 each omitted from uncotomy and medial temporal lobotomy because of receiving mid brain damage. These 2 cases each showed marked improvement.

disease are more pronounced following undercutting of the medial and orbital parts of the frontal lobes.

MACDONALD TOW and LEWIN (1953) tried orbital undercutting (called by them *orbital leucotomy*) in 20 patients followed from $1^1/_2$—3 years. 7 patients recovered, while 8 improved. Psychical defects were found considerably less frequent than in prefrontal lobotomy (table 11).

Table 11. *Cases and results of orbital leucotomy* (MACDONALD TOW and LEWIN).

| | Diagnosis | Duration of illness before operation (years) | Length of follow-up after operation (years) | Result |
|---|---|---|---|---|
| 1 | Chronic anxiety state | 14 | 3 | Improved slightly |
| 2 | Paranoid schizophrenia | 12 | 3 | Improved 2 months, relapsed |
| 3 | Paranoid schizophrenia | 9 | $1^1/_2$ | Improved (died later) |
| 4 | Aggressive psychopath | 11 | $2^3/_4$ | Recovered |
| 5 | Manic depressive psychosis | 4 | $2^3/_4$ | Improved |
| 6 | Schizophrenia, catatonic | 2 | $2^3/_4$ | Recovered |
| 7 | Manic-depressive psychosis | 22 | $2^3/_4$ | Recovered |
| 8 | Paranoid schizophrenia | 8 | $2^3/_4$ | Improved 6 months |
| 9 | Involutional melancholia | 11 | $2^1/_2$ | Improved |
| 10 | Agitated depression | 5 | $2^1/_2$ | Improved |
| 11 | Hebephrenic schizophrenia | 2 | $2^1/_2$ | Improved 9 months, relapsed |
| 12 | Hebephrenic schizophrenia | 7 | $2^1/_4$ | Recovered |
| 13 | Catatonic schizophrenia | 3 | 2 | Improved |
| 14 | Agitated depression | 3 | 2 | Recovered |
| 15 | Schizophrenia simplex | 6 | 2 | Improved |
| 16 | Agitated depression | 10 | $1^3/_4$ | Improved 2 months, relapsed |
| 17 | Hebephrenic schizophrenia | 13 | $1^1/_2$ | Improved slightly |
| 18 | Chronic anxiety state | 4 | $1^1/_2$ | Recovered |
| 19 | Agitated depression | 12 | $1^1/_2$ | Recovered |
| 20 | Catatonic schizophrenia | 6 | $1^1/_2$ | Unchanged |

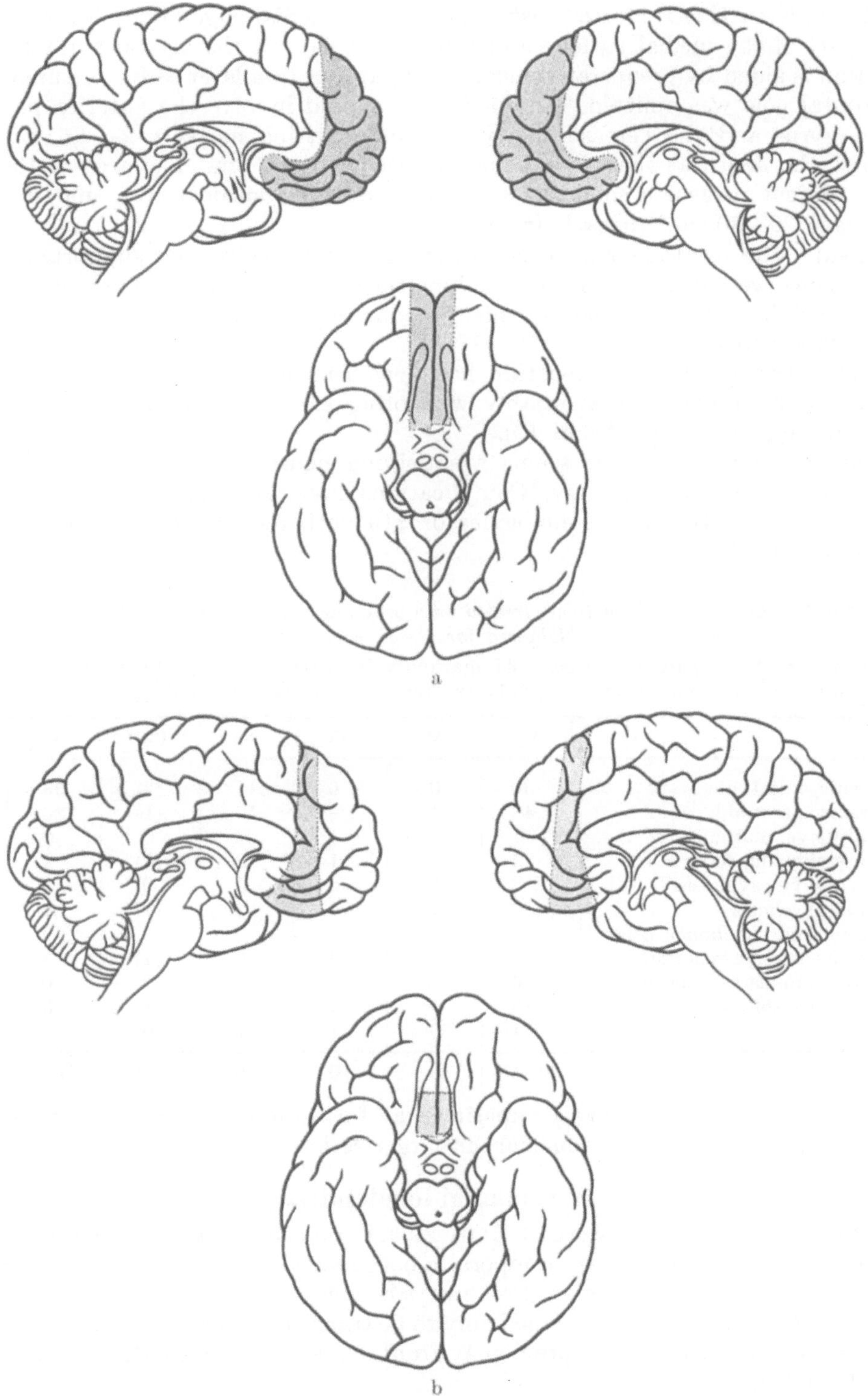


Fig. 13a and b. Orbitomedial undercutting a. m. Busch. a: as originally performed; b: as now performed.

## b) Orbitomedial undercutting (Busch).

In Copenhagen we have tried the undercutting technic in our orbitomedial operation: Through two parasagittal trephine holes 3 cm. in diameter just anterior to the coronal suture the undercutting is started just lateral to the medial edge of the frontal lobe and includes part of the medial surface and the medial part of the orbital surface (fig. 13). Localization is aided by preoperative encephalography. In a later series the undercutting of the frontal pole was omitted. The operation should involve the anterior part of the cingulate gyrus and the vertical leg of the undercutting measure 2—2,5 cm. antero-posteriorly, the depth at this place being between 6 and 7 cm. The area of the orbital surface undercut measures some $2 \times 3$ cm. and the total surface area undercut would thus average 20—30 cm.$^2$ in each frontal lobe.

**Comment.** The orbitomedial operation seems theoretically well supported by what scanty evidence we have. It seems to combine the advantages of the cingular operations with an effect in graver psychoses which in our experience is no less than in more extensive lobotomies.

**Results.** Orbitomedial undercutting has now been carried out in over 800 patients and results seem to compare favourably with other types of lobotomy as to effect on mental symptoms (see table 4 and 12).

The undercutting procedure seems a satisfying neurosurgical procedure and more exact than most forms of lobotomy. Complications have been singularly low in the series of SCOVILLE and of BUSCH—in our series of 810 patients (orbitomedial undercutting) mortality was 0,4%.

Table 12. *Results in 154 patients treated with orbitomedial undercutting (Copenhagen) followed for 1—3 years.*

No. number; AC apparently cured; MI markedly improved; SI significantly improved; (SH) improved patients postoperatively treated with shock; U unchanged; W worse.

| | No. | AC | MI | SI | (SH) | U | W |
|---|---|---|---|---|---|---|---|
| Schizophrenic, katatonic | 50 | 0 | 6 | 11 | (3) | 33 | 0 |
| Schizophrenic, paranoid | 48 | 1 | 9 | 17 | (1) | 20 | 1 |
| Manio-depressive, manic | 1 | 0 | 1 | 0 | 0 | 0 | 0 |
| Manio-depressive, depressive | 5 | 0 | 1 | 2 | (1) | 2 | 0 |
| Atypic depressive psychosis | 5 | 3 | 2 | 0 | 0 | 0 | 0 |
| Involutional psychosis | 10 | 1 | 5 | 3 | (1) | 1 | 0 |
| Psychopathia and psychoneurosis: | | | | | | | |
| Depressive-sensitive reaction | 9 | 1 | 5 | 0 | (1) | 3 | 0 |
| Obsessive-compulsive reaction | 6 | 2 | 3 | 1 | 0 | 0 | 0 |
| Emotional instability | 16 | 1 | 7 | 5 | (1) | 3 | 0 |
| Various | 4 | 0 | 1 | 1 | 0 | 2 | 0 |
| | 154 | 9 | 40 | 40 | (8) | 64 | 1 |

In the following various, mostly experimental, forms of lobotomy shall be mentioned. None of them have been made routinely in larger series.

## 8. Temporal lobotomies.

Based on the fundamental work of KLÜWER a. o. on the effect of temporal lobectomy, OBRADOR was the first to perform temporal lobotomy. With the idea of interfering with temporo-cingular and fronto-temporal pathways he made a cut, 4,5 cm. deep, just anterior to the temporal horn. The effect seemed only to be transient and as the temporal lobotomy in some cases was performed in previously frontally lobotomized patients, results were difficult to judge.

Similar experiments were made by CARILLO and by PIMENTA using the technic of OBRADOR. Out of PIMENTAS 42 chronic epileptics with troublesome psychical symptoms about $^2/_3$ showed some psychic alteration to the better, while the mental state of the patients made it difficult to judge psychical reduction.

The pioneer work of BAILEY and associates on anterior temporal lobectomy in psychomotor epilepsy showed that psychosis and severe personal disorders occur in 50% of patients with psycho-motor epilepsy with electroencephalographic discharges in the anterior temporal region, while psychosis was found in only 13% with medial temporal spike-focus. Following anterior temporal lobectomy improvement was found not only in epilepsy, but also in psychotic symptoms.

Recently some interesting experiences have been made by SCOVILLE and associates, who performed *medial temporal lobotomy* and *uncotomy*. Previously WALKER had performed *amygdaloidectomy* and resection of the uncus in deteriorated schizophrenics which resulted in temporary placidity, but with no lasting change in the psychosis.

*Uncotomy* (SCOVILLE) was done by lateral supra-orbital trephinations: When the dura is open, the frontal lobe is elevated and the arachnoid along the middle cerebral artery and lateral edge of the optic chiasm torn, permitting elevation of the posterior orbital cortex and lateral retraction of the tips of the temporal lobe. The uncus will be found just lateral to the third nerve, 3 cm. posterior to the tip of the temporal lobe. The uncal area is resected subpially by suction over an area approximately 3 cm. sagittally, 2 cm. vertically and 1,5 cm. in depth, thus including the uncal and periamygdaloid cortex, the pre-pyriform cortex and most of the amygdaloid nucleus, which lies some mm. deeper than the surface.

*Medial temporal lobectomy* includes a resection of the internal medial cortex of the temporal lobe, the anterior hippocampus and the nuclei and white matter lying medial to the medial wall of the temporal horn.

In the experiments these operations were in some cases combined with SCOVILLES *orbital undercutting*.

Results showed doubtful effect as to the psychosis, while the temporal operations seemed to cause less psychical deficit than undercutting of the lateral surfaces of the frontal lobes (table 10 B).

In 2 of SCOVILLES cases severe mid-brain damage occurred. Both showed *complete clinical remission* of the psychosis, which seems of considerable scientific interest.

WILLIAMS and FREEMAN reported effect on auditory hallucinations by bilateral amygdaloidectomy.

### 9. Parietal lobotomy.

In an attempt to cut the supra-longitudinal bundle without injuring thalamo-frontal tracts YAHN, PIMENTA and CETTE performed bilateral parietal lobotomy: The cut was made through an incision over the most prominent point of the parietal region (a little higher than PEETs point for ventriculography) on a line passing through the posterior border of the external ear; after opening the dura a ventricular needle was introduced perpendicularly towards the ventricle making a cut of 2—3 cm. in depth and length. 22 patients were operated in this way, mostly schizophrenics. Only 2 of the patients improved, but as 17 of them had had a previous, ineffective frontal lobotomy, results must have been difficult to evaluate.

### 10. Occipital lobotomy.

In a blind 30-year old patient with epilepsy and schizophrenia who under his hallucinations had destroyed both his eyes TORKILDSEN cut the whole of the white matter in the parieto-occipital region on both sides. No effect, either on the epilepsy or upon the schizophrenia, was noticed during the following 6 months, when a prefrontal lobotomy (FREEMAN-WATTS) was carried out—also without appreciable change.

## IV. Anesthesia.

In early psychosurgery *local anesthesia* was used by most neurosurgeons, whenever possible. As many patients, however, were non-cooperative and violent some sort of general anesthesia, frequently avertin, was sometimes necessary.

*Local anesthesia*, of course, has the advantage that one is able to follow the reactions of the patient during the procedure and some surgeons used to limit the cuts according to these reactions. Valuable information was gained by being in contact with the patient during the operation (FREEMAN and WATTS, SJÖQVIST and RYLANDER) and it was thought that the sudden lapse of the patient into torpidity or unconsciousness was of good omen for the ultimate result.

As operative procedures became more or less standardized, many neurosurgeons turned to *general anesthesia* as more convenient to both patient and surgeon. Penthotal (evipan) was used by many, endotracheal nitrous oxide with or without supplementary ether or penthotal by others. With the addition of trained anesthetists to the staff of most clinics these methods seem as safe as any and more convenient than most. In the "blind" lobotomies, where vomiting and venous congestion were common, endotracheal anesthesia with packing of the pharynx was found to be of definite advantage and was used routinely by FREEMAN and WATTS.

Personally we use intratracheal nitrous oxide supplemented by penthotal or trilene in most psychotic and violent patients, but may still use local anesthesia in other instances, especially in pain lobotomies, where the reactions of the patients may be of guiding or scientific interest. Ganglioplegics may be used in hypertensive patients, but may be dangerous in massive "blind" lobotomies.

*Preoperative medication* is commonly used—mostly atropine plus barbiturates, which are useful in guarding against an occasional epileptic fit, which, however, is mostly seen in cortical resections.

## V. Operative complications.

Operative complications in lobotomy are usually few and invariably due to some technical error causing hemorrhage or lesion of deep structures.

*Bleeding from the dura* is usually slight and easily controlled by diathermy or clips in the usual way. *Bleeding from veins crossing the subdural space* may be troublesome, but likewise easily controlled in the open operations. In atrophic brains in older patients several veins may have to be coagulated and this may be a cause of unspecificity of the intended operation, even if POOL experimentally found no effect on disease or psyche. *Bleeding from cortical vessels* is likewise easily controlled in the now used open operations. In the blind lobotomies bleeding may be due to lesion of branches of the anterior cerebral artery, when the cut has been carried too far medially, more seldom from anterior branches of the middle cerebral artery, when the burr hole is placed too far posteriorly (especially the FREEMAN-WATTS "radical" lobotomy). Arterial bleeding will then be seen in the cut and the brain may swell suddenly. FREEMAN and WATTS advocate irrigating the cut with saline for 5—15 minutes or packing the cut with cottonoid or gelfoam. Most neurosurgeons would probably prefer to enlarge the burr hole and make direct hemostasis in all but the most slight cases of arterial bleeding. If the bleeding can be stopped before blood has escaped into the basal cisterns or the ventricles and before brain swelling has become intense, no sequelae seem to follow and, as commonly known, no serious sequelae are seen following ligation of branches from the anterior cerebral artery on one side. This complication is unusual now, but occurred in several instances in the blind lobotomies and was then the most common cause of operative death—but, even so, surprisingly rare. In the now used open lobotomies (topectomy, undercuttings etc.) this complication is most rare and, if it occurs, easily dealt with.

*Lesion of deep structures* was mostly seen in the blind lobotomies due to faulty placing of the cut or to tugging on the brain by the blunt instruments used. Fall of blood-pressure and other signs of shock was sometimes noted, but more often symptoms set in later and belong to the postoperative complications. Lesion of the anterior horn was very frequent in the blind lobotomies, but seldom recognized until the postoperative Roentgen-examination, when contrast was found in the ventricles. Later symptoms were dependent on the contrast used, but mostly slight or non-demonstrable.

## VI. Postoperative complications.

With the introduction of modern forms of lobotomy (topectomy, undercuttings, decortications) postoperative complications have become extremely rare. The patient may be somewhat slow during the first days due to slight edema, but usually he is not. Sphincteric disturbances which were the rule following the blind and more extensive lobotomies likewise are exceptions and if present disappear during the first days. One might say that the immediate postoperative "lobotomy-syndrome" has disappeared following the introduction of partial and selective procedures. Even so

*postoperative intracerebral hematoma* may be seen. This complication was the most common one following the blind and extensive lobotomies. The patient may awaken after the operation, but during the following hours he becomes increasingly slow and torpid. Clinical signs of increased intracranial pressure may be seen, but are frequently slight or absent. If a patient does not awaken properly or, after having been awake, suddenly or progressively becomes more torpid, an intracerebral hematoma must always be thought of. Lumbar or, better, suboccipital, puncture will show bloody fluid, while pressure may or may not be significantly elevated. The safe course will be to open the wounds and remove the clot (or clots!) if present. FREEMAN and WATTS suggest the tapping of the cuts with a canula and have seen sudden improvement following the elapse of blood or xanthochromic fluid and this may be attempted in dubious cases. In all more serious cases most neurosurgeons will certainly prefer to open the wounds properly and evacuate the hematoma if present. In the open lobotomies postoperative hematomas are rare and if met with easily dealt with through the larger openings made. A clinical picture similar to that of postoperative hematoma may be met with in *postoperative edema* and the diagnosis may be impossible without exploration. The use of a contrast medium in all closed lobotomies may be of help as pointed out by SJÖQVIST, who described the bi-convex shadow of the contrast medium outlining the hematoma.

Even if bleeding and hematoma are the most common causes of death in the closed lobotomies, they are surprisingly rare in all larger materials: 3 cases in FREEMAN-WATTS' first 610 patients, 6 of 1000 patients in McKISSOCK's material, 4 out of our own FREEMAN-WATTS series of 400 patients. In the open lobotomies these complications are rarer still— one of POPPEN's 470 patients with open total lobotomy, one of our own 193 patients with the same technic, while out of our 800 patients with orbitomedial undercutting only one patient died from hematoma.

### 1. Immediate post-lobotomy syndrome.

As mentioned above many patients following the modern form of lobotomy (*topectomy, undercutting, decortication*) do not exhibit any special immediate post-lobotomy syndrome. This is particular evident when lobotomy has been performed for otherwise intractable pain and the patients' personalities are more or less intact.

In the blind and more extensive lobotomies this syndrome was, however, the rule: when the patient awoke, he was confused, blunted, and might be apathetic or violent. Micturition and defaecation were usually involuntary and even when these symptoms were transient, they in some cases persisted for weeks. False conclusions were drawn from such patients and it was commonly believed that they were necessary sequelae; likewise it was believed, that their appearance was a good omen for the ultimate result. The syndrome is still seen following total lobotomy, but even so less pronounced, when the lobotomy has been performed by open operation, than when performed by blind operation and by means of blunt instruments.

Another frequent cause of immediate post-lobotomy symptoms and even death in the blind, extensive lobotomies was incorrect placing of the cuts. That the anterior horn was opened in many cases is quite clear, but if no bleeding occurred this usually gave no definite symptoms except perhaps symptoms of cerebral oedema and some hypersecretion of cerebro-spinal fluid. If hypothalamic nuclei were damaged, however, vegetative symptoms occurred with disturbed metabolism, especially of water and sugar, general vasomotor paralysis with cutaneous bleedings in addition to prolonged unconsciousness. These symptoms sometimes disappeared after 2—3 weeks but it happened that patients died. Autopsy showed bleedings and oedema in the anterior part of the hypothalamus (3 personal cases).

Such symptoms might also appear because of secondary bleedings behind the cuts due to pulling on the brain by blunt instruments. Even nowadays such secondary softenings and thromboses may be met with, if only exceptionally in old and arteriosclerotic patients.

Postoperative confusion nowadays seems to be seen especially following operations on the convexities (*topectomy*, SCOVILLE's *undercutting of the lateral surface*) while it is the exception following operation on the medial surface (*orbito-medial undercutting, cingulectomy*).

A complication still met with is postoperative agitation with motor unrest, especially in some cases of schizophrenia. Barbiturates seem of no effect, while chlorpromazine may be useful.

## 2. The chronic post-lobotomy syndrome.

One of the most serious objections advanced against lobotomy is what has been called *the chronic post-lobotomy syndrome* or *post-lobotomy dementia*. This objection became important to us in the period when we tried *total lobotomy*. During this time many neurosurgeons felt that the reason for insufficient improvement in the patients' behaviour following lobotomy might be due to insufficient operation, and the tendency at that time was to make the lobotomy as complete as possible. In lobotomized patients where the operation is of benefit there is a *change in the patients' psychical manifestations* and this is, of course, the essential purpose of the operation. Whether this change however, means a *psychical defect* it has been extremely difficult to determine. Repeated tests (especially HALSTEAD) have mostly shown no or only doubtful intellectual defect, but it must be remembered that preoperative testing of these patients frequently was impossible. Most experienced investigators, however, agree, that some patients, especially totally lobotomized patients with arterio-sclerosis or other organic, especially atrophic, brain lesions, present psychical changes comparable to those which we in previous examinations (BUSCH) of psychical symptoms in patients with neurosurgical disease called *euphoric fatuity*—the patient's personality is flat with easily changed emotions, while responsibility, forethought and initiative are compromised. The syndrome is extremely difficult to describe as it varies with the individual personality but there is no doubt that some sort of *general primitivization* has taken place.

Even if these changes were a reasonable price to pay for improvement in violent and intractable schizophrenics they still were an extremely grave objection and is the reason why some psychiatrists and neurosurgeons show a negative attitude as to psychosurgery. It was, in addition, the most pressing motive in changing the technic of old-time lobotomy in the direction of less extensive and more selective operations.

We can now say that this massive syndrome only appears in some, mostly totally lobotomized, patients (table 13) and, as mentioned, especially in older patients with arteriosclerosis or other atrophic brain disease. In such patients we may even now with our selective operations see gross personality changes: one has the feeling that the operation compromises the last small margin, which conditions a certain amount of psychical life in such patients.

A personal experience: A 57 years old somewhat arteriosclerotic woman had been hospitalized for 10 years for schizophrenia. For 3 years she had been stuporous and impossible to contact. She did not speak, had to be fed by force and was continuously unclean. A series of insulin shocks were without effect. Following bilateral total frontal lobotomy (open method) it was possible to contact her, she spoke and was gradually able

*Table 13.* After O. ØDEGAARD: Personality Changes Following Leucotomy (1952).

| | Total leucotomy | | | | | | Lower quadrant leucotomy | | | | | |
|---|---|---|---|---|---|---|---|---|---|---|---|---|
| | No. | Result | | | Loss of initiative | Asocial traits developed | No. | Result | | | Loss of initiative | Associal traits developed |
| | | Remission | Improvement | No result | | | | Remission | Improvement | No result | | |
| Curative operations . . . . | 13 | 7 | 6 | | 2 | | 10 | 4 | 4 | 2 | | 1 |
| Palliative . . . | 10 | 8 | | 2 | | | 9 | 7 | | 2 | 1 | 1 |
| Total . . . . | 23 | | | 2 | 2 | | 19 | | | 4 | 1 | 2 |
| Curative . . . . | 15 | 8 | 7 | | 2 | 1 | 21 | 7 | 10 | 4 | | |
| Palliative . . . | 16 | 13 | | 3 | 5 | | 15 | 4 | | 11 | | |
| Total . . . . | 31 | | | 3 | 7 | 1 | 36 | | | 15 | | |
| Curative . . . . | 28 | 15 | 13 | | 4 | 1 | 31 | 11 | 14 | 6 | 3 | 3 |
| Palliative . . . | 26 | 21 | | 5 | 5 | | 24 | 11 | | 13 | 2 | 2 |
| Total . . . . | 54 | | | | 9 | 1 | 55 | | | 19 | 5 | 5 |

to learn the names of the nurses. She started to eat spontaneously and the first two months voraciously. Subsequently she ate normally, was able to be up and about in a quiet ward. She was, however, quite unemotional and without initiative, unquestioningly falling in with any suggestion. She chattered gaily with visiting relatives, but gave the impression that she lived exclusively in the moment. She was discharged fron the hospital, but was a continuous problem in her home, because of a complete lack of responsibility and after two months returned to the hospital, where she seems happy but "empty".

Compared with the preoperative condition this patient obviously improved, but there seems no doubt that lobotomy (total) in this patient was responsible for invalidating symptoms. Most neurosurgeons who have worked in this field in the time of total lobotomy will be able to reproduce similar experiences and the chronic postlobotomy syndrome must always be a memento in psychosurgery.

Many incorrect statements have, however, been made as to the frequency of this syndrome—incorrect because no due respect has been paid to two important factors: The type of operation performed and the particular brain operated upon. In the first years of psychosurgery, when quite hopeless, burned out, old and arteriosclerotic patients were submitted to primitive forms of lobotomy this syndrome was frequent. Even so, it was frequently impossible to be certain that the symptoms observed were due to operation and not were sequelae of disease. Growing experience with the same syndrome in different patients have now made it clear that the underlying pathology really is the operation performed—in particular brains.

With altered indications and with the introduction of the various forms of selective operations our percentage of invalidating postlobotomy syndrome is now less than 5% and the syndrome is practically only seen in patients with cerebral atrophy from some cause or other.

On the other hand this must not cause us to be lax in indications. It is quite clear that *any* form of interference with cerebral pathways *must* mean a potential reduction in cerebral function, even if we are unable to demonstrate this reduction. While some patients seem to be cured without any *demonstrable* psychical defect, other patients present symptoms which may or may not be due to the operation performed. In schizophrenic patients we have found it impossible to investigate this question satisfactorily. In 34 non-schizophrenic patients treated by orbito-medial undercutting no defect or conspicuous symptom was observed in 21. In 13 patients we found psychical changes, which, with due reservation, we have classified as post-operative sequelae: Lack of initiative, emotional blunting or inability to express otherwise "normal" emotions, slight euphoria, lack of restraint, failing comprehension and judgment and careless dispositions. In the majority of patients mentioned, however only one or a few of these symptoms were present and there was no "syndrome".

With the strict indications for lobotomy which we follow in Scandinavia these symptoms may seem a small price for recovery from an incapacitating disease, but it is certainly healthy for the psychiatrist as for well as the neurosurgeon to remember that even in patients where no pathological symptoms were demonstrated, potential cerebral reactions have certainly been limited. In other patients one has the indefinable feeling known to most investigators that there *is* some elusive change even when batteries of tests show no change. It seems that the introduction of the special tests of ROBINSON and FREEMAN may give us a chance of solving this question. Even if it is impossible in this place to go into details it must be mentioned that the investigations of ROBINSON and FREEMAN (1954) point to some change in what they call *self-continuity*. This has nothing to do with memory, but with the realization of the self between the past and the future—as a result of the first and as a possible factor in the second. Self-continuity is necessary for the feeling of responsibility for past, present and future acts and would seem necessary for correlated anxiety, hope and the sense of self-respect.

It may be that with the investigations of ROBINSON and FREEMAN we are at last in the way of tracking down the elusive symptoms in lobotomized patients without gross defects. However, most of the patients had been lobotomized by FREEMAN and WATTS standard lobotomy or by the blind transorbital operation. It would be of considerable interest to examine patients operated upon by selective operations by the tests of ROBINSON and FREEMAN.

## 3. Postoperative epilepsy.

While the modern selective operations as mentioned to a certain extent have eliminated the danger of gross psychical defects in most patients we must confess that one of the more serious complications of lobotomy, *postoperative epilepsy*, seems to be more frequent now than in the old-time blind lobotomy. The percentage of FREEMAN and WATTS of 12,3 % is one of the highest for this form of lobotomy—while the English Board of Controls 3,3 % seem to be the lowest. Usually the percentage for postoperative convulsions in the FREEMAN-WATTS lobotomy (lateral approach) has varied between 5—8%. A personal experience of 400 cases shows an incidence of fits of 7,2%. In *topectomy* the percentage seems to vary between 10—30%, while our own material of *orbito-medial undercutting* shows an all-over percentage of 14%. The fact that schizophrenic males, as pointed out by PARTRIDGE, seem especially liable to get postoperative epilepsy, is pronounced also in our material, where 35% of schizophrenic males had one or more postoperative fits as against only 10% for the other groups of orbitomedial undercutting. No certain explanation can be given for this—on the other hand it seems certain that atrophic brain lesions favour epilepsy and many of our schizophrenic patients, perhaps more males, had long histories and frontal atrophy on encephalography. This seems of interest in connection with the observation of FREEMAN and WATTS, who found 7,2% of convulsions in patients having one lobotomy, while no less than 47 % of patients having more than one operation developed fits.

Most of the patients have only one or two fits and are easily controlled by medication. Curiously enough it seems that patients having epilepsy before lobotomy usually have no more fits than before.

The interval between lobotomy and the first seizure is variable—in about one fourth the first seizure occurred during the first two month, in somewhat less than two thirds between 3—12 months, but fits have been known to start as late as two years after the operation.

Some authors think that preoperative electro-shock favours post-lobotomy epilepsy. We have seen no evidence of this. The EEG in many patients show dysrythmia preoperatively. Following lobotomy dysrythmia is the rule but tends to normalize itself after 1—2 months.

The seizures usually are universal, uncharacteristic and only exceptionally of focal character, except when unilateral hematoma or infection has occured. In these cases excision of the meningocerebral scar may have effect, but usually the fits are easily controlled by medication.

In order to cut down the percentage of fits various operative procedures have been tried—the placing of Gelfoam, spongostan and similar preparations over the cortical incision—in our hands, at least, without obvious gain. In a series of 100 undercuttings Gel-film was placed between the cortex-incision and the dura, without lowering the incidence of fits significantly.

Consequently, the risk of postoperative convulsions has to be reckoned with. Usually it plays no great rôle, but in some cases it may be a real complication and death in status epilepticus has been reported. A postoperative EEG with subsequent prophylactic medication may be of value.

Only in about 1 % of lobotomized patients postoperative epilepsy becomes a real problem—i.e. 1 % of the patients develop epilepsy with more than six fits a year. Still, also this complication has to be reckoned with when indications for psychosurgery is discussed.

## VII. Results and indications.

To anybody who has been working with psychosurgical problems it will be quite clear that it is extremely difficult to tabulate results in a statistical manner, because comparison between different series, even when the same technic and more or less comparable indications have been used, always will be difficult and not infrequently impossible. The tables cited above must therefore only be taken as examples of what has happened in particular series and must be taken with several grains of salt, not least because of differences in psychiatric classification and terminology in different places.

However, what evidence we do possess makes it abundantly clear that the introduction of psychosurgery in psychiatry has been of revolutionary importance performed as it for the most part was in otherwise intractable patients. Against these results stand the defects described and the theoretical, but therefore not less relevant, consideration that operations in which neuronal paths are severed *must* mean interference with the reaction possibilities of the brain operated upon.

While the indication for psychosurgery in the particular case always must be the responsibility of the psychiatrist, who alone has the necessary knowledge of the particular patient, some general lines can be laid down here, but it must be clearly understood that they only represent the point of view of the author. As a general rule we feel that psychosurgery should be considered an *ultimum refugium* and should never be resorted to until every other, less destructive, form of therapy has been tried. On the other hand most series seem to show that the best results are obtained if the history of the patient is not too long—PARTRIDGE finds the best results in patients with a history of less than five years and in our series also the best results (*apparently cured* and *much improved*) belong to this group. The experienced psychiatrist frequently will be able to make a prognosis of the particular case after some years of treatment and of observation and in this way valuable time may be saved (see a. o. KALINOWSKY).

### 1. Schizophrenia.

In many older materials schizophrenia was the only indication for psychosurgery and the group is still the most important one from a statistical point of view—in Scandinavia more than half of the beds in the psychiatric wards are occupied by schizophrenics.

It was by results in this, previously quite hopeless field, that psychosurgery established itself. Taking schizophrenia as a whole it may be said that psychosurgery in several large series has shown good results (i.e. *apparently cured* and *much improved*) in about one third, another third being *significantly improved*, while one third is unchanged or worse. In most larger materials 10—15% of the patients are able to work and live a normal life, while another 10—15% are able to live at home, but unable to do useful work.

Of the different groups of schizophrenia it seems established that *katatonic excitations* and the *paranoid* group show the best results, especially when personality is more or less intact, while results are less good in *katatonic stupors*, except in the group showing occasional bursts of excitement. In *simple schizophrenia* and in *hebephrenics* most series show only poor results and deterioration usually has progressed so far when psychosurgery comes into consideration that operation frequently has no purpose.

Generally it seems as if *pychnic constitutional type*, *premorbid adequate personality*, *sudden onset of illness* and some *response to shock-therapy* favour a good prognosis for psychosurgery, while malignant destruction of personality without tendency to remission reduces the chances of success.

The optimum time for psychosurgery in schizophrenia would seem to be within 3—5 years of onset of illness when other, less destructive therapies have failed. But it must be stressed that the experience of the psychiatrist *with the particular patient* must be the all-determining factor.

## 2. Affective disorders.

In *manic-depressive psychosis* the nearly specific effect of shock-therapy limits the number of candidates for psychosurgery, and there is no doubt that shock is the treatment of choice in these patients. There seems, however, to be a group of shock-resistant patients, mainly chronic, agitated endogenous depressions where psychosurgery is of definite help. Another group comprises those patients who relapse after a short time following shock. In both groups psychosurgery, especially the medial operations, shows good results some series having 50% of *much improved* and *apparently cured* with 30% *significantly improved*. Results seem better when *depression* dominates the clinical picture, while *manic* phases makes the prognosis worse and many investigators find psychosurgery contraindicated in *chronic manias*.

In *involutional depressive psychoses* as in *presenile depressions* results are impressive, especially when the picture is dominated by depression, anxiety, restlessness, hypochondriac and depressive delusions. Really good results *(apparently cured and much improved)* may be counted on in 70—80%. But even so indication must not be taken too lightly—patients have been known to suicide as a result of loss of inhibition. Partridge thinks that results in endogenous depressions are inferior to those with a more "reactive" background.

Consequently, in affective disorders, even more than elsewhere, psychosurgery is only indicated when *all* other treatments, especially *adequate* shock-therapy have been tried without avail.

## 3. Psychopathy and neurosis.

Among the chronic deviations of character and mood we have found it difficult to distinguish clinically between the predominantly constitutionally conditioned and the predominantly psychogenic or environmentally conditioned states. As, in addition, in our experience results of psychosurgery do not differ as regards the most psychopathy-resembling and the most neurosis-resembling pictures, they may perhaps be grouped together under three subdivisions: *Depressive-sensitive reactions*, *emotional instability* and *obsessive-compulsive reactions*.

In the first group, *depressive-sensitive reactions*, our *indications* have been incapacity and hospitalization for years on account of depressive basic mood, over-sensitiveness, dysphoria, anxiety, attempted suicide, irritability, dissatisfaction, grievance towards surroundings combined with feelings of inferiority and insufficiency etc. In this group, too all other forms of therapy must be tried before psychosurgery which, however, is of definite value—two thirds of our operated cases belong to the groups *apparently cured* and *much improved*.

In the *emotional instability-group* about half of our patients belong to these two groups. *Indications* have been prolonged, incapacitating, emotional instability manifested by violent affective reactions of varying sorts—aggressiveness on trifling provocation, shouting, obscene speech, negativism, attempts at suicide etc. With their in the main intact personalities these patients frequently make good recoveries and 40—50% become socially integrated and fit for work.

The group of *obsessive-compulsive reactions* has been one of the great successes of psychosurgery and several series show 80—90% good results. The *indications* are anguish and incapacity for years on account of obsessive phenomena with simultaneous anxiety, oversensitiveness, depressions or suicidal tendencies. When most series in spite of these good results are small the reason is that the risk of postoperative defects in these well-integrated, non-psychotic patients is of particular importance. Only the less destructive operations are indicated in this group.

## 4. Other indications.

Indication for psychosurgery may be found in various other forms of mental disease and derangement, especially when anxiety, emotional instability and tension dominates the picture.

In the deviations following in the wake of *chronic encephalitis* some authors have seen effect, while our own experience in this field is meagre. In *kryptogenic epilepsy* when accompanied by aggressive behaviour, emotional instability and other troublesome symptoms, psychosurgery not infrequently may be of help, especially in the form of medial operations (*orbito-medial undercutting*) or as LE BEAU's *cingulectomy*. As usual following craniotomy for any cause fits are less frequent in the time following lobotomy and epilepsy in itself is no contraindication for lobotomy—postoperative fits are *not* more frequent in epileptics than in other patients.

*Troublesome symptoms in oligophrenics* have been the indication in some series, but results seem conflicting. In our experience a certain pacification may be expected in about half of the patients, but the risk for postoperative further deterioration is considerable as in other patients with organic brain disease.

In *patients with otherwise intractable pain* the indication for psychosurgery is an old and well-founded one. It is well-known that lobotomy does not interfere with pain pathways, but serves to abolish or diminish anxiety and fear of pain—"the pain is still there, but it does not bother me" is the typical response of the patient following psychosurgery. The main indication is *intractable carcinoma* which cannot be relieved by the usual forms of pain surgery and where life-expectancy still is too long for the patient to be morphinized. Not a few patients with intractable carcinoma could be about their house and live a life of some joy and use to themselves and others, if it were not for pain. In most instances pain surgery (chordotomy etc.) is the answer. But in some cases, especially in carcinomas of the face and neck, these operations are not feasible, while in others the psychical situation is the decisive factor. In these cases psychosurgery undoubtedly serves a useful purpose, best performed as one of the selective operations. In our experience *orbito-medial undercutting* serves well in these patients and psychical reduction is usually slight or non-existant on tests. Curiously enough drugs, even in heavily addicted patients usually may be discontinued immediately after the operation, which fact has led to psychosurgery being tried in

*drug addiction and alcoholism*. Results have been conflicting, as might be expected, as the underlying psychopathology in these patients differs extremely. Also the attitude of the patient towards his affliction is of importance—PARTRIDGE found no effect in patients feeling no remorse for their action, while results were good in patients using drugs to combat anxiety and tension. In similar cases of alcoholism results have been noted, but extreme caution is necessary in this field as psychosurgery performed for other psychiatric conditions has been known to lead to alcoholism as a result of lack of inhibition and restraint. We have no personal experience in this field.

As might be expected psychosurgery has been tried in a number of conditions, which did not respond or responded adversely. In any form of *organic brain disease* caution is advisable because a destructive lesion already exists and the lesion of lobotomy superimposed thereon may mean a serious psychical deterioration. In some cases of *Parkinsonism* with depression the psychical situation has been improved.

## VIII. Which form of lobotomy should be used?

In the preceding pages the question posed in this chapter has been tentatively touched upon and it should be clear that our knowledge as yet is insufficient.

The ideal of a psychosurgical operation has been mentioned: *An operation combining a maximum of effect on pathological mental symptoms with a minimum of postoperative psychical defect.*

While belief in equipotentiality of the frontal cortex would reduce this problem to a purely quantitative one, the growing evidence that different parts of the frontal lobe have different functions makes *localization* of lobotomy of importance. In different neurosurgical centres different approaches have been made to solve this question, while blind, massive lobotomies are still performed in some quarters. The tendency, however, is clearly in the direction of more localized and selective operations. Which operation should then be chosen today? Is there a "standard" form of lobotomy to be used as a *passe-partout* key or should the operation be suited to the particular symptoms of the particular patient?

There is no doubt that this last-mentioned course would be the ideal one, but at present, it remains a counsel of perfection, On the other hand some lines of conduct may tentatively be mentioned as the personal opinion of the present writer:

1. It seems fairly certain that *cingulectomy* gives few recognizable psychical defects, while effect is insufficient in severe psychoses.

2. That operations involving *the lateral parts* of the frontal lobes (topectomy, undercutting of areas 9—10 etc.) have shown effect in even severe psychoses, while blunting of intellect, disturbances of mental balance and perhaps in "continuity of self" frequently have been noted.

3. That undercutting of *the orbital surface* has been effective in some series, especially in *psychoneuroses* and milder mood disturbances, but not infrequently has failed in *schizophrenia.*

4. That undercutting of *the medial surface* (orbitomedial undercutting of BUSCH medial lobotomy (POPPEN), LIVINGSTON's cingulate cortex isolation) has been as effective as any other form of lobotomy for relief in even severe psychoses, including schizophrenia, while personality changes seem rare.

Or, to use the words of MEYER and BECK (1954): "*The dorsal and, in particular, the dorsolateral sectors of white matter do not appear to be as significant for improvement as the mid-central, orbital and cingulate sectors. On the other hand involvement of the dorso-lateral and lateral white matter, and particularly cortex, appears to be one of the factors responsible for severe personality changes.*"

Consequently we *at the present moment* should feel inclined to answer the question posed in this chapter in the following way:

In *milder obsessional neuroses* and in *non-psychotic epileptic disorder* we would favour the use of *cingulectomy* as performed by LE BEAU.

In *all severe disorders* our method of choice would be *orbitomedial undercutting*, but other forms of medial lobotomy (POPPEN, LIVINGSTON) may be just as good. Others would prefer undercutting of the *orbital* surface (the extensive form of SCOVILLE), some few undercutting of the *superior* surface.

Personally we feel that *total lobotomy* (open method) nowadays seldom should be used as a primary operation, but it may be useful in *re-lobotomy* if this should be done at all. Actually, we have seen some few cases of schizophrenia responding to total lobotomy, while a previous orbitomedial undercutting had been in vain. Another indication for total lobotomy we find in *oligophrenics* with marked aggressiveness and gross deterioration, where one can hope for no intellectual improvement, and where the operation is performed for purely pacifying purposes. Even in such cases we not infrequently first perform our usual orbitomedial undercutting and only, when this has proved ineffective, total lobotomy is done.

With *transorbital lobotomy*, with which FREEMAN reports such good results, we have no experience and, consequently, no opinion.

At present we seem far from the ideal of suiting the operation to the particular patient. Still, evidence is accumulating and we now know that the present "selective" operations are less destructive than the blind, massive operations previously used. Still, this chapter should close on a warning note: To think that you can do even "selective" lobotomies without compromising at least potential reactions in that particular frontal lobe is, of course, mere foolishness. The astounding thing is that so few reactions actually are measuredly compromised. But even in "selective" operations—or what other self-deceiving names we may find—thousands of reaction possibilities are lost forever, and it is important never to forget that fact.

However, if the result of an admittedly destructive operation is the transformation of a shrieking, unclean, self-destructive demon into a more or less integrated and working personality, it is surely justified. And in other cases, where severe and distressing mental symptoms threaten to disintegrate a more or les intact personality and where *every other*, less destructive, therapy has been tried in vain, psychosurgery is the fully justified *faute de mieux*,—justified in a time of little or no understanding of the underlying pathophysiology.

## References.


ALMEIDA LIMA, P.: A technica cirurgica de leucotomia cerebrale. Med. contemp. Lisboa **67**, 267 (1949).

BAILEY, O. T., F. D. INGRAHAM, P. S. WEADON and A. F. SUSEN: Tissue reactions to powdered tantalum in the central nervous system. J. of Neurosurg. **9**, 83 (1952).

— P.: Treatment of psychomotor states by temporal lobectomy. Proc. Assoc. Res. Nerv. a. Ment. Dis. **31**, 341 (1953).

*Board of Control* (Great Britain): Results in 1000 leucotomies. H. M. Stationary Office, London 1947.

BRICKNER, R. M.: (a) The intellectual functions of the frontal lobes: a study based upon observation of a man after partial bilateral frontal lobectomy New York 1936.

— (b) Bilateral frontal lobectomy; follow-up report of case. Arch. of Neur. **41**, 580 (1936).

BURCKHARDT, G.: Über Rindenexcisionen, als Beitrag zur operativen Therapie der Psykosen. Allg. Z. Psychiatr. **47**, 463 (1891).

BUSCH, E.: Psychical symptoms in neurosurgical disease. Acta psychiatr. (Københ.) **15**, 257 (1940).

— O. HALMSTED, O. LUND, J. NEVIN and P. THELLE: Orbitomedial undercutting in mental disease. Danish Med. Bull. **2**, 10 (1955).

CARILLO, R., M. F. ORIBE y R. PARDALL: La leucotomia prefrontale. Dia. Med. (Buenos Aires) **19**, 2483 (1947).

CLARK, W. E. LE GG.: Connections of the frontal lobes of the brain. Lancet, **1948 I**, 353.

*Columbia Greystone Ass.*: (I) Selective partial ablation of the frontal cortex. New York 1949. (II) Psychosurgical problems. London 1952.

DAX, D. C., F. REILMAN et E. J. RADLEY-SMITH: Prefrontal leucotomy. Dig. Neur. et Psychiatr. **16**, 533 (1948).

—, and E. J. RADLEY-SMITH: The operation of prefrontal leucotomy. Brit. J. Surg. **36**, 74 (1948).

FERNÁNDEZ-MORÁN, H.: Leucotomia e enyectiones en los lobulos prefrontales por la via transorbitaria. Arch. Venezol. D. L. Soc. otolaryng., ophthalm., neurol. **7**, Nr. 4 (1946).

FIAMBERTI, A. M.: Transorbital lobotomy. Indicazioni e technica della leucotomia prefrontale transorbitaria. Rass. Neuropsichiatr. **1**, 3 (1947).
FRANZ, S. I.: Function of the cerebrum; the frontal lobes. Arch. Psychol. **1**, Nr. 2 (1949).
FREEMAN, W.: (I) Transorbital leucotomy. Lancet **1948**, 371.
— (II) Late results of prefrontal lobotomy, study of 200 patients followed 10—17 years. Congr. neurol. internat., Lisbonne **1954**, p. 452.
—, and J. W. WATTS: (I) Psychosurgery. London 1947.
— — (II) Psychosurgery, II. Springfield, Ill.: Ch. C. Thomas 1950.
FULTON, J.: Functional localization in the frontal lobes and cerebellum. Oxford 1949.
GLEES, P.: Effect or lesions on the cingular gyrus and adjacent areas. J. Neurol., Neurosurg. a. Psychiatry **13**, 178 (1950).
GRANTHAM, E. G.: Prefrontal lobotomy for relief of pain. Report of new operative technic. J. of Neurosurg. **8**, 405 (1951).
GREENBLATT, M., R. ARNOT and H. C. SOLOMON (Editors): Studies in lobotomy. New York 1950.
—, and H. C. SOLOMON (Editors): Frontal lobes and schizophrenia. New York 1953.
HAMLIN, H., J. M. R. DELGADO, W. P. CHAPMAN and H. E. ROSVOLD: Therapeutic interruption of frontal fibre tracts by electrolysis. V. Congr. neurol. internat., Lisbonne **1954**, p. 397.
HERRICK, C. J.: Brains of rats and men; survey of the origin and biological significance of the cerebral cortex. Chicago 1926.
HOFSTATTER, L.: Prefrontal lobotomy in treatment of chronic psychosis, with special reference to section of the orbital areas only. Arch. Neur. et Psychiatr. **53**, 125 (1945).
JONES, C. H., and J. G. SHANKLIN: Transorbital lobotomy. Northwest Med. **47**, 421 (1948).
KALINOWSKY, L. B., and P. H. HOCH: (I) Shock treatments, psychosurgery and other somatic treatment in psychiatry, 2. Edit. New York 1952.
— — (II) Shockbehandlungen. Psychochirurgie. Bern u. Stuttgart 1952.
KLÜWER, H., and P. BUCY: (I) Analysis of certain effects of bilateral temporal lobectomy in the rhesus monkey. J. of Psychol. **5**, 33 (1938).
— — (II) Preliminary analysis of funtions of temporal lobes in monkeys. Arch. Neur. et Psychiatr. **42**, 979 (1939).
LASHLEY, K. B.: Brain mechanism and intelligence: a quantitative study of injuries to the brain. Chicago 1929.
LE BEAU, J.: (I) Experience with topectomy for relief of intractable pain. J. of Neurosurg. **7**, 79 (1950).
— (II) Anterior cingulectomy in man. J. of Neurosurg. **11**, 268 (1954).
— (III) Psycho-chirurgie et functions mentales. Paris 1954.
LE GROS CLARK, W. G.: Connections of the frontal lobes of the brain. Lancet **1948 I**, 353.
LIVINGSTON, K. E.: Cingulate cortex isolation for treatment of psychoses and psychoneuroses. A. Proc. Assoc. Res. Nerv. a. Ment. Dis. **31**, 374 (1953).
LOVE, J. G.: Prefrontal lobotomy in treatment of mental diseases. Surg. technic. Proc. Staff, Meet. Mayo Clin. **18**, 372 (1943).
LYERLY, J. G.: (I) Transsection of deep association fibres of prefrontal lobes in certain mental disorders. South. Surgeon **8**, 426 (1939).
— (II) Surgical relief in pain. Florida M.A. J. **34**, 339 (1947).
MCGREGOR, J. S., and J. R. CRUMBIE: Improved leucotome. Lancet **1942 I**, 654.
MCKENZIE, K. G., and L. D. PROCTOR: Bilateral frontal lobe leucotomy in treatment of mental disease. Canad. Med. Assoc. J. **55**, 433 (1946).
MACKISSOCK, W.: Rostral leucotomy. Lancet **1951**, 91.
MCLARDY, T.: Thalamic projection to frontal cortex in man. J. of Neur. **13**, 198 (1950).
—, and A. MEYER: Anatomical correlates of improvement after leucotomy. J. Ment. Sci. **95**, 182 (1949).
MACLEAN, P. D.: (I) Psychiatric implication of physiological studies in fronto-temporal portion of the limbic system (visceral brain). Electroencephalogr. Clin. Neurophysiol. **4**, 407 (1952).
— (II) The limbic system and its hippocampal formation. Studies in animals and their possible application to man. J. of Neurosurg. **11**, 29 (1954).
MARIOTTI, E., e M. SCIUTI: Therapie intracerebrale nelle malatti mentale. Riv. sper. Freniatr. **61**, 870 (1937).
METTLER, F. A.: See Columbia-Greystone Ass.
MEYER, A.: Anatomical lessons from prefrontal leucotomy. Congr. internat. psychiatr., Paris 1950, III, 107.
MEYER, A., and E. BECK: (I) Neuropathological problems arising from prefrontal leucotomy. J. Ment. Sci., **91**, 411 (1945).
— — (II) Prefrontal leucotomy and related operations. Anatomical aspects of success and failure. London 1954.
—, and T. MCLARDY: Clinico-anatomical studies of frontal lobe functions based on leucotomy material. J. Ment. Sci. **95**, 403 (1949).
MONIZ, E.: (I) Premiere tentatives operatoires dans le traitment de certain psychoses. Paris.
— (II) How I came to perform prefrontal leucotomy. I. Internat. conf. of psychosurgery, Lisbon 1949.

MONIZ, E.: (III) Cirurgia das psicoses. Novos resultados terapeuticos. Bol. Acad. Cicuc. Lisboa **8**, 345 (1936).
— (IV) La psychochirurgie. Portugal Med. **21**, 1 (1937).
—, et P. ALMEIDA LIMA: Samptomes du lobe prefrontale. Revue neur. **65**, 582 (1936).
OBRADOR, M. S. ALCALDE: Temporal lobotomy. J. of Neuropath. **6**, 185 (1947).
ØDEGAARD, O.: Personality changes following leucotomy. I. Congr. mondial de psychiatrie, Paris 1950, IV, 388.
ODY, F.: Traitment de la demance precause par resection du lobe prefrontale. Arch. ital. Chir. **53**, 321 (1938).
PAPEZ, J. W.: (I) A proposed mechanism of emotion. Arch. of Neur. **38**, 725 (1937).
— (II) Cerebral mechanisms. J. Nerv. Dis. **89**, 145 (1939).
PARTRIDGE, M.: Prefrontal leucotomy. Oxford 1950.
PENFIELD, W.: Bilateral frontal gyrectomy and postoperative intelligence. Proc. Assoc. Res. Nerv. a. Ment. Dis. **27**, 519 (1947).
PETRIE, A.: Personality and the frontal lobes. London 1952.
PEYTON, W. T., H. H. NORAN, and E. W. MILLER: Prefrontal lobectomy (Excision of the anterior areas of the cerebrum). Amer. J. Psychiatr. **104**, 513 (1948).
PIMENTA, M., M. YAHN, e A. J. CETTE: Sobre a leucotomia parietale en 22 pacientes. II. Internat. conf. of psychosurg., Lisbon 1947.
POOL, J. L.: (I) The visceral brain of man. J. of Neurosurg. **11**, 45 (1954).
— (II) Topectomy, a surgical procedure for the treatment of mental illness. J. Ment. Dis. **110**, 144 (1949).
— R. HEATH, and J. WEBER: Topectomy, Surgical indications and results. N. Y. Acad. Med. **25**, 335 (1949).
POPPEN, J. C.: Technic of prefrontal lobotomy. J. of Neurosurg. **5**, 514 (1948).
RIECHERT, T.: Die stereotaktischen Operationen und ihre Anwendung in der Psychochirurgie. A Med. Contemp. **72**, 589 (1954).
RIZATTI, E., et G. BORGARELLO: Duecento malatti di mente operati di leucotomia prefrontale a la Moniz. Nevrasse **1**, 11 (1940).
ROBINSON, M. F., and W. FREEMAN: Psychosurgery and the self. New York a. London 1954.
RYLANDER, G.: (I) Personality analysis before and after lobotomy. Proc. Assoc. Res. Nerv. a. Ment. Diss. **27**, 691 (1948).
— (II) Relief of symptoms and personality changes of superior convexity and orbital undercutting. V. Congr. neurol. internat., Lisbonne 1952, II, 213.
SCARFF, J. E.: Unilateral prefrontal lobotomy for the relief of intractable pain, etc. Surg. etc. **89**, 385 (1948).
SCOVILLE, W. B.: (I) Selective cortical undercutting as a means of studying frontal lobe function in man. J. of Neurosurg. **6**, 65 (1949).
— (II) Selective cortical undercutting. Results in new method in fractional lobotomy. Amer. J. Psychiatr. **107**, 730 (1951).
— (III) Observation in medial temporal lobotomy and uncutomy in treatment of psychotic states. Proc. Assoc. Res. Nerv. a. Meut. Dis. **31**, 347 (1953).
SJÖQUIST, O. u. Mitarb.: Diagnosis of intracerebral haematomas following frontal lobotomy. I. Internat. conf. of psychosurgery, Lisbon 1947, p. 319.
SMITH, W. K.: Results of ablation of the cingulat region of the cingular cortex. Federat. Proc. **3**, 42 (1944).
SPIEGEL, E. A., and H. T. WYCIS: Stereoencephalotomy. New York 1952.
TALAIRACH, J., M. DAVID u. Mitarb.: Recherches sur la coagulation therapeutique des structures sous-corticales chez l'homme. Revue neur. **81**, Nr 1 (1949).
THORNDIKE, E. L. u. Mitarb.: Measurement of intelligence. New York 1927.
TORKILDSEN, A.: Experience with a case of bilateral occipital leucotomy. Acta psychiatr. (København.) **24**, 701 (1949).
TOW, P. M., and W. LEW: Orbital leucotomy. Lancet **1953 II**, 644.
VIANNA, J. M.: Lobotomia prefrontale; cadeira de technica operatorica e cirurgia experimentale. Thesis de faculd. de Med. Bahia 1946.
WALKER, E. A.: The primate thalamus. Chicago 1938.
WARD, A. A., and W. S. MACCULLOCH: Projection of frontal lobes on hypothalamus. J. of Neurophysiol **10**, 309 (1947).
WHITTY, C., J. DUFFIELD, P. M. TOW, and H. CAIRNS: Anterior cingulectomy in treatment of mental disease. Lancet **1952**, 475.
WILLIAMS, J. M., and W. FREEMAN: Amygdaloidectomy for the suppression of auditory hallucinations. J. Nerv. Dis. **116**, 456 (1952).
YAHN, M., PIMENTA e A. J. CETTE: Trattamento circurgico das molestias mentais (leucotomia). São Paulo 1951.

# Gezielte Hirnoperationen.

Von

LARS LEKSELL.

(Mit Abschnitten von K. LIDÉN und C. H. HERTZ.)

Mit 24 Abbildungen.

## A. Einleitung.

Für Operationen an tiefliegenden subcorticalen Teilen des Gehirns ist die gewöhnliche chirurgische Operationstechnik unter Leitung des Auges wenig geeignet. Der Mangel an deutlichen anatomischen Anhaltspunkten in der Hirnsubstanz erlaubt keine ausreichend genaue Lokalisation, und es läßt sich nicht vermeiden, daß oberflächlicher gelegene Strukturen erheblich geschädigt werden.

Im Jahre 1908 führten HORSLEY und CLARKE ihre stereotaktische Methode (στερεός: starr, räumlich, τάξις: Ordnung) für experimentelle Studien am Tier ein. Mit einem Richtinstrument, das am Kopf des Tieres befestigt wurde, konnten Nadelelektroden oder andere chirurgische Instrumente nach einem dreidimensionalen Koordinatensystem eingestellt werden, so daß sie jeden beliebig gewählten Punkt im Gehirn erreichen konnten. Diese Methode und verschiedene Modifikationen derselben haben eine ausgedehnte Verwendung für hirnphysiologische Studien gefunden.

Es dauerte auffallend lange, bis die stereotaktische Methode für Operationen am Menschen zur Anwendung kam. CLARKE (1920) war sich völlig darüber im klaren, welche Vorteile eine exakte mechanische Einstellung und Kontrolle der chirurgischen Instrumente gegenüber den gebräuchlichen Methoden hatte. Er schlug vor, die stereotaktische Methode zur Durchschneidung von Gehirnbahnen bei Neuralgien, zur Behandlung von Hirntumoren, zum Einführen von Radiumnadeln und zur Diagnose und Behandlung von Hirnblutungen und Abscessen zu verwenden.

Der erste, der eine genaue Zielmethode für intrakranielle Eingriffe am Menschen angewandt hatte, war indessen KIRSCHNER (1933). Unabhängig von HORSLEY und CLARKE arbeitete er seine Technik zur Elektrokoagulation des Ganglion Gasseri durch das Foramen ovale für die Behandlung der Trigeminusneuralgie aus. KIRSCHNERs Methode konnte mit unbedeutenden Modifikationen auch für andere intrakranielle Operationen übernommen werden. Er schlug vor, diese Technik zur Punktion von Hirnabscessen und der Hypophyse zu verwenden.

Für intracerebrale Operationen wurde die stereotaktische Methode zuerst von SPIEGEL, WYCIS und Mitarbeitern (1947, 1948) verwendet. Man versuchte damit in erster Linie die frontale Lobotomie bei psychischen Störungen durch einen mehr selektiven Eingriff im Thalamus zu ersetzen. Nach der Pionierarbeit von SPIEGEL und WYCIS sind an verschiedenen Orten Instrumente und Methoden für stereotaktische intrakranielle Operationen entwickelt worden (MEYERS und HAYNE 1948, BAUDOIN und REMOND 1949, 1951, JASPER und HUNTER 1949, LEKSELL 1949, TALAIRACH und Mitarbeiter 1949, 1950, 1951, HAYNE und MEYERS 1950, MONNIER 1950, 1951, UCHIMURA und NARABAYASHI 1950, BAILEY und STEIN 1951, RIECHERT und WOLFF 1951, PERTUISET 1951, DELGADO und

Mitarbeiter 1954, KÖBCKE 1954, LISTER und SHERWOOD 1955). Die meisten dieser Zielgeräte sind Varianten der von HORSLEY und CLARKE (1908) und CLARKE (1920) entwickelten rectilinearen oder äquatorialen Instrumente, doch sind zum Teil auch andere Lösungen gesucht worden. Die Lokalisation der gesuchten Struktur erfolgt in der Regel in drei verschiedenen Ebenen durch Röntgenaufnahmen, ausgehend von Beziehungspunkten im Gehirn oder am Schädel. Ein Teil der beschriebenen Methoden befindet sich noch in einem vorbereitenden experimentellen Stadium, während andere, wie z. B. diejenigen von SPIEGEL und WYCIS, TALAIRACH und RIECHERT klinisch in recht großem Umfang angewandt worden sind, insbesondere für die funktionelle Gehirnchirurgie: zur Zerstörung von Kernen und Bahnensystemen bei psychischen Krankheiten, chronischen Schmerzzuständen und Hyperkinesien. Die Methodik von SPIEGEL und WYCIS ist in einer Monographie mit einem stereotaktischen Atlas beschrieben worden (SPIEGEL und WYCIS 1952). Ausführliche Berichte über ihre eigenen Methoden sind auch von TALAIRACH und Mitarbeitern (1952), MONNIER (1952) und RIECHERT und WOLFF (1953) veröffentlicht worden. KIRSCHNERs Methode wird auch in KIRSCHNERs Chirurgischer Operationslehre behandelt (GULEKE 1950). HASSLER und RIECHERT (1954) haben kürzlich eine Übersicht über die gegenwärtigen Indikationsgebiete für gezielte Operationen gegeben.

In letzter Zeit wurden Versuche mit gezielten Hirnoperationen unter Anwendung von strahlender Energie gemacht (LEKSELL 1951, FRY 1953, LEKSELL und Mitarbeiter 1955). Mit der Ausarbeitung von zweckmäßigen stereotaktischen Methoden ist es möglich geworden, die Elektroden, die in das Gehirn eingeführt werden, durch ein Strahlenbündel zu ersetzen und durch Kreuzfeuerbestrahlung oder Focussierung der Strahlung in der gewünschten Struktur dieselbe zu zerstören oder funktionell zu beeinflussen. Grundsätzlich hat man damit den Schritt zu einer unblutigen intracerebralen Chirurgie getan. Von den verschiedenen Energieformen, welche die moderne Strahlenphysik zu bieten hat, kommen zunächst Ultraschall oder Röntgenstrahlen in Frage.

Die Versuche, Ultraschall für die Gehirnchirurgie zu verwenden, gehen auf die Experimente von LYNN und Mitarbeiter (1942) und LYNN und PUTMAN (1944) zurück, welche mit focussierter Ultraschallbestrahlung begrenzte Schädigungen am Tiergehirn erzielten. Der Effekt des Ultraschalles auf das Zentralnervensystem ist von mehreren Autoren studiert worden (PETERS 1949, WOEBER 1949, FRY und Mitarbeiter 1950, 1953, WALL und Mitarbeiter 1951, 1953, WULFF und Mitarbeiter 1951, ANDERSON und Mitarbeiter 1951, CICARDO 1951, ZUBIANI 1951, ALLEGRANZA 1952, HEYCK 1952, BUSNEL und Mitarbeiter 1953 u. a.). Kürzlich haben auch FRY und Mitarbeiter (1954, 1955) mit gezieltem Ultraschall umschriebene Schädigungen in der Tiefe des Katzenhirns erzeugt. LINDSTRÖM (1954) hat ohne Verwendung einer gezielten Methodik als Ersatz für die Lobotomie die Stirnlappen am Menschen beschallt. Die Anwendung des Ultraschalles zu unblutigen gezielten Operationen am Menschen wird indessen durch die Dämpfung des Schalles im Schädelknochen erschwert. Hinzu kommt die Schwierigkeit, die Tiefendosis genau zu berechnen. Bisher war es bei den meisten Versuchen notwendig, den Knochen vor Applikation des Ultraschalles zu entfernen.

Der Effekt der Röntgenstrahlung auf das Gehirn ist früher besonders in Zusammenhang mit der Strahlentherapie der Tumoren studiert worden (s. WARREN 1943, WACHOWSKI und CHENAULT 1945, PENNYBACKER und RUSSEL 1948, RUSSEL und Mitarbeiter 1949, ZEMAN 1949, HORNBERGER 1951, FOLTZ und Mitarbeiter 1953, HICKS und MONTGOMERY 1953, ROSS und Mitarbeiter 1953, MALAMUD und Mitarbeiter 1954 u. a.). Es hat sich dabei um große Bestrahlungsfelder gehandelt, und Versuche, einen örtlichen Effekt in der Tiefe des Gehirns zustande zu bringen, sind nicht gemacht worden. Durch intensive Kreuzfeuerbestrahlung mit schmalen Strahlenbündeln ist es indessen möglich, eine umschriebene Läsion in der gewünschten Struktur zu erzielen (LEKSELL 1951, CARPENTER und WHITTIER 1952, JEPPSSON und LEKSELL 1954). Die Möglichkeit, die ultraharte Strahlung der modernen Teilchenbeschleuniger zu verwenden, hat die Voraussetzungen für eine örtliche Bestrahlung von kleinen Gebieten im Gehirn verbessert. Bei Versuchen am Affen mit schmalen Strahlenbündeln eines Betatrons haben ARNOLD und Mitarbeiter (1954) kürzlich gezeigt, daß die Resistenz des Hirngewebes gegen Röntgenstrahlen weitaus geringer ist als bisher angenommen wurde.

Die gezielten Hirnoperationen können nun in zwei Gruppen eingeteilt werden. Einmal in solche, bei denen Nadelelektroden oder andere Instrumente ins Gehirn eingeführt werden: *offene gezielte Operationen*, und dann in solche, bei denen Bündel von strahlender Energie verschiedener Art verwendet werden: *gezielte Strahlenchirurgie*. Das ganze Gebiet dieser stereotaktischen Operationen befindet sich bislang noch in einem technischen Entwicklungsstadium und die klinischen Behandlungsresultate lassen sich zur Zeit noch nicht endgültig beurteilen.

In der folgenden Darstellung wird die Methode behandelt, mit der der Verfasser eigene Erfahrungen gemacht hat. Die physikalischen Grundlagen der Strahlenchirurgie werden von LIDÉN und HERTZ in besonderen Abschnitten behandelt. Ein ausführlicher Bericht über die gezielten Hirnoperationen bei verschiedenen Krankheitszuständen kann erst zu einem späteren Zeitpunkt gegeben werden. Zunächst gilt es, die technischen Hilfsmittel weiter zu verfeinern. "If our clumsy fingers are to unravel the mysteries or alleviate the disablements of the most exquisite instrument of which our imagination can conceive, it must be by a refined art, informed by a topographical accuracy not yet approached, aided by instruments whose delicacy and precision will tax our beggarly efforts at construction to their utmost limit, and inspired by a concern for the resources of the victim which will tolerate no scratch, nor jar, nor the waste of a drop of blood that any possible exercise of ingenuity can prevent" (CLARKE 1920).

# B. Methodik.

## I. Stereotaktisches Instrumentarium.

Die Konstruktion des stereotaktischen Instrumentes geht im Prinzip aus Abb. 1 hervor (LEKSELL 1949, 1955). Das Instrument besteht aus einem halbkreisförmigen Metallbogen $B$ mit einem Nadelführer oder Strahlrichter $C$, der entlang des Bogens $B$ gleitet und so eingestellt ist, daß die Nadel $N$ oder der entsprechend gerichtete Strahl, z. B. ein Röntgenstrahlenbündel, immer den Mittelpunkt des Bogens trifft. Der Bogen wird am Kopf des Patienten mit Hilfe eines Innenrahmens $D$ so befestigt, daß seine Achse durch den gesuchten Punkt $X$ geht. Entsprechend dem Abstand des Zielpunktes von der Mittellinie wird der Bogen seitwärts verschoben. Da der Bogen nach vorne und hinten geschwenkt und der Nadelführer an beliebiger Stelle fixiert werden kann, ist es möglich, die Nadel durch jedes beliebig angelegte Bohrloch in das Gehirn einzuführen. Wenn an Stelle der Nadel ein Strahlenbündel verwendet wird, kann die Struktur im Gehirn einer Kreuzfeuerbestrahlung ausgesetzt werden.

Ein stereotaktisches Instrument zur Einstellung von Nadelelektroden oder Kanülen ist in Abb. 2 dargestellt. Das Instrument besteht aus einem Außenbogen mit Nadelführer und einem rechtwinkligen Innenbogen mit eingravierten Koordinaten, die bei den Röntgenaufnahmen gleichzeitig als Markierungen auf den Film sichtbar werden. Der Innenbogen wird an drei Punkten am Kopfe des Patienten befestigt. Hierzu werden kleine Bohrlöcher in der Lamina externa angelegt. Das Instrument ist aus Aluminium hergestellt und wiegt etwa 1,5 kg.

Ein Instrument für die stereotaktische Strahlenchirurgie zeigt Abb. 3. Der massive Außenbogen ist so an der Röntgenröhre befestigt, daß das durch eine austauschbare Blende gelenkte Strahlenbündel den Mittelpunkt des Bogens trifft. Das Instrument kann als Ganzes um eine Achse rotiert werden, die dem zentralen Röntgenstrahl entspricht. Der Patient kann daher den Kopf etwas bewegen, ohne daß sich die Einstellung verändert.

Abb. 4 zeigt ein Instrument für Operationen mit Ultraschall. Ein starker Ultraschallgeber ist auf dem halbkreisförmigen Bogen befestigt und mit einem Spiegelsystem versehen, welches das Schallbündel auf einen Brennpunkt im Zentrum des Bogens konzentriert.

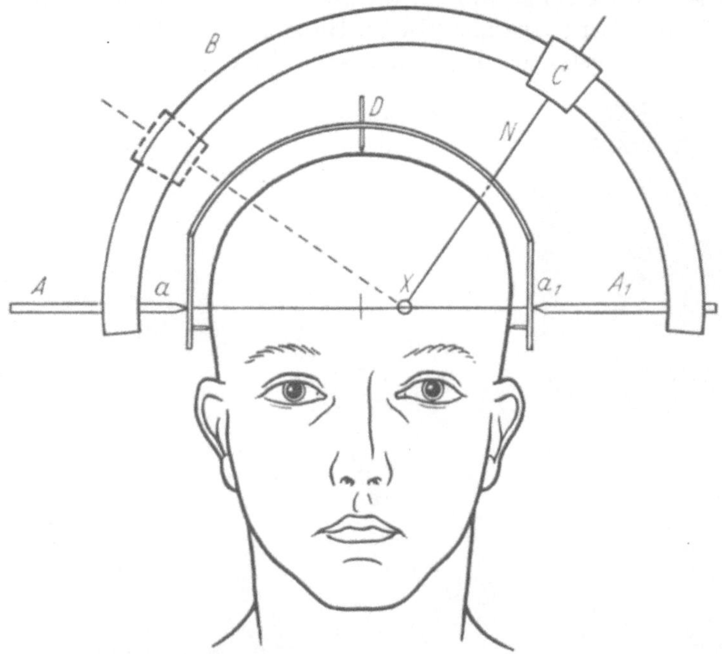


Abb. 1. Schematische Darstellung des stereotaktischen Instruments (s. Text).

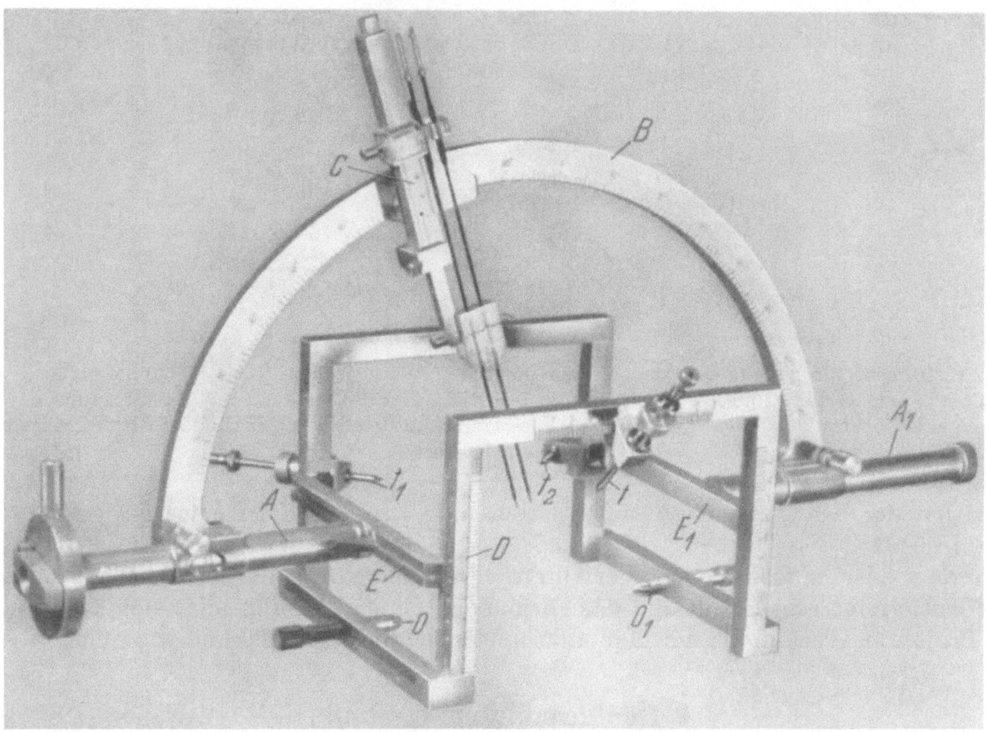


Abb. 2. Instrument für offene gezielte Operationen. Das Instrument besteht aus einem Außenbogen $B$ mit dem Nadelführer $C$, der in beliebiger Lage am Bogen befestigt werden kann. Die Achsen des Außenbogens $A$ und $A_1$ werden mit Hilfe zweier Querbalken $E$ und $E_1$ am Innenrahmen $D$ befestigt. Der Innenrahmen wird mittels der mit Stopphülsen versehenen Bohrer $f$, $f_1$ und $f_2$ im Schädelknochen befestigt. Die Ohrpflöcke $O$ und $O_1$ erleichtern ein symmetrisches Anbringen des Rahmens.

## II. Lokalisationsmethode.

Die stereotaktische Ortung gilt vornehmlich der Lagebestimmung normaler Hirnstrukturen, Kerne und Leitungsbahnen, die röntgenologisch nicht darstellbar sind. Die Lage dieser Strukturen wird vorzugsweise an Hand ihres Verhältnisses zu intracerebralen, encephalographisch dargestellten Bezugspunkten bestimmt. Die Ortung erfolgt durch

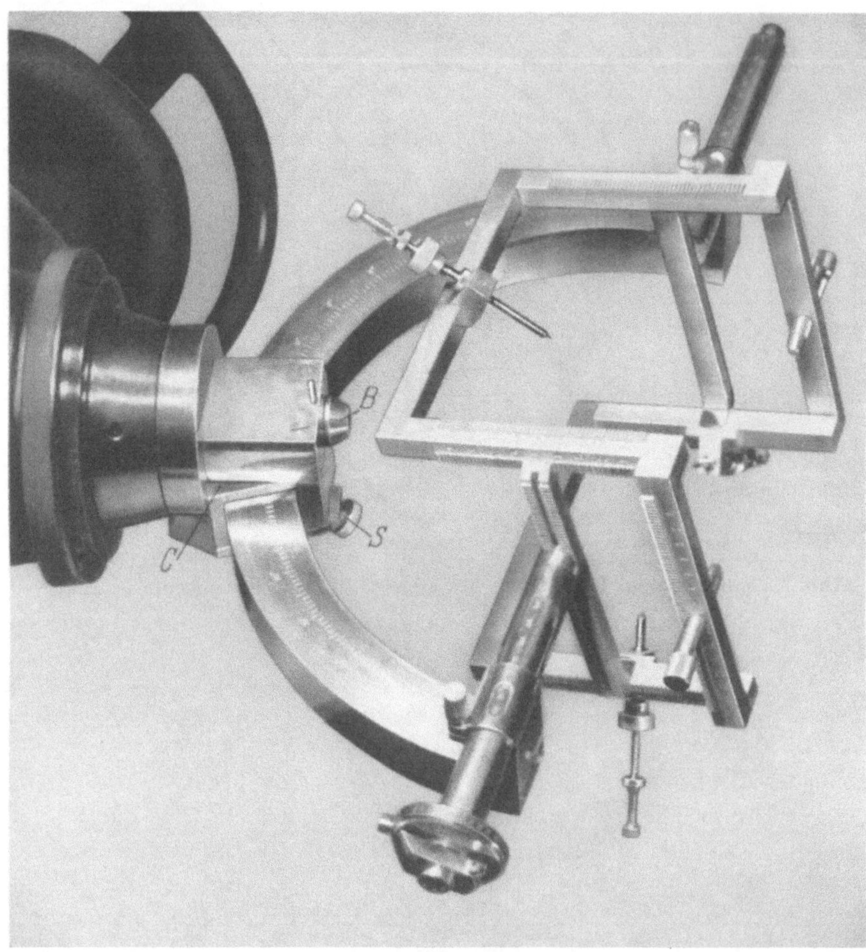


Abb. 3. Instrument für gezielte Strahlenchirurgie mittels Röntgenstrahlen. Der halbkreisförmige Außenbogen ist mit dem Halter *C* an der Röntgenröhre befestigt. Der Bogen kann mit der Schraube *S* in der gewünschten Lage befestigt werden. Das durch die Bleiblende *B* laufende Strahlenbündel trifft den Mittelpunkt des Außenbogens.

Korrelation der Röntgenbilder des Patienten mit Schnittbildern eines geeigneten Vergleichshirnes.

Bei dem hier beschriebenen Verfahren wird das Röntgenbild in verhältnismäßig kurzer Entfernung angefertigt und das gewonnene Perspektivbild mittels eines geometrischen Projektionsverfahrens mit dem anatomischen Bild in Beziehung gebracht.

### 1. Röntgenaufnahmetechnik.

Die Röntgenaufnahmen werden mit einer gewöhnlichen Röntgenapparatur angefertigt, die im Operationssaal eingebaut ist. Der am Kopf des Patienten befestigte Innenrahmen des Instrumentes ist mit der Röntgenröhre mechanisch verbunden. Mit dieser Anordnung (Abb. 5) lassen sich genaue Lateral- und Frontalprojektionen herstellen. Die

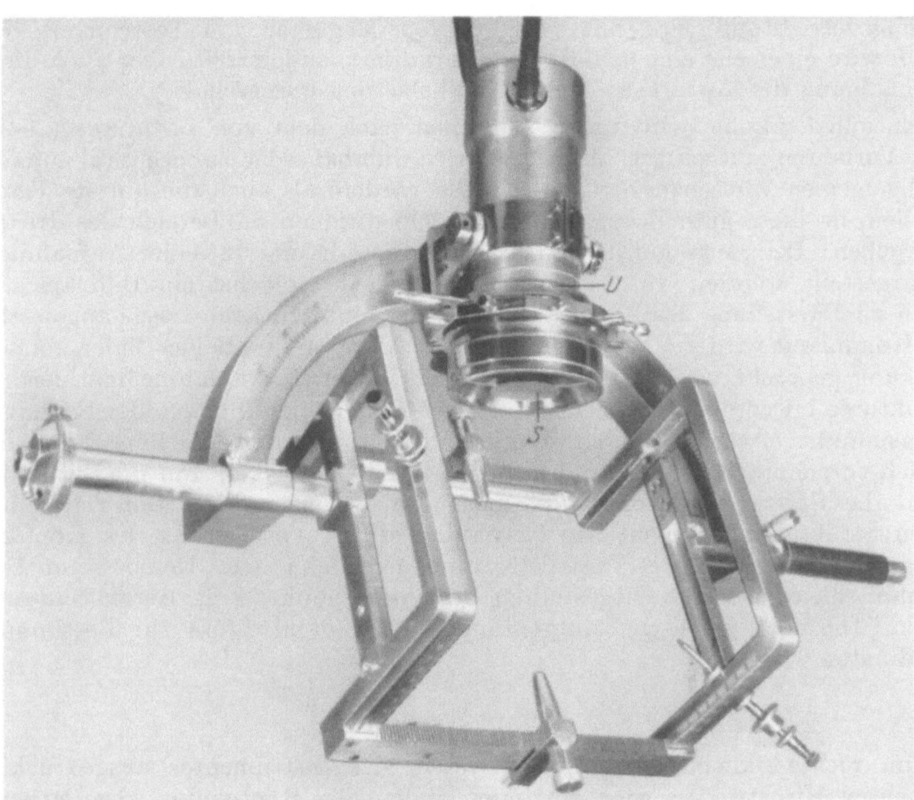


Abb. 4. Instrument für Strahlenchirurgie mittels focussiertem Ultraschall. Der Schallgeber ist mit einer Doppelspiegelvorrichtung *S* versehen, der die Strahlung zu einem Focus im Mittelpunkt des halbkreisförmigen Außenbogens konzentriert.

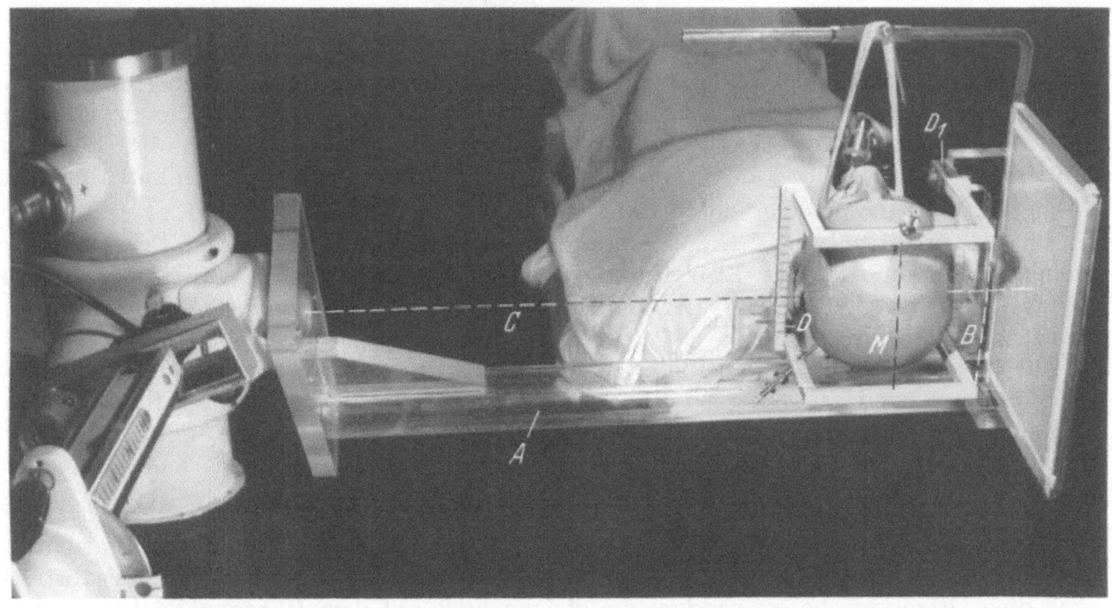


Abb. 5. Röntgenanordnung für den Ortungsvorgang. Die Röntgenröhre ist mittels einer Plexiglasröhre *A* mechanisch mit dem Innenrahmen des stereotaktischen Instrumentes sowie dem Kassettenhalter verbunden. Die Befestigung am Instrument geschieht mit Hilfe permanenter Magneten *D*, $D_1$. Der Zentralstrahl *C* (rechtwinklig zum Instrumentrahmen und zur Filmkassette) geht durch die Mitte des Rahmens. Der Abstand vom Focus der Röntgenröhre zur Mittelebene *M* des Rahmens ist im vorliegenden Falle 71 cm, zur filmnahen Rahmenebene *B* 80 cm.

Verbindungsvorrichtung wird mit permanenten Magneten am Instrument befestigt. Hierdurch wird einerseits eine exakte Lage garantiert, andererseits aber auch die Gefahr einer Schädigung der Apparatur durch Überbelastung ausgeschaltet.

Die Encephalographie wird im wesentlichen nach dem von LINDGREN (1949) empfohlenen Verfahren ausgeführt. Das Gas wird lumbal oder suboccipital injiziert. Es ist im allgemeinen wünschenswert, sowohl die vordere als auch die hintere Kommissur darzustellen, da diese gute Bezugspunkte bei Operationen im Bereich des dritten Ventrikels ergeben. Bei geeigneter Technik können diese häufig auf einer Aufnahme gleichzeitig dargestellt werden. In der Regel wird jedoch zunächst ein Bild am sitzenden Patienten zu Darstellung des Aquäduktes und der hinteren Kommissur angefertigt. Die vordere Kommissur wird am liegenden Patienten dargestellt. Beide Bilder können dann zur Deckung gebracht und beide Kommissuren auf einer Aufnahme markiert werden. Für Strukturen im vorderen Bereich des Gehirnes können die Spitzen der Seitenventrikel als Bezugspunkte verwendet werden. Für das Mesencephalon und die hintere Schädelgrube eignen sich vornehmlich der Aquädukt und der vierte Ventrikel. Für die seitlichen Hirnteile sind die Spitzen der Temporalhörner gute Bezugspunkte. Die Darstellung der jeweiligen Strukturen geschieht wie gewöhnlich durch Verlagerung des Kopfes, wobei sich die gewünschten Teile des Ventrikelsystems mit Gas füllen. Der besseren Übersicht wegen empfiehlt es sich, die dargestellten Beziehungspunkte z. B. durch Nadelstiche zu markieren. Die noch feuchten Röntgenfilme werden dann direkt zur Bestimmung der Zielkoordinaten verwandt.

## 2. Ortungsverfahren.

Die im rechtwinklichen Koordinatensystem des Instrumentes ausgedrückte Lage der gesuchten Hirnstruktur wird bestimmt, indem das Röntgenbild des Patienten mit Photographien frontaler und sagittaler Hirnschnitte in Beziehung gebracht wird. Ein Beispiel für die anatomischen Bezugsbilder ist in Abb. 6 und 7 dargestellt. An dem *in situ* fixierten Gehirn wurde mit einem Focus-Objektabstand von 15 m eine Ventrikulographie vorgenommen. Der das Gehirn treffende Teil des divergenten Strahlenbündels ist dann annähernd parallel und alle Teile des Gehirnes werden somit in natürlicher Größe wiedergegeben. Das auf transparentem Film angefertigte Bezugsventrikulogramm wird genau auf das anatomische Schnittbild superponiert, welches die gewünschte Struktur zeigt. Die Lage des gesuchten Punktes X, auf dem Hirnschnitt wird auf dem transparenten Ventrikulogramm markiert, das dann mit der Röntgenaufnahme des Patienten in Beziehung gebracht wird.

Die beiden Bilder werden aufeinandergelegt und mit Hilfe geeigneter Bezugspunkte zueinander orientiert. Zur Ermittlung der $x$—$y$-Koordinaten des Operationspunktes dienen die Seitenbilder und es wird dabei vorzugsweise von Bezugspunkten der Mittelebene, z. B. den Kommissuren des dritten Ventrikels, ausgegangen.

Zur Orientierung der beiden Bilder zueinander dient ein geometrisches Hilfsdiagramm (Abb. 8), bestehend aus einer Vielzahl von Radien und konzentrischen Kreisen. Die Radiuslängen zwischen den Kreisen bilden eine geometrische Reihe, deren Quote $k$, gleich ist dem Verhältnis zwischen den Abständen des Röntgenfocus zum filmnahen Plan $B$, und zur Mittelebene $M$ des Instrumentes ($k = \frac{FB}{FM}$, siehe Abb. 5). Der Origo des Diagramms entspricht dem Zentralstrahl auf der Röntgenaufnahme des Patienten. Einfache Berechnungen[1] zeigen, daß Punkte der Mittelebene $M$, die einen Kreisabstand nach dem Origo verschoben werden, die gleiche Lage auf dem Röntgenbild bekommen, als wären sie parallel zum Zentralstrahl auf die Instrumentebene $B$ projiziert worden. Die Koordinaten ($x$, $y$) können dann auf den Skalen dieser Instrumentebene abgelesen werden.

[1] Eine ausführliche Beschreibung des Lokalisationsvorganges wird an anderer Stelle veröffentlicht.

Die Seitenaufnahme des Patienten mit den darauf abgebildeten Instrumentskalen wird also als erstes auf der geometrischen Figur so ausgerichtet, daß der Zentralstrahl, d. h. der Punkt des Filmes, dessen focusnahe und filmnahe Koordinaten übereinstimmen,

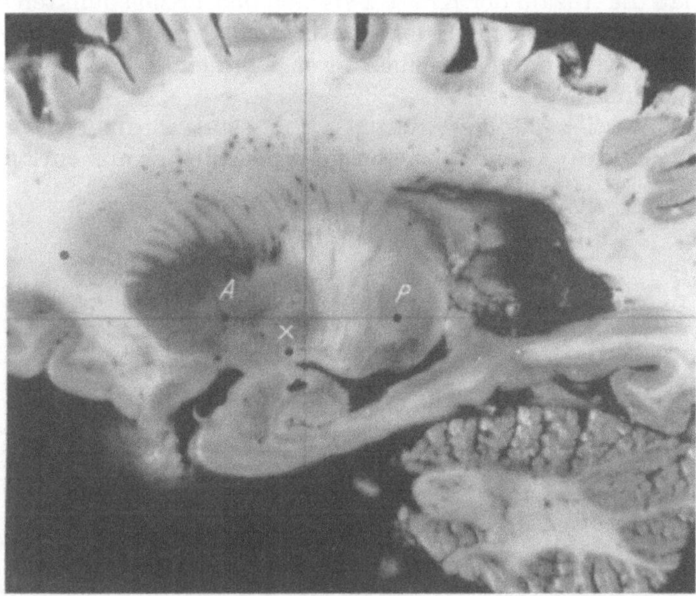


**Abb. 6.** Beispiel eines anatomischen Bildes eines Bezugshirnes. Auf das Schnittbild wurde das dazugehörige mit Parallelstrahlen angefertigte transparente Ventrikulogramm (Abb. 7) genau superponiert. *A* vordere, *P* hintere Kommissur. Die Lage der gesuchten Struktur *X* ist auf dem superponierten Ventrikulogramm markiert.

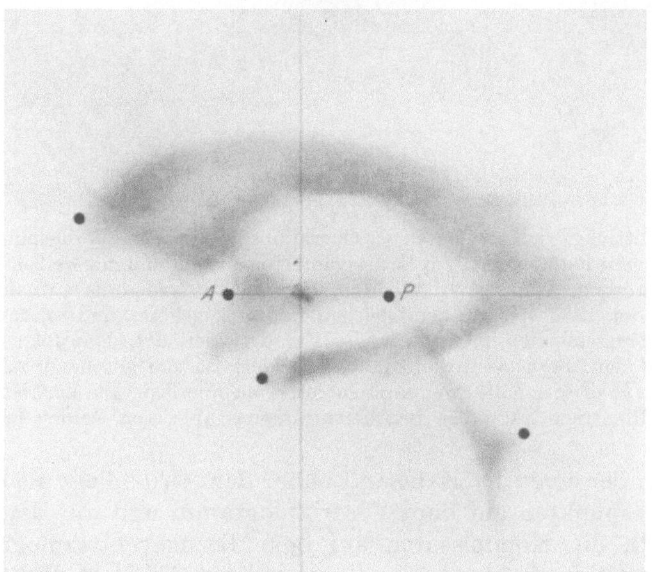


Abb. 7. Ventrikulogramm eines Bezugsgehirns mit bezeichneten Beziehungspunkten. *A* vordere, *P* hintere Kommissur. Diese Aufnahme kann genau auf die die gesuchte Struktur zeigende Photographie des Hirnschnittes superponiert werden und die Lage der Struktur *X* in ihrem Verhältnis zu den Bezugspunkten markiert werden. Das Bild wird darauf mit der Röntgenaufnahme des Patienten entsprechend Abb. 8 korreliert.

im Origo liegt. Das Ventrikulogramm (Abb. 7) mit der gewünschten, darauf markierten Struktur *X* wird dann so auf die Röntgenaufnahme gelegt, daß die korrespondierenden Bezugspunkte in der Mittelebene, z. B. die Kommissuren, dem gleichen Radius zugehören (Abb. 8). (An Stelle von Punkten in der Mittelebene kann der Mittelpunkt zwischen zwei zur Mittelebene symmetrischen Punkten benutzt werden. Der hierbei entstehende geometrische Fehler kann vernachlässigt werden.) Bei der Orientierung wird darauf geachtet, daß die Anzahl der Kreise zwischen den Bezugspunkten auf der Röntgenaufnahme des Patienten und denen des Ventrikulogramms die gleiche ist. Die korrespondierenden Punkte sind dann bezüglich ihrer Lage einander ähnlich mit dem Origo als Ähnlichkeitszentrum.

Die Lage des Operationspunktes, dessen $x$- und $y$-Koordinaten, erhält man durch Verschiebung des Punktes $X$ auf dem Bezugsventrikulogramm entlang seines Radius

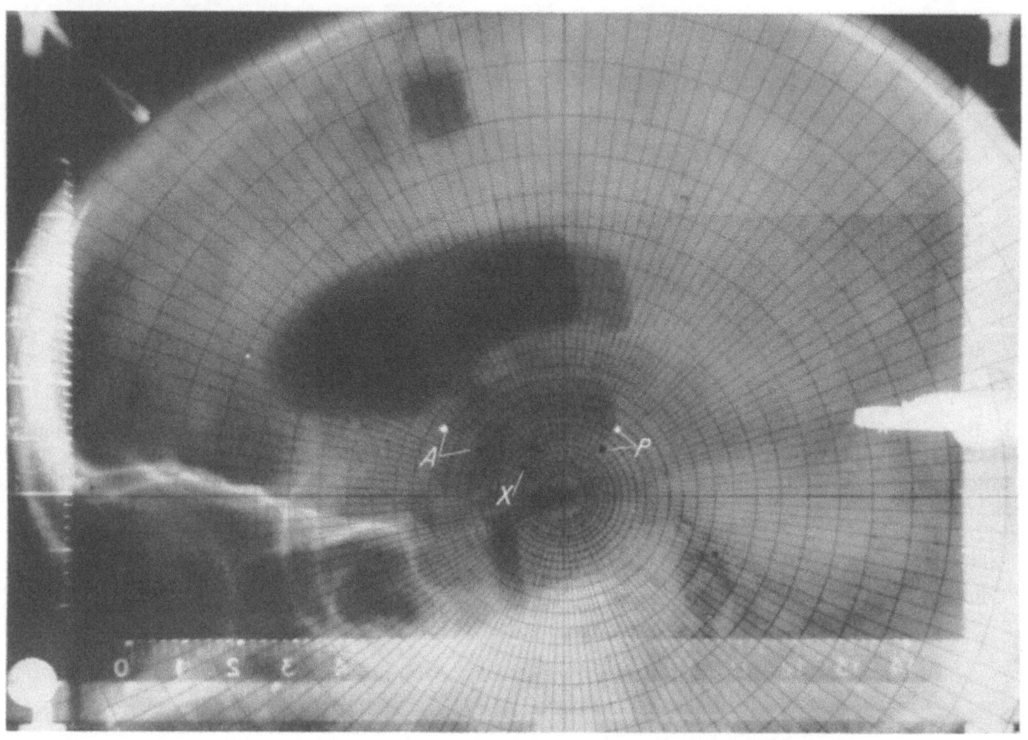


Abb. 8. Beispiel für Ermittlung der Koordinaten des Operationspunktes. Die Bezugspunkte, die Kommissuren $A$ und $P$, sind mit schwarzen Punkten auf dem Bezugsventrikulogramm und mit weißen auf dem Röntgenbilde des Patienten markiert worden. Wie aus der Abbildung hervorgeht, werden die Aufnahmen derart orientiert, daß die korrespondierenden Bezugspunkte dem gleichen Radius zugehören und so, daß sich zwischen ihnen die gleiche Anzahl von Kreiseinheiten, im vorliegenden Fall drei, befindet. Man folgt dann dem Radius des Punktes $X$, welcher auf dem Bezugsventrikulogramm markiert ist, die gleiche Anzahl von Kreiseinheiten minus einer Einheit, also in diesem Falle zwei Kreiseinheiten, nach außen. Die Zielkoordinaten können dann auf der kleineren, filmnahen Skala des Instrumentrahmens abgelesen werden ($x = 6{,}8$, $y = 2{,}6$).

bis zu einem Punkt, der einen Kreisabstand näher dem Origo liegt als der Anzahl Kreise zwischen den Bezugspunkten auf dem Ventrikulogramm und auf dem Patientbild entspricht. Wenn z. B. die Kommissuren auf dem Bezugsventrikulogramm drei Kreiseinheiten näher am Origo liegen als die Kommissuren auf dem Patientbilde, wird der Punkt $X$ zwei Kreise nach außen vom Origo aus verschoben. Die $x$- und $y$-Koordinaten können dann mit Hilfe eines Winkellineals direkt auf den Skalen der filmnahen Rahmenebene abgelesen werden.

Zur Feststellung des Abstandes des Operationspunktes von der Mittelebene, der $z$-Koordinate, werden die entsprechenden Frontalbilder benutzt. Man kann hierbei genau so wie bei der lateralen Projektion vorgehen. Das frontale Bezugsventrikulogramm wird auf dem Patientbilde mit Hilfe geeigneter Referenzpunkte wie z. B. die Spitzen des einen Temporalhornes und der Mittellinie orientiert. Liegen die Bezugspunkte, wie es mit dem vorderen Teil der Temporalhörner der Fall ist, in ungefähr dem gleichen Abstand von der filmnahen Rahmenebene wie die Mittelebene $M$ bei der Seitenprojektion, wird ein und dasselbe geometrische Hilfsdiagramm benutzt. Der auf dem Bezugsventrikulogramm markierte Punkt $X$ wird in der gleichen Weise wie bei Anwendung der Seitenbilder verschoben und die $z$-Koordinate wird auf der Skala des filmnahen oberen Rahmenbalken des Instrumentes abgelesen.

Der Vorgang ist für jeden beliebigen Focus-Objekt und Filmabstand verwendbar. Die konzentrischen Kreise auf dem geometrischen Hilfsdiagramm werden in Übereinstimmung mit dem Abstand vom Focus zu den Bezugspunkten und zu den Rahmenplänen konstruiert, auf welchen die Koordinaten abgelesen werden.

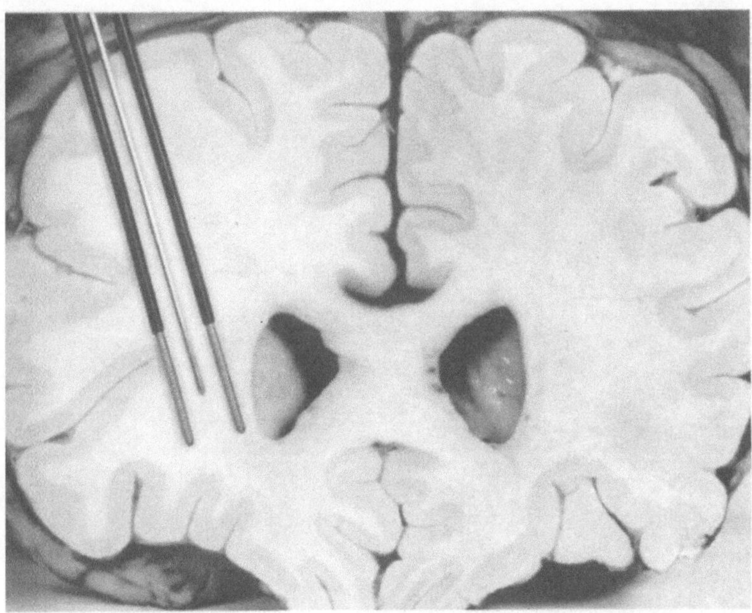

Abb. 9. Bipolare Elektrodenanordnung mit Thermoelement zwischen den Elektroden. Auf den Spitzen der Elektroden dünne Spiralen aus Tantaldraht, die nach durchgeführter Erwärmung als Röntgenindicatoren zurückgelassen werden.

## III. Offene gezielte Operationen.

Die offenen Operationen sind in erster Linie für die Einstellung von Kanülen oder Elektroden zur Punktion von Hirntumoren oder zur Zerstörung intracerebraler Strukturen durch Erwärmung vorgesehen.

### 1. Die temperaturkontrollierte Wärmeläsion.

Für die Erzeugung der Wärmeläsionen wird hochfrequenter Wechselstrom (1,75 MHz) eines chirurgischen Diathermieapparates mit symmetrischem Ausgang angewandt. Die Erwärmung findet zwischen zwei doppelten, mit Ebonitröhrchen isolierten Stahlelektroden statt. Die Temperatur im Gewebe wird mit einer Thermoelementnadel gemessen, die so eingeführt wird, daß sie zwischen den beiden Elektrodenspitzen liegt.

Die Elektrodenanordnung geht aus Abb. 9 hervor. Auf die Elektrodenspitzen werden kleine Spiralen aus dünnem Metalldraht aufgeschoben, die später als Röntgenindicatoren zurückgelassen werden. Die Temperatur wird auf einem Galvanometer abgelesen und das Gewebe wird bis auf 55—60° C erwärmt. Die beabsichtigte Ausdehnung der Läsion wird durch Veränderung der Länge der Elektrodenspitzen sowie des Elektrodenabstandes bestimmt.

## 2. Ausführung der Operation.

Die Operation wird im allgemeinen zusammen mit dem Ortungsvorgang in einer Sitzung durchgeführt. Der Innenrahmen des Instrumentes wird symmetrisch am Kopfe des Patienten befestigt, wonach die Ortung nach dem oben beschriebenen Verfahren vorgenommen wird. Nachdem nun die Zielkoordinaten des Operationspunktes ermittelt

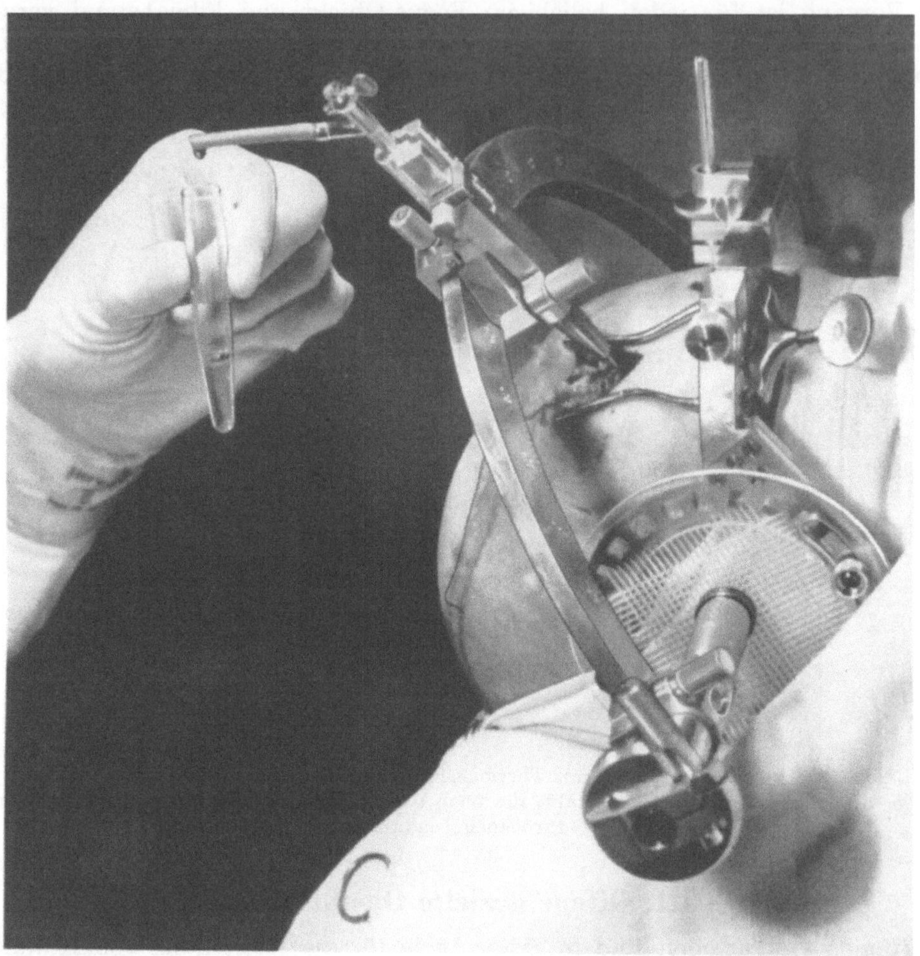

Abb. 10. Gezielte Punktion eines cystischen Kraniopharyngeoms zur Injektion radioaktiver Isotope. (Im vorliegenden Falle wurde ein Innenrahmen älterer Konstruktion benutzt.)

sind, wird an einer geeigneten Stelle der Konvexität ein Bohrloch angelegt. Die Querbalken ($E$ und $E_1$ in Abb. 2) werden entsprechend den $y$-Koordinaten des Operationspunktes am Innenrahmen befestigt. Danach werden die Achsen des Außenbogens an den Querbalken, entsprechend der $x$-Koordinate, angebracht. Zuletzt wird der Außenbogen je nach Abstand des Zielpunktes von der Mittellinie seitwärts verschoben ($z$-Koordinate). Der Mittelpunkt des Außenbogens ist dann so eingestellt, daß er dem gesuchten Punkt im Gehirn entspricht.

Der Bogen wird in einem der Lage des Bohrloches entsprechenden Winkel eingestellt und der Nadelführer über demselben am Bogen fixiert. Dann werden die Kanülen oder die Elektroden auf eine dem Mittelpunkt des Bogens entsprechende Tiefe eingeführt.

Die Punktion eines cystischen Kraniopharyngeoms und gleichzeitige Injektion von radioaktiven Isotopen zeigt Abb. 10.

Zur Erzeugung einer Wärmeläsion werden die mit den Drahtspiralen versehenen Elektroden und die Thermoelementnadel eingeführt und der Diathermiestrom langsam eingeschaltet. Die Erwärmung nimmt gewöhnlich 1—2 Minuten in Anspruch. Danach werden zunächst die Stahlelektroden und dann die Ebonithülsen entfernt, wobei die Drahtspiralen in der Läsion zurückgelassen werden. Nachdem das Bohrloch geschlossen ist, werden Röntgenaufnahmen zur Lagekontrolle der Spirale angefertigt (Abb. 11).

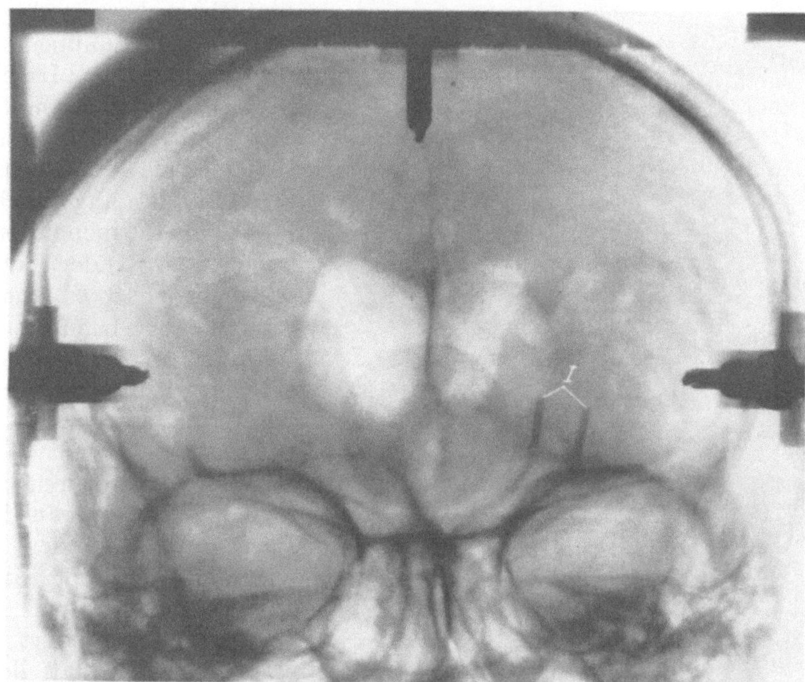

Abb. 11. Postoperative Röntgenkontrollaufnahme. (Pallidotomie bei Parkinsonismus). Die Lage der Wärmeläsion wird durch die zurückgelassenen Metallspiralen *I* markiert.

## IV. Gezielte Strahlenchirurgie.

Die stereotaktische Bestrahlung ist hauptsächlich für die funktionelle Hirnchirurgie vorgesehen. Die Operationen können teils mit Ultraschall und teils mit Röntgenstrahlen ausgeführt werden.

### 1. Gezielte Operationen mit Ultraschall.

#### a) Apparatur.

Zwei handelsübliche Ultraschallgeräte für Industriezwecke mit planen Quarzkristallschwingern sind benutzt worden (200 Watt, 10 cm² und 800 Watt, 30 cm²). Die Frequenz der Geräte ist 800 bzw. 500 kHz und es ist mit Schallintensitäten bis zu etwa 20 Watt/cm² am Kristall gearbeitet worden. Die Fokussierung des Schallbündels geschieht mit Hilfe einer Doppelspiegelanordnung, wie sie BARONE (1952) angegeben hat (Abb. 4). Der Abstand vom Rande des Spiegels zum Zentrum des Brennflecks beträgt 7 cm. Zur Kupplung zwischen dem Sender und dem Kopf des Patienten dient ein wassergefüllter Plastikbehälter (Abb. 13).

#### b) Die Ultraschalltransmission durch den Schädelknochen.

Beim Durchgang durch den menschlichen Schädelknochen wird der Ultraschall erheblich geschwächt (GÜTTNER und Mitarbeiter 1952, HÜTER 1952). Bei hohen Frequenzen ist ein dicker Schädelknochen ein nahezu völliges Hindernis. Mit der hier benutzten Frequenz von 800 kHz dürfte nach HÜTER die Dämpfung etwa 7 Dezibel/cm Knochendicke betragen, d. h. nur etwa 20 % des Schalls dringt durch den Knochen hindurch. Bei Anwendung des gezielten Schalls muß auch mit Veränderungen der Konfiguration des Brennflecks auf Grund der Reflexion im Knochen gerechnet werden.

Um festzustellen, ob es trotz dieser ungünstigen Bedingungen möglich ist, Ultraschall zu Erzeugung von Hirnläsionen durch den Schädelknochen hindurch zu benutzen, sind Versuche mit der in Abb. 12 gezeigten Anordnung gemacht worden. Die Form und Lage des Brennflecks wurde mit einem Thermoindicator ($Ag_2HgJ_4$) untersucht, wobei verschiedene Knochenstücke im Schallbündel angebracht wurden. Bei dicken spongiösen Schädelknochen wird der Schall so geschwächt, daß es ausgeschlossen ist, mit der benutzten Frequenz Läsionen in der Hirnsubstanz zu erzeugen. Bei dünnen Knochen der Temporalgegend ist die Schwächung jedoch nicht so groß, daß sie die Verabreichung einer ausreichenden Dosis ausschließt. Größe, Form und Lage des Brennflecks wird in gewissem Grade durch Interposition verschiedener Knochenproben verändert. Unter der Voraussetzung, daß der Knochen keinen allzu schrägen Winkel zum Schallbündel bildet, sind diese Variationen nicht von derartiger Größenordnung, daß sie eine ausreichende genaue Einrichtung des Focus verhindern. Die Schallintensität im Brennfleck variiert jedoch unter verschiedenen Bedingungen so erheblich, daß es nicht möglich ist, die verabfolgte Dosis anzugeben.

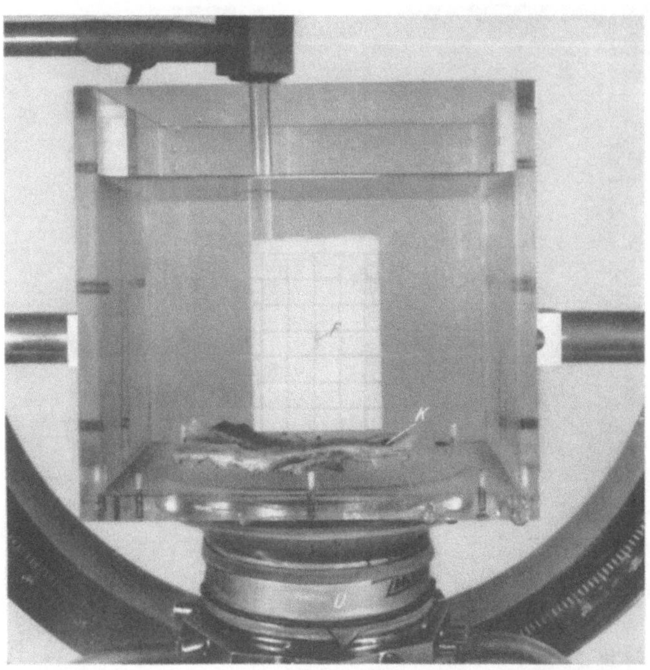


Abb. 12. Anordnung zur Untersuchung eines Ultraschallfocus bei der Transmission von Schall durch den Schädelknochen. Schallkopf *U* mit Focussierungsanordnung. Darstellung des Focus *F* mit Hilfe eines Thermoindicators, der in einer dünnen Schicht zwischen zwei Plexiglasscheiben angebracht ist. *K* Knochenstück (temporaler Knochenlappen).

Ohne Entfernung des Schädelknochens kann der Ultraschall also vorläufig nur in gewissen Fällen benutzt werden, nämlich wenn der Knochen dünn ist und wenn der Operationseffekt als Indicator für die Dosierung dienen kann.

### c) Ausführung der Operation.

Eine Anordnung zur Operation mit Ultraschall geht aus Abb. 13 hervor. Die Lokalisation der gewünschten Hirnstruktur geschieht nach der oben beschriebenen Methode. Die Operation wird der Encephalographie nicht direkt angeschlossen, sondern findet erst etwa 1 Woche später statt, wenn das Gas völlig resorbiert ist. Der Innenrahmen des Gerätes wird dann wieder exakt in den alten Bohrlöchern befestigt. Das Instrument ist in diesem Falle so ausgeführt, daß die Beschallung über die Temporalregion ausgeführt werden kann, wo der Knochen am dünnsten ist. Der Ultraschallkopf wird an einer geeigneten Stelle längs des Außenbogens angebracht, so daß die Spiegelanordnung ungefähr parallel zu der Fläche der Schläfengegend steht und die Schallstrahlung den Knochen so senkrecht wie möglich trifft. Während der Beschallung wird der Sender mit dem Instrumentbogen um dessen Achse hin und her bewegt. Auf diese Weise wird das Eintrittsfeld bedeutend vergrößert, während der Focus sich dauernd im eingestellten Operationspunkt befindet.

Die in Abb. 13 abgebildete Operation wurde an einem Patienten mit schwerem doppelseitigem Parkinsonismus ausgeführt. Bei der Beschallung war der Schallfocus auf den rechten Globus pallidus eingestellt. Postoperativ war die Rigidität im linken Arm und Bein verbessert; komplizierende neurologische Symptome wurden nicht beobachtet.

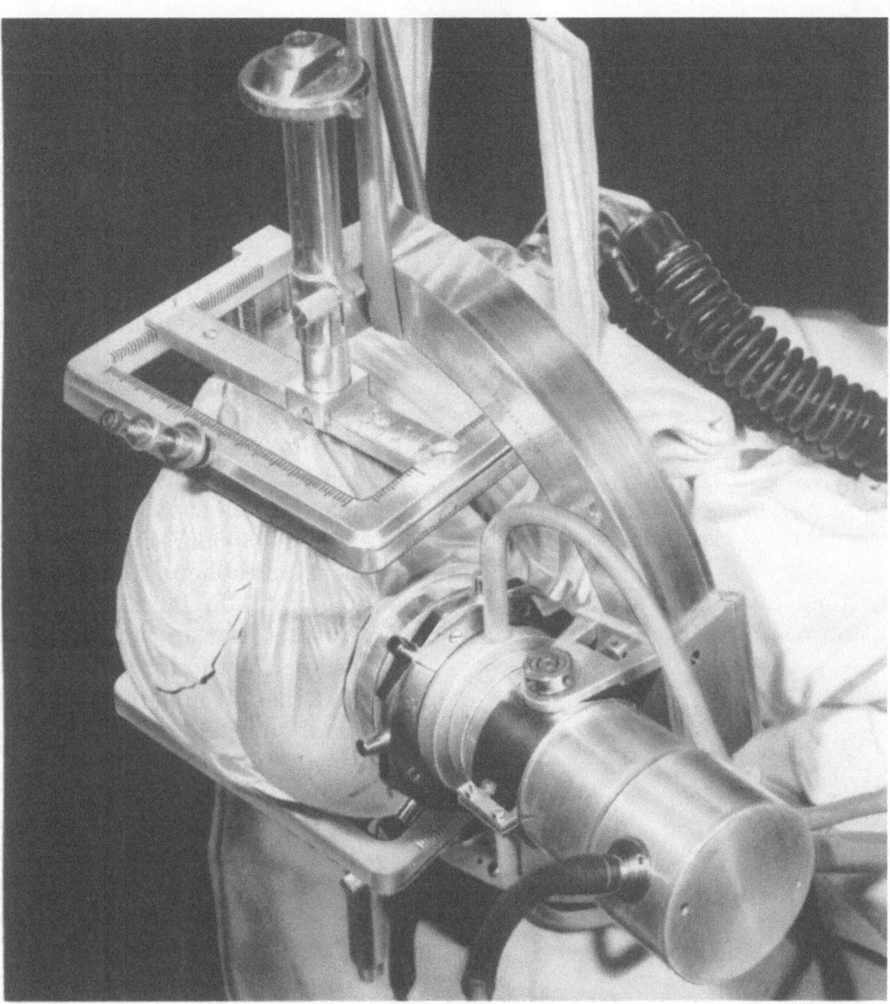

Abb. 13. Stereotaktische Ultraschallpallidotomie bei Parkinsonismus. Das focussierte Schallbündel wird über der Temporalregion, wo der Schädelknochen am dünnsten ist, angebracht. Ein Plastikbehälter mit entgastem Wasser dient zur Kuppelung zwischen dem Schallgeber und der Haut.

## 2. Gezielte Operationen mit Röntgenstrahlen.

### a) Strahlenquelle.

Die Methode ist für hochenergetische Strahlung vorgesehen. Als Strahlenquelle eignet sich hierfür einer der modernen Teilchenbeschleuniger, z. B. ein Betatron oder ein linearer Accelerator. Auch bei den äußerst kleinen Bestrahlungsfeldern, um die es sich hier handelt, kann dann eine zufriedenstellende Tiefendosis und eine scharfe Begrenzung des Strahlenbündels erhalten werden. Bestrahlung mit schweren Teilchen wie Protonen oder Deuteronen dürfte besonders vorteilhaft sein. Sie ermöglichen die Verwendung sehr dünner Strahlenbündel mit einer beträchtlichen Dosisleistung (Tobias und Mitarbeiter 1952). Indessen kann die stereotaktische Methodik auch für

Strahlung geringerer Energie verwendet werden und für die grundlegenden Versuche ist der herkömmliche 200—400 kV-Bereich anwendbar. Die bisherigen klinischen Versuche sind zum größten Teil mit einer 300 kV-Apparatur durchgeführt worden (280 kV-Gleichstrom, 10 mA, HWS 2 mm Cu, Anode 5×5 mm).

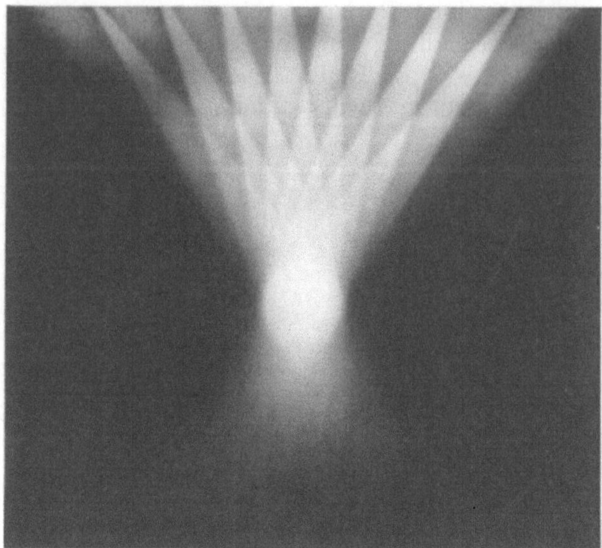

Abb. 14. Beispiel für die Strahlenverteilung und den focussierenden Effekt bei Bestrahlung in einer Ebene mit der in Abb. 3 gezeigten Vorrichtung. Blendendurchmesser 10 mm, 9 Felder mit 10° zwischen jedem Strahlenbündel.

**b) Technik der stereotaktischen Kreuzfeuerbestrahlung.**

Wie aus den Abb. 3 und 16 hervorgeht, ist das stereotaktische Instrument fest mit der Röntgenröhre verbunden und der Kopf des Patienten ist im Instrument aufgehängt. Der Operationspunkt im Gehirn kann einer Kreuzfeuerbestrahlung durch Fixation des Außenbogens in verschiedenen Lagen im Halter an der Röntgenröhre und durch Einstellung des Kopfes des Patienten in verschiedenen Winkeln um die Bogenachse ausgesetzt werden. Durch Anwendung einer ausreichenden Felderzahl bekommt man auch im 250—300 kV-Bereich im Herd eine mehrfach höhere Dosis als auf der Haut. Eine Vorstellung des Effekts der Kreuzfeuerbestrahlung gibt Abb. 14. Eine stereotaktische Röntgenläsion des Katzengehirns wird in Abb. 15 gezeigt (JEPPSON und LEKSELL 1954).

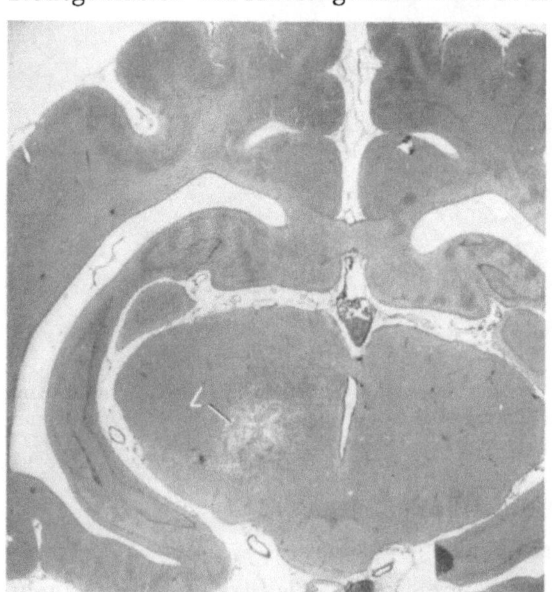


Abb. 15. Stereotaktische Röntgenläsion *L* im Thalamus der Katze 38 Tage nach der Bestrahlung. Herddosis etwa 20000 r.

Bei dieser Methodik ist der Focus-Herdabstand konstant; der Focus-Hautabstand der Bestrahlungsfelder der Schädelkonvexität dagegen ändert sich. Mit der hier verwendeten 280 kV-Spannung und den übrigen physikalischen Faktoren hängt die Herddosis für jedes Bestrahlungsfeld in hohem Maße von der Tiefe der bestrahlten Struktur ab. Die Felder werden daher nicht gleichmäßig über die Schädelkonvexität verteilt, sondern am zweckmäßigsten innerhalb eines Gebietes, in welchem die Struktur der Oberfläche am nächsten liegt. Die Größe der Blendenöffnung wird der Größe der gewünschten Läsion angepaßt. Die Behandlung wird durch Verwendung eines Dosierungsdiagramms erleichtert, aus welchem die Behandlungszeit und die Tiefendosis für verschiedene Haut-Herdabstände bei einer bestimmten maximalen Hautdosis abgelesen werden kann (s. LIDÉN).

Abb. 16 zeigt eine gezielte Strahlenoperation mit dieser Technik. Es handelt sich in diesem Falle um eine Abschneidung der thalamofrontalen Bahnen im vordersten Abschnitt der Capsula interna an Stelle der frontalen Lobotomie (LEKSELL und Mitarbeiter 1955). Eine Tiefendosis von gut 4000 r (Einzeldosis) wurde auf beiden Seiten durch insgesamt 32 Felder in der Frontalregion verabfolgt.

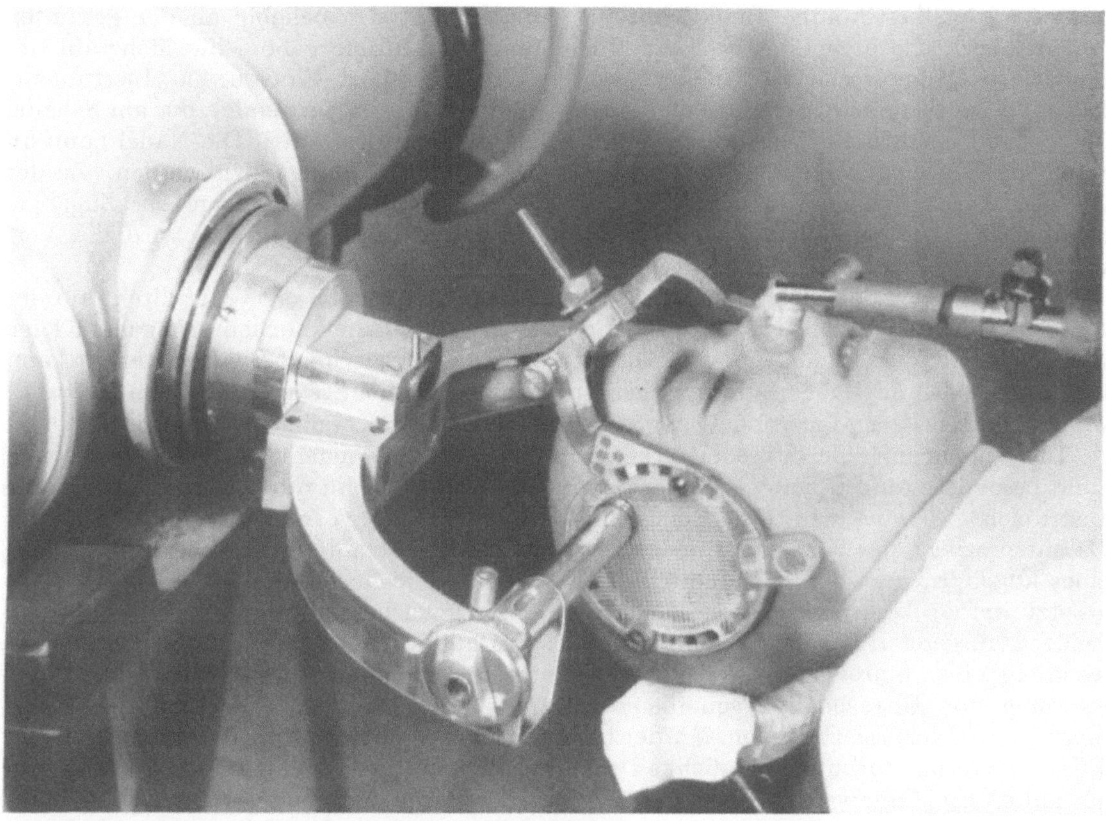

Abb. 16. Stereotaktische Operation mit Röntgenbestrahlung. Fall einer schizophrenen Psychose, bei der die Läsionen im vordersten Teil der Capsula interna zur Durchtrennung der thalamofrontalen Verbindungen angelegt wurden.

## C. Diskussion.

**Stereotaktische Instrumente und Lokalisationsmethoden.** Die Konstruktion stereotaktischer Instrumente kann auf verschiedene Arten variiert werden, aber im Prinzip gibt es nur eine begrenzte Anzahl geometrischer Lösungen. Die für Tierexperimente verwendeten Instrumente sind in rectilineare und äquatoriale Instrumente sowie in verschiedene Mikromanipulatoren eingeteilt worden (CLARKE 1920, CARPENTER und WHITTIER 1952). Die für Operationen am Menschen verwendeten Instrumente können, wenn man so will, in gleicher Weise zusammengefaßt werden. Ein Beispiel für ein Instrument von rectilinearem Typ ist das Stereoencephalotom von SPIEGEL und Mitarbeiter (1947, 1951, 1953), das eine Abwandlung der Apparatur von HORSLEY und CLARKE ist. Ein Beispiel für äquatoriale Instrumente ist der Apparat von RIECHERT und WOLFF (1951, 1953) (vgl. CLARKE 1920). Das hier beschriebene Instrument kommt auch dem äquatorialen Typ am nächsten. Da im Gegensatz zu den meisten tierexperimentellen Methoden röntgenologische Lokalisationsverfahren verwendet werden, müssen die Instrumente diesen angepaßt werden. Eine in dieser Hinsicht gut durchgearbeitete Technik ist die von TALAIRACH (1954).

Von praktischer Bedeutung bei der Handhabung der Instrumente ist es, welche Möglichkeiten bestehen, den gesuchten Punkt auf verschiedenen Wegen durch verschiedene Strukturen zu erreichen. Bei einem Teil der Instrumente ist der Zugangsweg nach Abschluß der Einstellung auf den gesuchten Operationspunkt festgelegt, andere lassen hierbei jedoch eine größere Wahlfreiheit zu. Nach diesen Gesichtspunkten können die Instrumente in drei Typen eingeteilt werden: die Nadel kann nach fertiger Einstellung nur an einem bestimmten Punkt, entlang einer Linie, oder beliebig an der gesamten Schädeloberfläche eingeführt werden. Zu der ersten Gruppe gehört die Mehrzahl der beschriebenen Instrumente. Zu der zweiten Gruppe gehört Kirschners Instrument. Bei seiner Methode wird bekanntlich ein rechtwinkliger Bogen verwendet, der am Schädel fixiert wird, so daß die Achse durch den gesuchten Punkt verläuft. Die Nadel kann an beliebiger Stelle entlang einer sagittalen Linie auf dem Kopf eingeführt werden. Zu der letzten Gruppe gehört das hier beschriebene Instrument. Da die Lage der Zugangsöffnung von der Einstellung auf den Operationspunkt unabhängig ist, wird die Verwendung des Instrumentes erleichtert.

Das Befestigen der Instrumente am Kopf des Patienten kann entweder direkt auf der Haut und den Weichteilen oder durch Bohrlöcher im Schädelknochen erfolgen. Kleine Bohrlöcher in der Lamina externa geben eine exakte Fixierung. Das Instrument kann bei Operationen mit mehreren Sitzungen an genau derselben Stelle wie vorher angebracht werden und bei langdauernden Eingriffen hat der Patient weniger Beschwerden.

Die Verwendung der stereotaktischen Technik für strahlenchirurgische Operationen stellt besondere Anforderungen an die Apparatur. Bisher scheint nur das hier beschriebene Instrument für eine derartige Einstellung von Strahlung verwendet worden zu sein. Da entsprechend der Konstruktion des Instrumentes die Strahlungsquelle überall entlang einer kugelförmigen Oberfläche mit ihrem Mittelpunkt in der eingestellten Struktur angesetzt werden kann, kann diese leicht einer Kreuzfeuerbestrahlung von verschiedenen Feldern ausgesetzt werden. Die Röntgenbestrahlung wird am einfachsten durch Verwendung einer hinreichend großen Anzahl stationärer Felder durchgeführt. Bei Verwendung von Ultraschall liegen die Verhältnisse etwas anders. Die Strahlung kann hierbei direkt fokussiert werden. Mit der beschriebenen Vorrichtung wird der fokussierende Effekt weiterhin durch die Möglichkeit erhöht, die Struktur von einem größeren, passend gewählten Einfallsgebiet her zu bestrahlen. Der Schallkopf kann manuell über dem ganzen Gebiet in ständiger Bewegung gehalten werden, ohne daß die Einstellung auf den Focus geändert wird. Dadurch werden auch Ungleichheiten im Ultraschallfeld ausgeglichen, die sich bei stationärer Anbringung des Schallkopfes störend auswirken.

Bei Operationen am Menschen ist es nicht wie bei kleinen, gleichmäßig gebauten Tierschädeln geglückt, durch Bezugspunkte am Schädel eine zufriedenstellende Genauigkeit der Lokalisation zu erreichen. Auf Grund anatomischer Messungen konnte Kirschner allerdings das Foramen ovale auf diese Weise lokalisieren. Topometrische Untersuchungen über die Lage einiger intracerebralen Strukturen, wie Nucleus dorso-medialis, Centrum medianum und Nucleus ruber, im Verhältnis zu den Schädelknochen, sind von Delmas und Pertuiset (1952) und Schmiedt (1952) ausgeführt worden. In der Regel ist es jedoch nötig, für eine exakte Lokalisation von normalen Hirnstrukturen Bezugspunkte im Gehirn heranzuziehen.

Nach der Methode von Spiegel und Wycis wird die Lage der gesuchten Struktur im Verhältnis zu einem intracerebralen Bezugspunkt, Corpus pineale oder der hinteren Kommissur, durch Messungen an anatomischen Bildern parallel und senkrecht zur Horizontalebene bestimmt. Die Röntgenbilder werden mit einem relativ kleinen Focus-Filmabstand angefertigt, die vergrößerten Maße werden jedoch mit Hilfe eines gleichzeitig photographierten Maßstabes korrigiert (vgl. Wolff 1952). Talairach und Mitarbeiter (1949, 1950, 1952) wenden teilweise andere Prinzipien an. Das Ventrikelsystem des Patienten wird mittels Ventrikulographie dargestellt und mit praktisch paralleler Röntgenstrahlung im Verhältnis zu Metallgittern auf dem Instrument abgebildet. Der Focus-Filmabstand beträgt 4 m. Die Röntgenbilder, auf denen das Ventrikelsystem und die Gitterlöcher abgebildet sind, werden danach auf anatomische Sagittal- bzw. Frontalschnitte gelegt und diejenigen Löcher ermittelt, welche der gesuchten Struktur entsprechen.

Die anatomische Korrelation wird erleichtert, wenn die Röntgenbilder mit parallelen Strahlen gemacht werden, so daß keine Vergrößerungsunterschiede auftreten. Hierfür muß aber der Focus-Objektabstand beträchtlich sein. Das stellt große Anforderungen an die Röntgenapparatur und an die Geräumigkeit des Operationssaales. Methoden, die diese Nachteile vermeiden, wurden unter anderem von SCHALTENBRAND (1953) und MARK und Mitarbeiter (1954) vorgeschlagen. SCHALTENBRAND verwendet eine orthoröntgenographische Technik, bei der sich die Röntgenröhre mit einer Spaltblende während der Exponierung parallel zur Kasette bewegt; hierdurch werden die Objekte ohne Vergrößerung in der Bewegungsrichtung der Röhre abgebildet. MARK und Mitarbeiter korrigieren die Vergrößerungsunterschiede an Hand einer graphischen Methode. Hierbei werden die auf der Röntgenaufnahme vergrößerten Abstände zwischen den Indicatoren des Instrumentes und den entsprechenden Punkten im Gehirn auf Diagramme übertragen, auf denen die Röntgenstrahlen durch divergierende Linien veranschaulicht sind. Mit Hilfe dieses Liniensystems kann die wirkliche Lage der Punkte im Schädel ermittelt werden.

Bei der hier benutzten Methode sind zwei verschiedene Lokalisationstechniken zur Anwendung gekommen. In der einen (LEKSELL 1955) diente die Verbindungsvorrichtung zwischen Röntgenröhre und Instrument etwa als eine optische Bank, und der Kopf des Patienten wurde mit Hilfe wiederholter Röntgenaufnahmen so eingestellt, daß die Bezugspunkte des Gehirns mit denen eines an der Kasette angebrachten anatomischen Schnittbildes übereinstimmen. Die Korrelation zwischen den intracerebralen Bezugspunkten und dem anatomischen Vergleichsbild wurde also direkt im divergenten Röntgenstrahlbündel vorgenommen.

Das hier beschriebene Verfahren mit geometrischer Projektion stellt eine einfache Lösung des Lokalisationsvorganges dar. Die Einstellung der Röntgenröhre ist durch die mechanische Verbindung zwischen Röhre und Instrumentrahmen am Kopfe des Patienten festgelegt. Die Methode kann bei jedem röntgenologisch und praktisch geeigneten Focus-Objektabstand angewandt werden. Auf Grund des geometrischen Projektionsverfahrens ist die Lage des Röntgenzentralstrahles innerhalb des Rahmens gleichgültig und ein besonderer Einstellungsvorgang erübrigt sich. Eine Korrelation zwischen dem Röntgenbild des Patienten und dem anatomischen Bild kann leicht durchgeführt werden, wobei etwaige Größenunterschiede zwischen dem Gehirn des Patienten und dem Bezugshirn ausgeglichen werden können.

Die angeführten Methoden sind Beispiele dafür, wie die stereotaktische Ortung unter Verwendung von sehr verschiedenen Verfahren gelöst werden kann. Alle Lokalisationsmethoden sind mit Fehlerquellen behaftet. Diese sind verschiedener Natur, wie mangelnde mechanische Genauigkeit des Instrumentes selbst, ungenaue Röntgenprojektionen mit hieraus folgender Verzerrung der Bilder und individuelle anatomische Verschiedenheiten. Die auf individuellen anatomischen Variationen beruhenden Fehler sind am schwersten auszuschalten. Es hängt dabei viel von der Wahl geeigneter Bezugspunkte ab. Im Prinzip müssen Punkte gewählt werden, die so nahe der gesuchten Struktur wie möglich liegen. Die Frage geeigneter Bezugspunkte ist bisher nur unvollständig bearbeitet worden und es sind weitere Studien über die Beziehungen verschiedener Kerne und Leitungsbahnen zu den röntgenographisch auf verschiedene Weise darstellbaren Bezugsstrukturen erforderlich.

**Offene gezielte Operationen und stereotaktische Strahlenchirurgie.** Die zur Zeit gebräuchlichste Indikation für stereotaktische Eingriffe liegt auf dem Gebiete der funktionellen Hirnchirurgie. Von größter Bedeutung für die klinischen Resultate ist dabei die Verwendung einer geeigneten Methode zur Durchführung der Läsionen in der Hirnsubstanz. Der von CARPENTER und WHITTIER (1952) am Affen gemachte Vergleich zwischen verschiedenen Läsionen, die unter anderem mit Elektrolyse, Implantation radioaktiver Substanz und Elektrokoagulation hervorgerufen wurden, hat gezeigt, daß die elektrolytischen Schädigungen in Größe und Form unberechenbar variierten. Das gleiche wurde bei Operationen am Menschen beobachtet (SWEET und MARK 1953). Die Implantation von Radonnadeln ergab runde, wohlbegrenzte Destruktionen von konstanter

Konfiguration und gleichförmigem histologischem Charakter (s. CAMPBELL und NOVICK 1949, STEIN und PETERSON 1950, BORISON und WANG 1951, McCLURE und Mitarbeiter 1953, DE AJURIAGUERRA und Mitarbeiter 1954). Auch Hochfrequenzdiathermie ergab ziemlich gut begrenzte Läsionen, jedoch machte die Isolierung der Elektroden Schwierigkeiten. Bei Operationen am Menschen werden nun neben der Elektrolyse oder Elektrokoagulation auch radioaktive Isotopen, vor allem Gold angewandt (TALAIRACH und Mitarbeiter 1952, AMADOR und BAILEY 1953, RONDEPIERRE und TALAIRACH 1953).

Mit dieser stereotaktischen Methode sind seit 1952 nur Wärmeläsionen mit hochfrequentem Wechselstrom gesetzt worden. Wie DUSSER DE BARENNE und ZIMMERMANN (1935) und SILVER und WALKER (1947) mit Thermokoagulationsversuchen am Cortex zeigten, ist eine Erwärmung zwischen 55 und 80$^0$ ein schonendes Verfahren zur Ausschaltung von Hirngewebe. Die Schwierigkeiten bei der Erwärmung mit Diathermie können bei geeigneter Technik beseitigt werden. Durch Kontrolle der Erwärmung mit einem Thermoelement kann der Gewebeschaden genau abgestuft werden.

Die stereotaktische Strahlenchirurgie befindet sich noch im Anfangsstadium. Hinsichtlich des Ultraschalls zeigten schcn die Arbeiten von LYNN und PUTNAM (1944), daß es mit focussierter Beschallung möglich ist, begrenzte Hirnnekrosen hervorzurufen. Die Dämpfung des Schalls beim Durchgang durch den Schädelknochen bildet jedoch ein erhebliches Hindernis für die Benutzung dieser Energieform. Wenn der Knochen entfernt und der Schall direkt auf die Dura appliziert wird, gestalten sich die Verhältnisse bedeutend günstiger. Mit einer derartigen Technik wäre es ohne Zweifel möglich, hinreichend exakte therapeutische Läsionen herzustellen. Durch die genauen tierexperimentellen Untersuchungen von FRY und Mitarbeitern (1953, 1954, 1955) ist gezeigt worden, daß man auf diese Weise gut kontrollierbare fokale Hirnläsionen bekommen kann. Wenn ein Knochenlappen angelegt werden muß, ist es jedoch zweifelhaft, ob der Ultraschall Vorteile bietet, da man praktisch den gleichen Effekt durch das Einführen von Elektroden in ein kleines Bohrloch erzielen kann. Möglicherweise kann der selektive Effekt auf das Myelin unter Schonung der Blutgefäße und Nervenzellen die Anwendung dieser Energieform indizieren. Vermutlich kann der Ultraschall für die Hirnchirurgie jedoch nur dann praktische Bedeutung gewinnen, wenn eine Applikation durch den Knochen hindurch möglich ist.

Untersuchungen mit Ultraschall für diagnostische Zwecke in der Form von Echoencephalographie (LEKSELL 1955) haben ergeben, daß es möglich ist, diagnostische Befunde durch den Schädelnkochen hindurch zu erheben, obgleich die physikalischen Messungen auf das Gegenteil hindeuten (GÜTTNER 1952, U.S. A.E.C. 1955). Erfahrungen mit der hier beschriebenen Operationstechnik zeigen auch, daß es in gewissen Fällen möglich ist, durch Beschallung des Schädelknochens an seinen dünnsten Stellen klinisch gesehen ausreichend genaue Läsionen in der Hirnsubstanz zu erhalten. Da die Tiefendosis in so hohem Maße von der Knochendicke abhängt und nicht exakt berechnet werden kann, sind diese Operationen solchen Fällen vorbehalten worden, in denen im Anschluß an die Beschallung während der Operation entschieden werden kann, wann der gewünschte Effekt erreicht ist. Dieses gilt z. B. für die Pallidotomie beim Parkinsonismus, da Rigidität und Tremor in den Extremitäten gewöhnlich unmittelbar nach Erzeugung der Läsion aufhören. Bei der funktionellen Hirnchirurgie am Menschen sind häufig Läsionen von recht bedeutendem Ausmaß notwendig und die Forderung nach Erzeugung genauer, kleiner Läsionen soll nicht übertrieben werden.

Von den zugänglichen Strahlungsformen bietet zunächst die ionisierende Strahlung, wenn es sich um die Erzielung von umschriebenen Läsionen in verschiedenen Hirnstrukturen handelt, gewisse Vorteile. Die Messung der Dosis für diese Art von Strahlung ist gut entwickelt und die Herddosis kann genau bestimmt werden. Bei einem Vergleich mit der Methode durch Applikation einer radioaktiven Substanz, z. B. $Au^{198}$, eine tiefliegende Hirnläsion zu erzielen, scheint diese Methode mit äußerer Kreuzfeuerbestrahlung sicher überlegen zu sein. Die Größe der Läsion kann durch Änderung der Blendengröße leicht geändert werden und sie kommt zustande, ohne daß ein Instrument ins Gehirn eingeführt werden muß.

Die genaue Strahlendosis, welche zur Zerstörung von Gewebe in verschiedenen Hirnabschnitten beim Menschen notwendig ist, ist bisher nicht bekannt. Mit einer sehr hohen Röntgendosis wird eine Totalnekrose des Hirngewebes erzeugt und der Effekt tritt beinahe unmittelbar auf. Mit niedrigen Dosen kann es sehr lange Zeit dauern, bis der Gewebeschaden manifest wird. Nach den interessanten Untersuchungen an Affen von ARNOLD und Mitarbeitern (1954), kann man mit Dosen der 23 MeV-Betatronröntgenstrahlen bis hinunter auf 1500 r nach einem halben Jahr oder später auftretende Effekte beobachten. Bei Dosen zwischen 1500 r und 3000 r bei 23 MeV wurde eine selektive Wirkung auf das Myelin unter Schonung der Blutgefäße erzielt. Der Röntgeneffekt gilt also in erster Linie der weißen Hirnsubstanz und nicht, wie die meisten früheren Untersucher angaben, den Blutgefäßen. Wenn die Verhältnisse beim Menschen gleichartig sind, spricht dieser Umstand für die Anwendung ionisierender Strahlung zum Abschneiden von Leitungsbahnen im Gehirn, trotz des Nachteiles der eventuell langen Latenzzeit. Vom klinischen Gesichtspunkt kann übrigens eine Verzögerung des Effektes in gewissen Fällen von Vorteil sein. Durch die langsame Ausbildung der Läsion wird eine initiale Schockwirkung vermieden.

Ein Nachteil bei der Benutzung ionisierender Strahlung ist die Ungewißheit, was im Laufe sehr langer Zeit in den zerstörten Gewebsstrukturen geschieht, ob nämlich eine Gefahr für Spätblutungen, Ödem oder andere Komplikationen vorliegt. Klinische Beobachtungen von spät auftretenden Radionekrosen im Gehirn nach Behandlung von Tumoren (FISCHER und HOHLFELDER 1930, MARKIEWIECZ 1935, O'CONNELL und BRUNSCHWIG 1937, PENNYBACKER und RUSSEL 1948, FOLTZ und Mitarbeiter 1953 u. a.) deuten darauf hin, daß hier gewisse Gefahren vorliegen können. In diesen Fällen hat es sich jedoch um Bestrahlung großer Felder gehandelt, und die Ergebnisse können nicht direkt auf die sehr kleinen bestrahlten Bezirke übertragen werden, um die es sich hier handelt. Bei der Auswahl von Fällen für derartige Operationen mit Röntgenläsionen muß jedoch auf diesen Unsicherheitsfaktor Rücksicht genommen werden. Dieses gilt auch für die Applikation von Radiogold oder einer anderen radioaktiven Substanz im Gehirn. Von besonderem Interesse in diesem Zusammenhang ist die Anwendung sehr dünner Bündel der ionisierenden Strahlung zum Abschneiden der gewünschten Hirnverbindungen. Werden schlitzförmige Felder von nur 1—2 mm Breite hierzu benutzt, sind die Heilungsverhältnisse wahrscheinlich andere. Hierüber sind weitere Untersuchungen notwendig. Präliminäre Beobachtungen bei Verwendung eines Synchro-cyclotronen in Upsala (LARSSON und Mitarbeiter 1956) deuten an, daß millimeterdicke Protonenbündel ein zweckmäßiges Werkzeug für diese Form der Hirnchirurgie sind.

**Klinische Anwendung.** Das erste stereotaktische Operationsverfahren am Menschen, KIRSCHNERs Ganglion Gasseri-Koagulation, wurde seinerzeit ziemlich viel angewandt, konnte aber die gebräuchlichen Trigeminusoperationen nicht verdrängen.

Bei intracerebralen Eingriffen sind die offenen stereotaktischen Methoden, nach ihrer Einführung durch SPIEGEL und WYCIS, jetzt in einer recht großen Anzahl von Fällen angewandt. Die Operationen haben aber noch vielfach den Charakter vorläufiger klinischer Versuche mit verschiedenen Methoden und die Resultate hängen in hohem Maße von verschiedenen technischen Umständen ab.

Die Entwicklung auf dem Gebiete der Psychochirurgie wurde mit Läsionen am Thalamus eingeleitet (SPIEGEL und Mitarbeiter 1948, 1949, 1950, 1951, 1952, FREED und Mitarbeiter 1949, TALAIRACH und Mitarbeiter 1949, WYCIS und SPIEGEL 1949, ORCHINIK und Mitarbeiter 1950, BAIRD und Mitarbeiter 1951, TALAIRACH 1952, RONDEPIERRE und TALAIRACH 1953). Eine stereotaktische Durchschneidung von Leitungsbahnen in den Stirnlappen wie bei der Lobotomie ist von TALAIRACH und Mitarbeiter (1949), RIECHERT und WOLFF (1951) und HAYNE und Mitarbeiter (1952) ausgeführt worden. Chronische

Schmerzzustände sind mit einer Durchschneidung der spinothalamischen Bahnen im Mesencephalon oder mit Läsionen in den sensiblen Thalamuskernen behandelt worden (SPIEGEL und Mitarbeiter 1948, 1949, 1952, 1953, WYCIS und Mitarbeiter 1949, 1950, 1951, TALAIRACH und Mitarbeiter 1949, 1952, HÉCAEN und Mitarbeiter 1949, DAVID und Mitarbeiter 1949, MONNIER und FISCHER 1950, 1951, MURTAGH und Mitarbeiter 1951). Versuche, Epilepsie, petit mal zu behandeln, sind in einzelnen Fällen mit Läsionen im Nucleus dorsomedialis gemacht worden, ohne jedoch zu überzeugenden Resultaten geführt zu haben (SPIEGEL und Mitarbeiter 1948, 1950, 1951, 1952). Hyperkinesien sind mit Erfolg mittels Läsionen im Pallidum, in der Gegend der Ansa lenticularis und im oralen Ventralkern des Thalamus behandelt worden (TALAIRACH und Mitarbeiter 1950, WYCIS und SPIEGEL 1951, 1952, 1953, SPIEGEL und WYCIS 1952, 1954, GUIOT und BRION 1953, NARABAYASHI und OKUMA 1953, HASSLER und RIECHERT 1954).

Die hier beschriebene Technik kam hauptsächlich bei psychochirurgischen Eingriffen und bei Parkinsonismus zur Anwendung. Wärmeläsionen im vorderen Teil der Capsula interna wurden in 110 Fällen von Angstzuständen und Schizophrenien erprobt. Durch die Möglichkeit der genauen Kontrolle von Größe und Lage der Läsion und wegen der geringen Gefahr chirurgischer Komplikationen und nachfolgender Epilepsie konnte diese Methode hier bis auf weiteres die Standardlobotomie ersetzen. Gezielte Eingriffe im Gebiet des Pallidum haben in 56 Fällen von Parkinsonismus zu einer eindeutigen Besserung sowohl des Tremors als auch besonders der Rigidität geführt. Für gewisse Tumoren ist auch die Punktion und Isotopeninjektion eine brauchbare Behandlungsmethode (LEKSELL und LIDÉN 1953, TALAIRACH und Mitarbeiter 1954, 1955, WYCIS und Mitarbeiter 1954).

Die gezielte Strahlenchirurgie mit ionisierender Strahlung befindet sich noch in einem Stadium, in dem es darauf ankommt, die Wirkung der verschiedenen Strahlungsformen auf die verschiedenen Hirnstrukturen am Menschen festzustellen und eine optimale Dosierung bei möglichst schmalen Bestrahlungsfeldern zu erreichen. Bezüglich des Ultraschalls müssen besonders Fragen über optimale Schallfrequenzen im Hinblick auf Knochendicke und erforderlicher Focusschärfe weiter bearbeitet werden. Mit der hier beschriebenen Technik für gezielte Röntgen- und Ultraschallbestrahlung sind bis jetzt nur wenige Operationen ausgeführt worden. Es ist deshalb verfrüht, ein Urteil über die klinischen Resultate abzugeben. Die technische Weiterentwicklung wird noch viele Jahre in Anspruch nehmen. Soviel ist jedoch sicher, daß die stereotaktische Strahlenchirurgie sowohl mit ionisierender Strahlung als, in mehr begrenzter Ausdehnung, mit Ultraschall ein anwendbares Operationsverfahren darstellt. Eingriffe in der Tiefe des Gehirns können nun unblutig ohne Schädigung der oberflächlichen Gewebestrukturen durchgeführt werden.

## D. Zusammenfassung.

In einem einleitenden Abschnitt wird ein kurzer Rückblick über die Geschichte der gezielten Hirnoperationen gegeben. Die stereotaktischen Eingriffe werden in offene Operationen mit Nadelelektroden und anderen chirurgischen Instrumenten und in gezielte Strahlenchirurgie eingeteilt.

Die vom Verfasser benutzte Operationsmethode wird beschrieben. Das stereotaktische Instrument kann in verschiedenen Ausführungen für offene gezielte Operationen und für die gezielte Strahlenchirurgie angewandt werden.

Die Lage des gesuchten Punktes im Gehirn wird durch seine Beziehung zu encephalographisch dargestellten Hirnstrukturen ermittelt. Die Röntgenaufnahmen des Patienten werden durch ein geometrisches Projektionsverfahren mit anatomischen Schnittbildern eines Bezugshirns in Korrelation gebracht.

Ein Verfahren für offene gezielte Operationen mit temperaturkontrollierten Wärmeläsionen wird beschrieben.

Versuche über die Durchlässigkeit des Schädelknochens für Ultraschall werden kurz beschrieben. Es wird hierbei gezeigt, daß es unter gewissen Voraussetzungen trotz der ungünstigen physikalischen Bedingungen möglich ist, hinreichend genaue therapeutische Ultraschalläsionen durch den Schädelknochen hindurch zu erzeugen.

Die Verwendung verschiedener Arten ionisierender Strahlung für die stereotaktische Strahlenchirurgie wird kurz behandelt.

Schließlich wird die Methode beschrieben, die in den ersten Fällen von unblutigen gezielten Operationen am Menschen, mit Hilfe von fokussiertem Ultraschall oder Röntgenstrahlung zur Anwendung kam.

Im Anschluß an die Beschreibung dieser stereotaktischen Methode werden einige andere Verfahren für gezielte Operationen kurz besprochen. Technische Fragen im Hinblick auf verschiedene Instrumente und Lokalisationsmethoden sowie einige weitere Fragen über die Verwendung gezielter Strahlung werden diskutiert.

Die klinischen Ergebnisse der gezielten Hirnoperationen bei den verschiedenen Krankheitszuständen werden nicht im einzelnen mitgeteilt, da der Zeitpunkt für eine Beurteilung als verfrüht angesehen werden muß. Die physikalischen Grundlagen der gezielten Strahlenchirurgie mit ionisierender Strahlung sowie mit Ultraschall werden nachfolgend in besonderen Abschnitten von K. LIDÉN und H. HERTZ behandelt.

# E. Physikalische Grundlagen für die Verwendung ionisierender Strahlung bei gezielter Hirnchirurgie.

Von

KURT LIDÉN.

## I. Einleitung.

Ein gezielter Operationseffekt in einem gut abgegrenzten und verhältnismäßig kleinen Gebiet, dem Operationspunkt, kann im Gehirn im Prinzip dadurch erreicht werden, daß man mit Hilfe einer äußeren Strahlenquelle eine geeignete Dosis einführt. Dabei ist exakte Lokalisation des Operationspunktes, gegen den das Strahlenbündel sorgfältig gerichtet werden muß, erforderlich. Gleichzeitig muß die Wirkung des Bündels auf das Operationsgebiet begrenzt werden können. Dies kann prinzipiell auf verschiedene Weise erreicht werden. Die benutzte Strahlung kann so beschaffen sein, daß sie selektiv von den Zellen oder Zellteilen der Gewebsabschnitte, die bestrahlt werden sollen, absorbiert werden. Es gibt Strahlenarten, deren spezifische Energieabgabe in gewisser Tiefe der zu bestrahlenden Substanz am größten ist. Eine hinreichende Strahlendosis eines Strahlungstypus mit relativ schlechter Tiefenwirkung kann in das betreffende Gebiet dadurch eingeführt werden, daß man die benutzte Strahlung auf dieses konzentriert (Kreuzfeuerbestrahlung).

Mehrere Formen elektromagnetischer, corpusculärer und akustischer Energietransporte können für eine derartige gezielte Strahlenchirurgie verwendet werden. Versuche zeigen, daß ein focusiertes Ultraschallbündel für gezielte operative Effekte ausgenutzt werden kann; wie im Abschn. F (Die Anwendung von Ultraschall für gezielte Hirnoperationen) erwähnt wurde, setzt dies gewöhnlich voraus, daß eine Öffnung im Schädelknochen vorliegt, da dieser sonst die Ultraschallwellen stark absorbiert und reflektiert. OLDENDORF (1949) hat in der Cortex des Kaninchengehirnes mit Hilfe von elektromagnetischen Mikrowellen (Wellenlänge 12 cm), begrenzte Läsionen erzeugt. Sein Bericht ist leider etwas kurz, jedoch dürfte eine Tiefenwirkung mit derartiger Strahlung unter keinen Umständen erzielt werden können. Dagegen können verschiedene Arten von Röntgen- und Gammastrahlen, sowie schnelle Corpuscularstrahlen benutzt werden, ohne daß mechanische Eingriffe in außerhalb des Gehirns liegende Gewebsschichten erforderlich sind. Derartige ionisierende Strahlenarten, die eine unblutige gezielte Strahlenchirurgie zulassen, sind von besonderem Interesse. Der physikalische Hintergrund für die Möglichkeiten der ionisierenden Strahlung wird unten näher diskutiert.

## II. Allgemeine Eigenschaften der ionisierenden Strahlung, unter besonderer Berücksichtigung der gezielten Strahlenchirurgie.

Die biologische Wirkung der ionisierenden Strahlung entsteht durch die bei der Absorption der Strahlung gebildeten Ionen. Die elektromagnetische Strahlung vom Typus der Röntgen- oder Gammastrahlung wirkt durch die bei den Absorptionsprozessen entstandenen Elektronen. Schnelle Elektronen, Protonen, α-Teilchen usw. ionisieren die Moleküle, die sie direkt passieren. Die Röntgeneinheit, 1 r, entspricht der Bildung von etwa 1,6 Ionpaaren in einem Wasservolumen von $10^{-12}$ cm$^3$ (= 1 $\mu^3$).

Bei Benutzung obengenannter Strahlung zur gezielten operativen Methode ist man offenbar bestrebt, im Operationspunkt kräftig genug zu ionisieren, um eine für den beabsichtigten Zweck adäquate Strahlendosis zu erhalten, und um gleichzeitig und möglichst sicher die Bestrahlung angrenzender Gewebe zu vermeiden. Dabei treten Verschiedenheiten im Absorptionsmechanismus bei der Benutzung von Strahlenbündeln mit kleinem Querschnitt sowohl in der elektromagnetischen als auch in der corpusculären Gruppe bedeutend stärker hervor als bei der Bestrahlung großer Felder.

Bei der Absorption von Photonen mit etwa *100 KeV* Energie, z. B. in Wasser oder Hirnsubstanz, geschieht die Absorption hauptsächlich durch Comptonprozesse, bei denen durchschnittlich 14 % der Photonenergie auf ein Elektron übergeht, während das Comptonphoton aus der Richtung des Primärphotons mit einer mittleren Energie von 86 KeV abweicht. Die Herabsetzung der Intensität in einem schmalen Strahlenbündel von 100 KeV geschieht also derart, daß nur ein kleiner Teil des Energieverlustes als Strahlendosis abgegeben wird. Die gestreuten Photonen, deren Richtungsverteilung bei 100 KeV relativ isotrop ist, können danach in neuen Comptonprozessen absorbiert werden usw. Eine derartige Mehrfachstreuung kann die Strahlendosen bei Benutzung großer Strahlungsquerschnitte wesentlich erhöhen, wie z. B. bei der normalen Radiotherapie; bei sehr kleinen Feldern, Nullfeldern, ist sie kaum noch von Bedeutung.

Die Absorption von 1 MeV Photonen im lebenden Gewebe verschiedener Art geschieht ausschließlich über Comptonprozesse. Die Richtungsverhältnisse und der Energieumsatz unterscheidet sich jedoch ziemlich wesentlich von den Verhältnissen bei 100 KeV. Die Comptonstreuung geschieht so, daß die gestreuten Photonen in 75 % sämtlicher Prozesse im Winkelgebiet 0—90° und 40 % innerhalb von 45° liegen, welches eine markierte Vorwärtsstreuung und eine beginnende Gleichrichtung mit den Primärstrahlen bedeutet. Die Intensitätsherabsetzung eines 1 MeV-Strahlenbündels ist bedeutend kleiner als für 100 KeV, aber die prozentuelle Energie, die jedes comptongestreute Photon durchschnittlich abgibt, ist 45 %, und damit bedeutend größer als für 100 KeV. Schließlich bedeutet die Mehrfachstreuung nicht so viel für die Verbesserung der Tiefenwirkung bei großen Feldern im Verhältnis zum Nullfeld wie bei 100 KeV.

Bei Photonenergien von 10 MeV ist die Comptonstreuung mehr nach vorwärts gerichtet als bei 1 MeV; im Winkelgebiet 0—45° liegen jetzt reichlich 60 % aller Comptonphotonen. Aber bei Energien über 1,02 MeV kommt zum Absorptionsprozeß die *Paarbildung*, wobei ein Elektron-Positron-Paar in die Richtung des Primärphotons emittiert wird, hinzu. Bei 10 MeV werden in einem Paarbildungsprozeß annähernd 9 MeV direkt in Ionisationsenergie umgesetzt. Der Anteil der Paarbildungsabsorption in der Strahlendosis in weichem Gewebe, wie z. B. des Gehirns, ist ebenso groß wie der der Comptonabsorption bei etwa 20 MeV und nimmt dann mit steigender Energie zu. Für Photonenergien über 10 MeV werden die einzelnen primären und sekundären Absorptionsprozesse immer mehr gleichgerichtet.

Die andere Gruppe ionisierender Strahlung, die schnellen Corpuscularstrahlen, bieten einige interessante Möglichkeiten, weil ihre spezifische Ionisation am Ende der Bahn stark zunimmt und weil sie zum Unterschied von den Röntgen- und Gammaphotonen eine relativ definierte Reichweite haben. Ein schmaler Strahl monoenergetischer Elektronen mehrerer MeV's Energie hat sich als weniger anwendbar erwiesen, da die geringe Masse des Elektrons Streuung mit sich bringt, wodurch das Strahlenbündel erweitert wird (LAUGHLIN und Mitarbeiter 1953; LAUGHLIN 1954).

Die schweren Teilchen — Protonen, Deuteronen, $\alpha$-Teilchen usw. — verhalten sich bei hohen Energien anders. Sie schlagen relativ unbehindert durch alle Moleküle und Elektronenhüllen hindurch und bewegen sich ohne nennenswerte Streuung in geraden Bahnen. Die Ionisation ist am Ende der Bahn am größten. Hierdurch erhält man ein Dosismaximum in einer Tiefe, die der Reichweite nahezu gleich ist. Auch schmale Strahlenbündel bleiben nach dem Durchschnitt durch mehrere Zentimeter Materie gut beieinander und die Reichweiteschwankungen sind im Vergleich zu den Elektronen unbedeutend (TOBIAS und Mitarbeiter 1952). Die Energie, die via Kernreaktionen mit $p$, $d$ und $\alpha$ absorbiert wird, ist im Vergleich zu den Ionisationsenergien minimal.

## III. Absorption und prozentuelle Tiefendosis.

Die praktisch zugängliche elektromagnetische Strahlung von Röntgenaggregaten, VAN DE GRAAFF-Maschinen und Beschleunigungsgeräten verschiedener Art hat eine kontinuierliche spektrale Verteilung. Ihre Härte kann darum nicht durch die Energie der wenigen Photone angegeben werden, welche der von der Maschine gelieferten maximalen Energie entspricht. Man benutzt gewöhnlich die Halbwertschicht (HWS) als Maßstab für die Qualität der zusammengesetzten Strahlung zusammen mit den Daten für die Höchstenergie. Experimentelle Untersuchungen über die Absorption derartiger Strahlung in Wasser bei Nullfeldern zeigt, wie die prozentuelle Tiefendosis $(D_d)_0$ ($d$ ist der Abstand von der Oberfläche) mit zunehmender HWS der Strahlung zunimmt. In Abb. 17 zeigt das Diagramm den Verlauf der prozentuellen Tiefendosis für verschiedene Strahlenqualitäten.

Die Röntgenstrahlung mit einer HWS von 0,5 bzw. 5 mm Cu hat ihr Maximum an der Oberfläche (100%) und in 10 cm Tiefe ist $(\mathrm{D}_{10})_0 = 8$ bzw. 19%. Das bedeutet, daß mit einer HWS von 5 mm Cu eine mehr als doppelt so große Strahlendosis in 10 cm Tiefe gegeben werden kann als mit einer HWS von 0,5 mm Cu. Aber die für den einzelnen Fall maximal zugelassene einmalige Bestrahlung der Haut begrenzt offenbar die Dosis, die mit einer HWS von 5 mm Cu in 10 cm Tiefe appliziert werden kann. Wenn man annimmt, daß die maximale Hautdosis, $(R_{\mathrm{H}})_{\max}$, 1000 r beträgt, ist es für Erreichung einer Tiefendosis von 10000 r erforderlich, die Einfallsfläche der Strahlung auf der Haut über ein Gebiet $A$ auszubreiten, das mindestens 50mal größer ist als der eigene Querschnitt der Strahlung auf der Haut. Das bedeutet, daß die Bestrahlung entweder von 50 voneinander getrennten Feldern geschehen muß oder daß eine kontinuierliche Verschiebung des Strahles auf der Haut entlang einer Kreis- oder Spiralbahn stattfindet, bei der die bestrahlte Hautoberfläche gleich Fläche $A$ ist. Könnte die Gammastrahlung von $\mathrm{Co}^{60}$ ausgenutzt werden, wäre $(\mathrm{D}_{10})_0 = 38\,\%$ und die Anzahl der Felder könnte in dem geschilderten Falle auf 25 reduziert werden.

Bei einer Röntgenstrahlung von z. B. 20 MeV Höchstenergie treten ganz andere Verhältnisse auf. Die von JOHNS (1953) angegebene Tiefendosiskurve für 22 MeV hat ein flaches Maximum (100%) bei $d = 4$ cm, und bei $d = 10$ cm ist $(\mathrm{D}_{10})_0 = 82\,\%$ von $(\mathrm{D}_4)_0$. Die relative Hautdosis oder $(\mathrm{D}_0)_0$ beträgt nur $^1/_4$ der Dosis in 10 cm Tiefe. Das oben gegebene Beispiel mit 10000 r im Operationspunkt könnte dann mit etwa 10 Feldern erreicht werden. Die Höchstdosen erhält man dabei in 4 cm Tiefe mit etwa 1200 r je Feld. Der Austrittspunkt des Strahlenbündels kann bei gewissen Richtungen in der Mundhöhle liegen; die Dosis im Ausgangspunkt wird jedoch dabei niemals größer als für *ein* Feld im Operationspunkt, d. h. in diesem Falle weniger als 1200 r.

Für ein Deuteronstrahlenbündel von 190 MeV Energie hat man eine für gezielte Hirnchirurgie interessante Tiefendosisverteilung gefunden (Abb. 17). Durch Herabsetzung dieser Energie kann man das Dosismaximum z. B. in 10 cm Tiefe verlegen und dort in einem sehr begrenzten Gebiet mit einem einzigen Strahl eine 4mal höhere Dosis erhalten als an der Oberfläche. Von 3 Feldern könnten also bei einer Hautdosis von nur etwa 800 r je Feld theoretisch 10000 r in 10 cm Tiefe eingeführt werden. Praktisch ist dies schwer zu erreichen, und man hat mit dem 100%-Teil des Strahlenbündels zu arbeiten. Versuche mit einem Strahlenbündel von 12 mm Durchmesser haben gezeigt, daß der Querschnitt auch nach Durchdringung von z. B. 6 cm Al unverändert bleibt (Tobias und Mitarbeiter 1952, 1955).

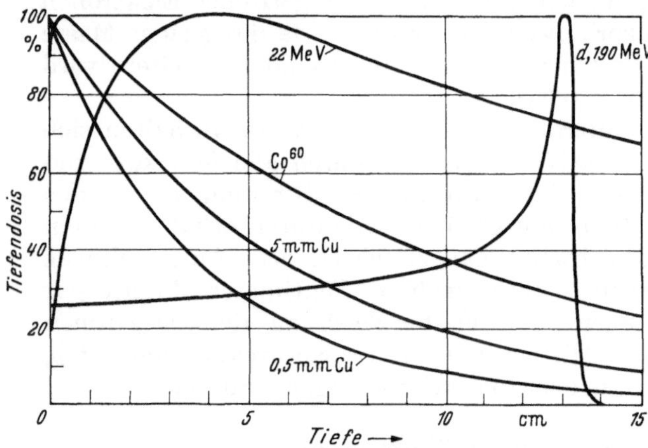


Abb. 17. Relative Tiefendosis für Nullfelder. Für Röntgenstrahlung mit einer HWS von 0,5 und 5,0 mm Cu sowie für Gammastrahlung von $Co^{60}$ ist der FHA = 50 cm. Für 22 MeV Röntgenstrahlung vom Betatron sowie für 190 MeV Deuteronen ist der FHA = 100 cm.

Bei gezielten Hirnoperationen mit Hilfe ionisierender Strahlung wird eine Durchstrahlung des Schädelknochens vorausgesetzt. Hierbei ist es von Bedeutung, eventuelle Unterschiede im Absorptionsvermögen für verschiedene Strahlenqualitäten z. B. zwischen Knochen und Hirnsubstanz und die damit zusammenhängenden Variationen der Energieabsorption klarzulegen. Spiers (1946, 1949) hat gezeigt, daß Knochengewebe auf Grund seines Gehaltes an schweren Elementen besonders bei weicher Strahlung viel mehr Energie je Gramm und je Röntgeneinheit absorbiert als z. B. Muskelgewebe. Bei einer Halbwertschicht von 0,5 mm Cu ist die Energieabsorption und damit die biologisch wirksame Ionisation mehr als viermal größer im Knochen als im Muskelgewebe. Mit größerer HWS wird dieser Faktor kleiner; für Strahlung im Gebiete von 400 KeV bis 10 MeV ist die Energieabsorption für Knochen, Muskel und andere Gewebe annähernd gleich. Bezüglich der Hirnsubstanz sollte man nach Wachsmann-Vetterlein (1949) bei einer HWS von 0,5 mm Cu im Gehirn eine etwa zweimal größere Energieabsorption als im Muskelgewebe erhalten. Neuere Untersuchungen (Cederlund und Mitarbeiter 1954; Balz und Mitarbeiter 1955) zeigen jedoch, daß dieses nicht der Fall ist, sondern daß das Gehirn bezüglich der Energieabsorption nahezu mit Wasser oder Muskelgewebe äquivalent ist. Mit Rücksicht auf das Cranium ist es jedoch wünschenswert, härtere Strahlung anzuwenden.

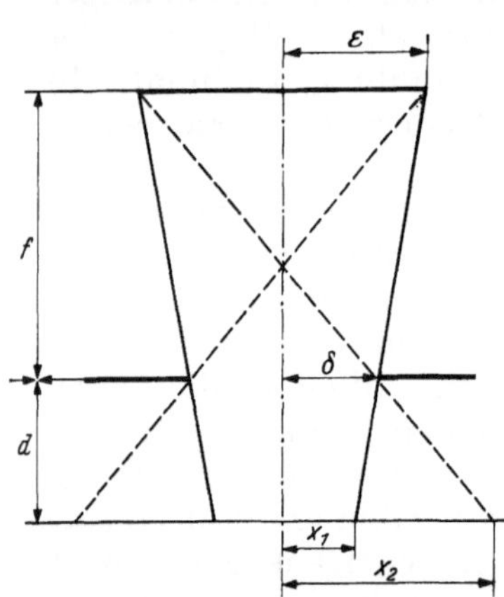


Abb. 18. Schematische Skizze zur Berechnung der Intensitätsverteilung des Halbschattens.

## IV. Dosierungsprobleme der Strahlenchirurgie.

Aus dem Obigen geht hervor, daß die Einführung einer großen Strahlendosis in ein kleines, gut abgegrenztes Gebiet des Gehirns Strahlung mit ausreichender Tiefenwirkung und ausreichender Intensität erfordert. Außerdem muß die benutzte Strahlung zu einem engen Bündel abgeblendet werden können und schließlich muß dieses Strahlenbündel während der Bestrahlungszeit exakt auf den aktuellen Operationspunkt gerichtet werden können. Die Erfüllung der letzten Forderung ist natürlich von großer Bedeutung. Die von LEKSELL (s. oben) beschriebene stereotaktische Methode dürfte eine gute Lösung dieses Problems darstellen.

1. Zur effektiven Abblendung der Strahlung muß *der Focus* der Strahlenquelle klein sein. Die Blende, welche die Feldgröße im Operationspunkt (OP) bestimmt, kann diesem nicht näher als bis zur Haut gebracht werden. Hierbei ergibt sich die Frage, welchen Einfluß der Halbschatten auf die Bestrahlung des Operationspunktes hat. Geht man von einem runden, gleichförmig emittierenden Focus und einer dünnen, aber völlig effektiven Blende mit runder Öffnung aus, so kann man die Intensitätsverteilung im Halbschatten leicht berechnen. Das Gebiet um den Operationspunkt in der Tiefe $d$, das vom ganzen Focus bestrahlt wird, bzw. die Außenkante des Halbschattens, sind von Kreisen mit den Radien $x_1$ bzw. $x_2$ begrenzt (Abb. 18):

$$x_1 = \delta - \frac{d}{f}(\varepsilon - \delta) \tag{1}$$

$$x_2 = \delta + \frac{d}{f}(\varepsilon + \delta) \tag{2}$$

Aus (1) erhält man $x_1 = 0$ für $\delta' = \varepsilon/(f/d + 1)$, d. h. für $\delta < \delta'$ wird kein Teil des OP mit voller Intensität bestrahlt.

Der Intensitätsverlauf im Halbschatten ist für verschiedene Blenden ziemlich gleichartig. Dem Idealfall mit punktförmigem Focus ohne jeden Halbschatten nähert man sich, wenn $\varepsilon/\delta$ kleingehalten werden kann; für praktische Zwecke sollte man anstreben, daß $\varepsilon/\delta$ kleiner als 1 ist.

Wenn es die Intensität der disponiblen Strahlenart zuläßt, ist eine Erhöhung von $f$ zur Verringerung des Halbschatteneinflusses möglich.

2. Die Schwächung eines sehr engen Strahlenbündels beim Durchtritt durch Gewebe wird ausschließlich durch die Absorptionsprozesse bestimmt. Erhöht man jedoch den *Querschnitt* der Strahlung, wird die relative Tiefendosis für primäre Energie unterhalb von etwa 10 MeV durch den Zuschuß an Sekundärstreuung von dem bestrahlten Gebiet um den Meßpunkt herum mehr oder weniger verbessert; dieser Zuschuß stammt hauptsächlich von Comptonphotonen. Da diese Steigerung am schnellsten im Gebiet 0—20 cm² geschieht, ist es von Interesse, die Bedeutung dieses Effektes für Dosierungsfragen der Strahlenchirurgie zu untersuchen.

Die üblichen Tabellen für relative Tiefendosen enthalten als kleinstes Feld oft 20 cm² (Brit. J. Radiol. 1953, Suppl. 5; GREBE und WIEBE 1950). MAYNEORD und LAMERTON (1941) geben eine empirische Formel für Variationen von $(D_d)_A$ mit der Feldgröße $A$ an, die ziemlich gut mit den experimentellen Befunden übereinstimmt. Berechnete Werte aus dieser Formel, deren Konstanten aus den Tiefendosiswerten von $A = 100$ cm² und $A = 400$ cm² gefunden sind, und die experimentellen Tabellenwerte für einige Feldgrößen, wie 20 und 35 cm², zusammen mit einigen hier ausgeführten Tiefendosismessungen für kleine Felder und einer HWS von weniger als 5 mm Cu, sind zur Konstruktion des Diagrammes in Abb. 19 benutzt worden. Diese Abbildung zeigt die Abhängigkeit der relativen Tiefendosis von der Feldgröße $A$ bei $d = 5$ cm und $d = 10$ cm für verschiedene Strahlenqualitäten. Der Streustrahlenzuschuß ist bei niedriger HWS am größten; er hat jedoch ein Maximum bei HWS $\sim 1$ mm Cu und nimmt also sowohl mit weicher als auch härter werdender Strahlung ab. Bei Multimillionvoltqualitäten wie 22 MeV Beschleunigerstrahlung, wo die Streustrahlung fast völlig mit der Primärstrahlung gleichgerichtet ist, erhält man hingegen bei großen und kleinen Feldern die gleiche relative Tiefendosis. Bei der Strahlenqualität HWS = 3 mm Cu, 300 kV, welche von LEKSELL (s. oben) für Strahlenchirurgie im Gehirn benutzt worden ist, ist der Streustrahlenzuschuß bei einem 2 cm² großen Feld und bei $d = 10$ cm etwa 25%. Hieraus geht hervor, daß die Feldgröße bei der Berechnung von Tiefendosiswerten berücksichtigt werden muß, wenn ähnliche Strahlenqualitäten zur Anwendung kommen, d. h. im Gebiet HWS = 0—10 mm Cu.

Die Dosisleistung im Operationspunkt, $(L_d)_A^f$, ist für die Anzahl der Felder, die angewendet werden müssen, entscheidend. Sie wird in der Praxis teils durch die maximale Leistung der Strahlungsquelle und teils durch die zulässige Hautdosis, $(R_H)_{max}$, bestimmt. Für Qualitäten mit einer HWS $< 5$ mm Cu nimmt die Tiefenwirkung ziemlich schnell mit zunehmendem $d$ ab. Aber die Apparate für derartige Strahlen geben keine besonders hohe Röntgenausbeute. Eine Verkleinerung des FHA $f$ zur Erhöhung der Dosisleistung wird jedoch durch $(R_H)_{max}$ begrenzt. Eine Abwägung dieser Faktoren ist notwendig. Das Verhältnis $F$ der relativen Tiefendosiswerte $(D_d)_A^{f_1}$ und $(D_d)_A^{f_2}$ für den FHA $= f_1$ bzw.

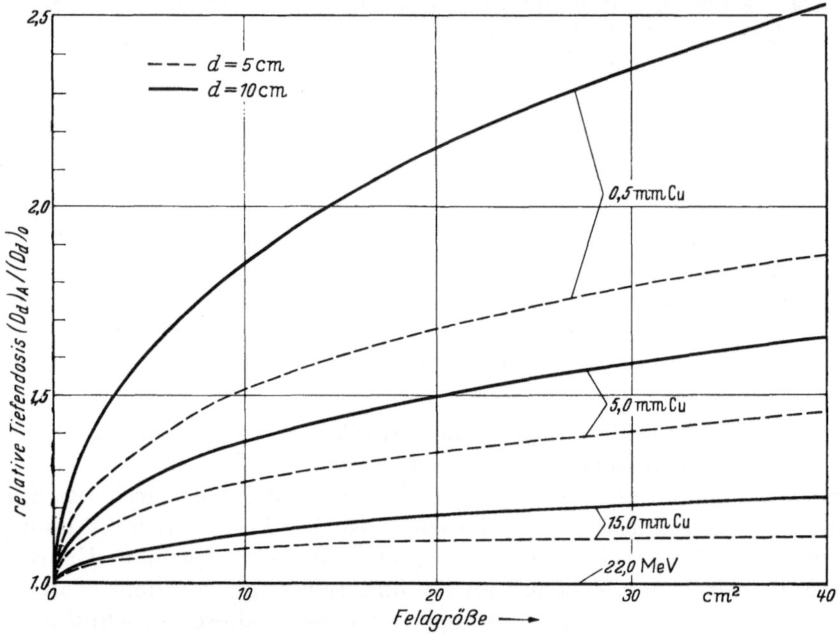


Abb. 19. Die Abhängigkeit der relativen Tiefendosis von der Feldgröße $A$ bei d = 5 cm und d = 10 cm und einem FHA von 50 cm für eine HWS von 0,5 mm, 5,0mm, 15,0 mm Cu sowie für 22 MeV.

$f_2$ unter ausschließlicher Berücksichtigung der Absorption der Primärstrahlung wird leicht berechnet.

$$F = \frac{(D_d)_A^{f_2}}{(D_d)_A^{f_1}} = \left[\frac{f_1 + d}{f_2 + d} \times \frac{f_2}{f_1}\right]^2 \tag{3}$$

Durch den Streustrahlenzuschuß bei großen Feldern wird der Faktor $F$ zu groß. Für sehr kleine Felder $A$ gilt der $F$-Faktor jedoch mit guter Annäherung. Abb. 20 zeigt $F$ für $d = 10$ cm, 5 cm und 2 cm bzw. mit $(D_d)_0^{50}$ als Einheit für jede Kurve.

Für die praktische Anwendung ist die Variation der Dosisleistung $(L_d)_A^f$ mit dem FHA von Interesse. Berechnungen von $L$ für $d = 15$ cm, 10 cm, 5 cm und 0 cm sind in Abb. 21 zusammengestellt worden, in der $(L_d)_0^{50} = 1$ ist. Aus dem Diagramm in Abb. 21 geht z. B. hervor, daß $(L_{10})_0^{20}$ 4,0mal größer ist als $(L_{10})_0^{50}$, während $(L_{10})_0^{100}/(L_{10})_0^{50} = 0{,}3$ ist. Das gleiche Diagramm kann auch dazu benutzt werden, schnell zu schätzen, wie z. B. eine Erhöhung der Dosisleistung in der Tiefe $d$ von einer höheren Hautdosis gefolgt ist. So erhält man z. B., daß $(L_{10})_0^{30}/(L_{10})_0^{50} = 2{,}25$ ist, während das entsprechende Hautdosisverhältnis $(L_0)_0^{30}/(L_0)_0^{50} = 2{,}78$ wird, d. h. die Erhöhung der Hautdosis ist 24% größer als die Zunahme der Operationspunktdosis.

3. Die kleinste *Anzahl der Felder*, die zur Einführung einer beabsichtigten Dosis in einen Operationspunkt mit einer gewissen Strahlenart benutzt werden muß, wird hauptsächlich von der maximal zulässigen Hautdosis $(R_H)_{max}$ bestimmt. Wenn hierbei die disponible Strahlungsintensität z. B. bei einem FHA von 50 cm verhältnismäßig klein ist, so erhebt

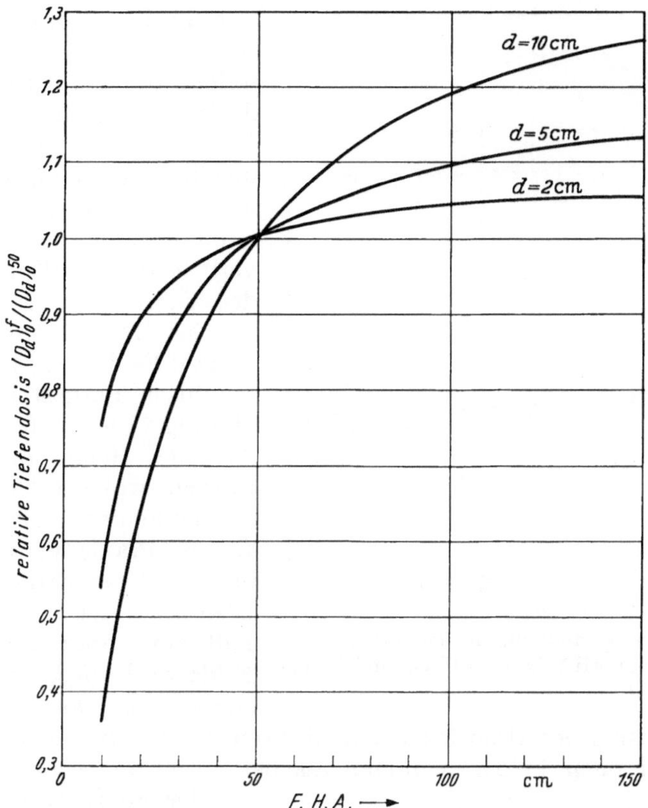


Abb. 20. Die relativen Veränderungen der Tiefendosis, $F = (D_d)_0^f/(D_d)_0^{50}$ mit variierendem FHA für d = 10 cm, 5 cm und 2 cm.

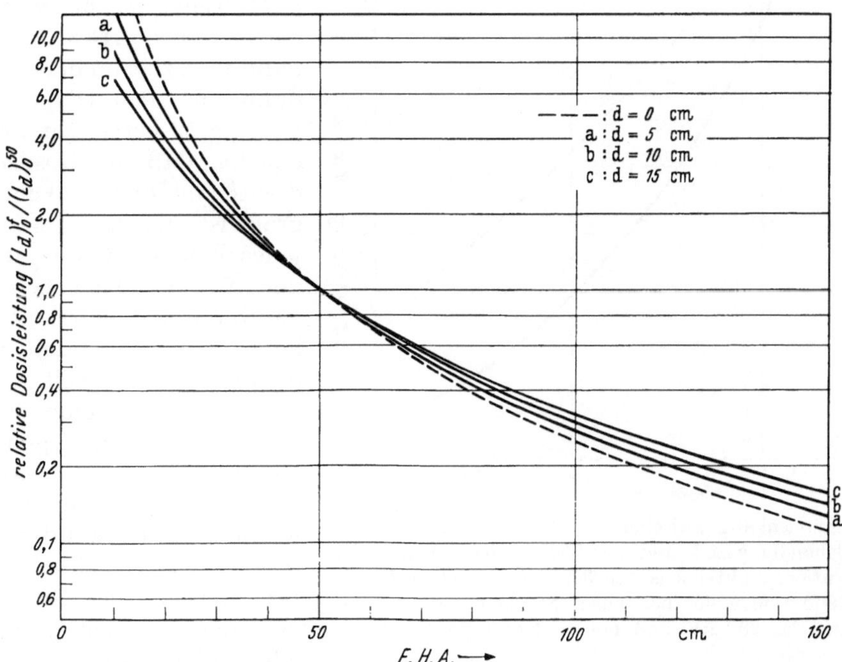


Abb. 21. Die relativen Veränderungen der Dosisleistung $(L_d)_0^f/(L_d)_0^{50}$, mit variierendem FHA für d = 15 cm, 10 cm, 5 cm und 0 cm.

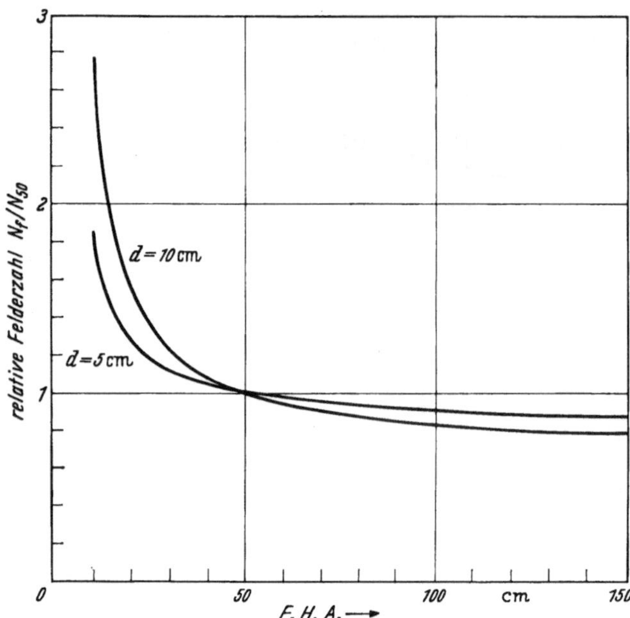


Abb. 22. Die relativen Veränderungen der Felderzahl, $N_f/N_{50}$, mit variierendem FHA für d = 10 cm und 5 cm.

sich die Frage, wie sich eine Verkleinerung des FHA auf die Felderzahl, durch welche die geplante Operationspunktdosis eingestrahlt werden soll, auswirkt. Eine Erhöhung der Felderzahl zur Ermöglichung einer größeren Dosisleistung und damit kürzerer Behandlungszeit kann nützlich sein, solange der Zeitverlust für die Einstellung kleiner als der Gewinn an Bestrahlungszeit ist.

Der Zusammenhang zwischen der Anzahl Felder $N_f$ und dem FHA $f$ kann graphisch dargestellt werden. In Abbildung 22 ist $N_f/N_{50}$ als Funktion von $f$ für $d = 10$ cm und 5 cm dargestellt worden, wobei man voraussetzt, daß $d$ für alle Felder 10 cm bzw. 5 cm beträgt. In der Praxis wird $d$ im allgemeinen immer etwas variieren, aber aus dem Diagramm kann für einen aktuellen Fall eine präliminäre Schätzung der Felderzahl vorgenommen werden. Um eine gewisse Dosis in 10 cm Tiefe (unter maximaler Ausnützung der Hautdosis) einzuführen, muß man bei $f = 20$ cm nach dem Diagramm 1,56mal mehr Felder benutzen als bei $f = 50$ cm, welches eine Vermehrung der Felderzahl um 56% bedeutet. Die Verlängerung des FHA $f$ führt keinen größeren Vorteil im Verhältnis zu $f = 50$ cm mit sich; $f = 100$ cm gibt 16% weniger Felder als $f = 50$ cm. Der Gewinn an Behandlungszeit im ersten Falle kann dann aus dem Diagramm in Abbildung 22 berechnet werden; man ersieht, daß die Dosisleistung bei $d = 10$ cm für $f = 20$ cm viermal so groß ist als bei $f = 50$ cm, d. h. jedes Feld wird mit einem Viertel der für $f = 50$ cm benötigten Behandlungszeit bestrahlt. Die wirkliche Behandlungszeit wird dann, in Prozent der Zeit bei $f = 50$ cm ausgedrückt, gleich $0{,}25 \times 1{,}56 \times 100 = 39\%$. Der Zeitgewinn beträgt also 61%. Hierzu muß jedoch in der Praxis die Mehrzeit addiert werden, die notwendig ist, um weitere $0{,}56 \times N$ Felder einzustellen. Ist hierbei die Bestrahlungszeit von der gleichen Größenordnung oder kleiner als die Einstellungszeit, nimmt der wirkliche Zeitgewinn schnell mit zunehmendem $N$ ab. Für Apparate, die im Operationspunkt geringe Dosisleistung ergeben, kann der Zeitgewinn jedoch für die Durchführung der Behandlung von Bedeutung sein.

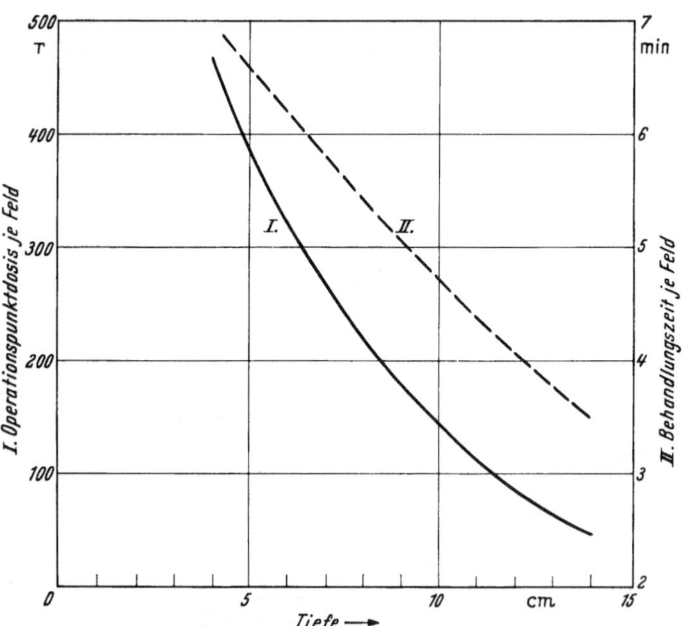


Abb. 23. Zusammenhang zwischen der Dosis im Operationspunkt, der Behandlungszeit und der Tiefe $d$ bei konstantem Abstand Operationspunkt-Focus von 37,5 cm und einer Hautdosis von 1000 r je Feld bei einer Strahlenqualität von HWS = 2 mm Cu, 280 kV und einem 1 cm² großen Feld.

4. Bei der *praktischen Durchführung* eines gezielten strahlenchirurgischen Eingriffes mit Hilfe einer stereotaktischen Methode ist es notwendig, die Verteilung der Bestrahlungsfelder im Voraus zu bestimmen. Da diese Methode einen konstanten Abstand zwischen Focus und Operationspunkt hat, wird die Tiefe $d$ auf Grund der verschiedenartigen Krümmung des Craniums für die verschiedenen Felder variieren und damit tritt auch eine Variation des FHA auf. Für Röntgenstrahlung bis zu 1000 kV nimmt $(D_d)_0$ verhältnismäßig schnell mit zunehmender Tiefe $d$ ab; es ist deshalb vorteilhaft, die Behandlungsfelder so zu wählen, daß kleinstmögliche Werte für $d$ ausgenutzt werden. Zur Erreichung einer konstanten (eventuell maximalen) Hautdosis muß die Bestrahlungszeit je Feld variiert werden. Als Beispiel wird eine in Lund benutzte Röntgenapparatur, die mit 280 kV Gleichspannung, 10 mA und einer HWS von 2 mm Cu arbeitet, angegeben. Der Abstand vom Focus zum OP war 37,5 cm. In Abb. 23 zeigt das Diagramm den Zusammenhang zwischen Operationspunktdosis und der Tiefe $d$ für eine Hautdosis von 1000 r je Feld; die entsprechende Behandlungszeit ist ebenfalls daraus ersichtlich. Mit Hilfe dieses Diagramms konnten alle für einen klinischen Fall notwendigen Berechnungen ausgeführt werden. Die vorliegenden Werte stammen von direkten, mit kleinen Ionisationskammern ausgeführten Tiefendosismessungen bei 1 cm² Feldgröße. Derartige Daten können auch mit den üblichen Tiefendosistabellen berechnet werden, wenn man die oben angeführten Resultate berücksichtigt und von Nullfeldwerten ausgeht. Hierbei darf man auch den Einfluß des Schädelknochens nicht übersehen (SPIERS 1946).

## V. Strahlenquellen.

Aus den oben besprochenen Daten für Absorption, Streuung usw. von Röntgen-, Gamma- und Corpuscularstrahlung geht hervor, daß Photonen mit hoher Energie, 10 bis

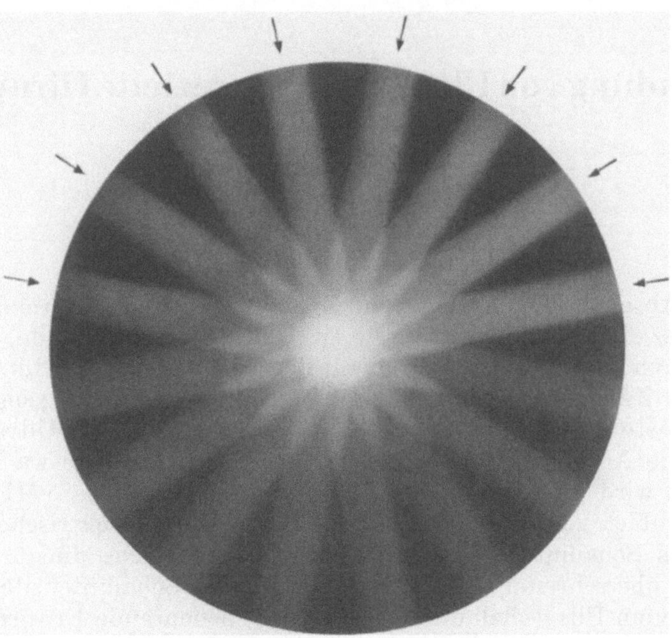

Abb. 24. 25 MeV Röntgenstrahlung von einem Synchrotron. Felddurchmesser 8 mm; 8 Felder. $f = 100$ cm. Der tangential bestrahlte Film wurde zwischen Perspexscheiben von 2,5 cm Dicke und 12 cm Durchmesser gelegt.

20 MeV, oder hochenergetische schwere Teilchen wie Protonen oder Deuteronen in physikalischer Hinsicht am besten für Strahlenchirurgie im Gehirn geeignet sein dürften. Die zur Herstellung dieser Strahlenarten erforderliche Apparatur ist jedoch erheblich schwerer zu handhaben als die übliche Röntgentherapieausrüstung. Besonders gilt dies natürlich für Cyclotrone und ähnliche Maschinen zur Herstellung von schweren

Teilchen mit Energien von mehreren Hundert MeV. Ein Betatron oder ein linearer Beschleuniger für 5—20 MeV ist beweglicher und es ist ohne weiteres möglich, die hier beschriebene stereotaktische Technik z. B. zusammen mit einem Betatron anzuwenden. Hierbei muß jedoch eine ausreichend große Dosisleistung zur Verfügung stehen. Die Emission von Photonen von einem Beschleunigungsgerät z. B. bei 20 MeV geschieht in einem sehr kleinen Raumwinkel mit einer Halbwertbreite von $5^0$; dieser Umstand macht diesen Strahlentypus besonders vorteilhaft im Vergleich z. B. mit der 300 kV Röntgenstrahlung, die gleichförmiger im Raum emittiert wird.

Da es beabsichtigt ist, die hier beschriebene stereotaktische Methode für Strahlenchirurgie zusammen mit einer fixierten oder beweglichen Strahlenquelle anzuwenden, sind alle derartigen Typen von Interesse. Eine Apparatur mit hoher Dosisleistung und kleinem Focus verdient hierbei den Vorzug. Synchro-cyclotrone und ähnliche Maschinen für schwere corpusculäre Strahlung dürften nicht allgemein zugänglich werden. Für gewisse Fälle kann die vorteilhafte Dosisverteilung dieser Strahlungen jedoch sehr wertvolle Erfolge geben. Die Dosisleistungen kommerzieller Betatrone und Synchrotrone im Energiegebiet von 10—40 MeV sind zur Zeit nicht ganz zufriedenstellend. Der lineare Beschleuniger kann für hohe Dosisleistungen konstruiert werden, aber bisher hat man die Frage der Herstellung handlicher Maschinen für z. B. 20—30 MeV noch nicht gelöst. Eine für Strahlenchirurgie ideale Apparatur gibt es also im Augenblick nicht, aber die Entwicklung auf dem Gebiete der Beschleunigungsgeräte wird in absehbarer Zeit bedeutende Verbesserungen bringen. Eine sehr vorteilhafte strahlenchirurgische Dosisverteilung mit kleinen Feldern ergibt z.B. die 25 MeV-Röntgenstrahlung. Die Abb. 24 stammt von einem Versuch mit einem 35 MeV-Synchrotron. Hierbei wurde der Film zwischen zwei 25 mm dicke Perspexscheiben von 12 cm Durchmesser gelegt und längs 8 verschiedenen Durchmessern mit zirkulären Feldern von 8 mm Durchmesser bestrahlt.

# F. Die Anwendung von Ultraschall für gezielte Hirnoperationen.

Von

Carl Hellmuth Hertz.

## I. Einleitung.

Wie schon im Abschnitt E (Physikalische Grundlagen für die Verwendung ionisierender Strahlung bei gezielter Strahlenchirurgie, S. 199) erwähnt wurde, ist energiereiche Strahlung, die durch das Gehirn hindurch auf den Operationspunkt hin gerichtet werden kann, ein für die Zwecke der gezielten Hirnchirurgie besonders geeignetes Werkzeug. Eine hierfür geeignete Strahlenform ist deshalb der Ultraschall. Als Ultraschall bezeichnet man allgemein jede Art von Schall, dessen Frequenz größer als etwa 20 kHz ist (obere Hörgrenze), meist wird jedoch mit Frequenzen von 100 kHz bis 5 MHz gearbeitet. In diesem Frequenzgebiet können unter Anwendung des piezoelektrischen oder magnetostriktiven Effektes Schallintensitäten erhalten werden, welche die für hörbaren Schall erreichbaren weit überschreiten. Auf Grund der hohen Schallintensitäten kann in dem Material, welches vom Ultraschall durchlaufen wird, bedeutende Erwärmung stattfinden, wodurch z. B. biologisches Gewebe zerstört werden kann. Weiterhin kann der Ultraschall ähnlich wie Licht durch Linsen oder Spiegel auf eine Stelle hin focussiert werden, an welcher dann lokalisiert eine besonders hohe Erwärmung auftritt. Da sich schließlich die weiße Gehirnsubstanz als besonders empfindlich für Schädigung durch Ultraschall erwies, war zu erwarten, daß mit Hilfe von focussiertem Ultraschall streng lokalisierte Läsionen tief im Gehirn hergestellt werden könnten, ohne die Gehirnsubstanz im übrigen zu schädigen. Versuche an Tieren haben dies bestätigt, und es ist zu erwarten, daß mit dieser Methode noch weitere wesentliche Fortschritte erreicht werden können.

Die Erzeugung des Ultraschalles geschieht meist mit Hilfe von piezoelektrischen Kristallen (z. B. Quarz), welche durch eine elektrische Wechselspannung, deren Frequenz mit der Resonanzfrequenz des Kristalls übereinstimmt, zu lebhaften mechanischen Schwingungen angeregt werden können. Eine ausführliche Behandlung des Ultraschalles samt reichhaltigem Literaturverzeichnis findet sich bei BERGMANN (1954).

## II. Physikalische Eigenschaften des Ultraschalles.

Die Geschwindigkeit, mit der sich der Schall fortpflanzt, ist für alle praktischen Fälle unabhängig von seiner Frequenz und Intensität und nur von den Eigenschaften des Materials, durch welches er sich hindurchbewegt, abhängig. In tierischen Geweben ist die Schallgeschwindigkeit sehr ähnlich der Schallgeschwindigkeit in Wasser, für Gehirn z. B. 1515 m/sec (Wasser 1497 m/sec). Die Unterschiede der Schallgeschwindigkeit in den Geweben verschiedener tierischer Organe sind nur klein (LUDWIG 1950).

Für eine longitudinale Schallwelle berechnet sich die Intensität des Schalles $I$ (erg/cm² = $10^{-7}$ Watt/cm²) nach der Gleichung

$$I = \frac{1}{2} \varrho v (2 \pi f)^2 \cdot A^2 . \quad (1)$$

wobei $\varrho$ die Dichte des Materials (gr/cm³) ist, welches vom Schall durchlaufen wird, $v$ die Schallgeschwindigkeit (cm/sec), $f$ die Frequenz (Hz) und $A$ die Schallamplitude (cm). Die Schallwechseldruckamplitude $P$, welche den größten Über- und Unterdruck angibt, welcher sich in der Schallwelle ausbildet, findet man aus der Gleichung

$$P = 2 \pi f \varrho v A . \quad (2)$$

Für eine Schallwelle in Wasser mit einer Intensität von 2 W/cm² und einer Frequenz von 1 MHz findet man hieraus $A = 0{,}026\ \mu$ und $P = 2{,}5$ Atm., es ist also zu erwarten, daß solcher Schall unter Umständen erhebliche Wirkungen auf die Materie, welche er durchläuft, ausüben kann.

Durchläuft ein Schallstrahl in einer bestimmten Materie die Strecke $x$, so nimmt seine Intensität $I$ auf Grund der immer stattfindenden Absorption des Schalles nach der Gleichung

$$I = I_0 \cdot e^{-\alpha x} \quad (3)$$

ab, wobei $I_0$ die Intensität an der Stelle $x = 0$ ist. Die durch Absorption verlorene Schallenergie ist dabei in Wärme umgewandelt worden, d. h. die durchlaufene Materie wird erwärmt. Die meisten Wirkungen des Ultraschalles auf tierisches Gewebe muß auf solche Erwärmung zurückgeführt werden, welche so weit getrieben werden kann, daß irreversible Schäden entstehen (PÄTZOLD und Mitarbeiter 1947).

HÜTER (1948) hat gezeigt, daß die Größe $\alpha$ in Gl. (3) in tierischen Geweben proportional mit der Frequenz wächst. Bei einer Frequenz von 1 MHz wurde für Gehirnsubstanz der Wert 0,15 (HÜTER 1952) bis 0,2 (FRY und Mitarbeiter 1953A) ermittelt.

Für gezielte Hirnoperationen ist es einerseits wünschenswert, daß der Schall an der Operationsstelle möglichst stark absorbiert wird, um dort eine starke Erwärmung oder andere Schädigung hervorzurufen. Aus diesem Grunde wäre die Verwendung einer hohen Frequenz (großes $\alpha$) anzustreben. Dies führt jedoch den Nachteil mit sich, daß ein relativ großer Teil des Schalles bereits auf dem Wege zur Operationsstelle absorbiert wird, wodurch eventuell andere Teile des Hirnes geschädigt werden. Weiterhin muß bei der Wahl der Frequenz beachtet werden, daß die Wellenlänge des Schalles wesentlich kleiner als der Durchmesser der Schallquelle sein muß, da man sonst wegen Beugungserscheinungen keinen gut definierten Schallstrahl erhält, was für gezielte Hirnoperationen unerläßlich ist. Bei der Wahl der Frequenz muß also eine Kompromißlösung gesucht werden. Untersuchungen über die Wahl der günstigsten Frequenz liegen noch nicht vor, die meisten Versuche wurden jedoch mit Schallfrequenzen von 1 MHz durchgeführt.

Da das endgültige Ziel der gezielten Hirnoperationen mit Ultraschall die Operation ohne Öffnung des Schädelbeines ist (also durch den Knochen hindurch), müssen schließlich auch noch die Effekte, die bei der Reflektion des Schalls an der Grenze Gewebe–Knochen und Knochen–Gehirn entstehen, betrachtet werden. Falls ein Schallstrahl senkrecht auf eine ebene Grenzfläche zwischen zwei Materialien 1 und 2 fällt, welche die Dichten $\varrho_1$ und $\varrho_2$ haben, und in welchen der Schall die Geschwindigkeiten $v_1$ und $v_2$ hat, so ergibt sich für die reflektierte Schallintensität $I_R$

$$I_R = I_0 \left( \frac{\varrho_2 v_2 - \varrho_1 v_1}{\varrho_2 v_2 + \varrho_1 v_1} \right)^2 \tag{4}$$

und für die durchgehende Intensität $I_D$

$$I_D = I_0 - I_R = I_0 \frac{4 \varrho_1 v_1 \varrho_2 v_2}{(\varrho_2 v_2 + \varrho_1 v_1)^2} \,. \tag{5}$$

Fällt der Schallstrahl schräge auf die Grenzfläche, so gelten komplizierte Ausdrücke (Bergmann 1954).

Da das Produkt $\varrho \cdot v$ (Schallwellenwiderstand) für Gewebe und Knochen recht verschieden ist (Hüter 1952) und außerdem eine kräftige Erwärmung an der Grenzfläche Gewebe–Knochen stattfindet, die nach Lehmann (1951, 1953 A) darauf zurückzuführen ist, daß im Knochen auch transversale und Scherungsschallwellen erzeugt werden, geht ein nicht unbeträchtlicher Teil der Ultraschallintensität hier verloren. Der letztgenannte Effekt tritt um so stärker hervor, je höher die Frequenz des angewandten Ultraschalles ist (Lehmann und Mitarbeiter 1951). Hinzu kommt noch, daß der Knochen selbst einen relativ großen Absorptionskoeffizienten aufweist (Hüter 1952, Theismann und Mitarbeiter 1949). Aus diesen Gründen ist es bisher weder an Versuchstieren noch an Menschen gelungen, Ultraschalläsionen im Gehirn durch das Schädelbein hindurch zu erzeugen, da dieses dabei entweder zu stark erwärmt oder sogar zerstört wurde (Fry und Mitarbeiter 1955 A, Lindström 1954).

Das wichtigste Ziel der Hirnoperationen mit Ultraschall ist, an bestimmter Stelle im Gehirn begrenzte Läsionen bekannter Größe herzustellen. Dies kann entweder dadurch erreicht werden, daß man den Schallgeber auf einem Kreise, welcher den Operationspunkt zum Mittelpunkt hat, hin und her bewegt und auf diese Weise die vom Ultraschall am Operationspunkt hervorgerufene Wirkung gegenüber der im umgebenden Gewebe wesentlich erhöht. Ein einfacheres und besseres Verfahren erhält man aber durch Fokussieren des Ultraschalles auf den Operationspunkt hin mittels geeigneter Linsen bzw. Spiegel. Da der Ultraschall in verschiedenen Materialien verschiedene Geschwindigkeiten hat und also beim Durchgang durch eine Grenzfläche zwischen zwei Materialien mit verschiedener Schallgeschwindigkeit ähnlich wie Licht eine Brechung erleidet, kann man ihn ähnlich wie Lichtstrahlen durch Linsen in einem Brennpunkt sammeln. Solche Linsen werden meist aus Plexiglas hergestellt (vgl. Bergmann 1954), da wegen der relativ ähnlichen Schallwellenwiderstände von Wasser oder Öl und Plexiglas die Reflexionsverluste an den Linsenoberflächen nicht zu groß sind. Auf diese Weise können Schallintensitäten von mehreren 100 W/cm² im Brennpunkt der Linse erreicht werden. Bei größeren Schallintensitäten erwärmen sich diese Linsen jedoch so stark (Esche 1952), daß sie leicht zerstört werden. Linsen aus Aluminium zeigen dagegen große Verluste durch Reflexion an den Linsenoberflächen. — Eine alternative Lösung ergibt sich entweder durch ein von Barone (1952) angegebenes Doppelconus-Spiegelsystem (vgl. auch Bergmann 1954, Fry und Mitarbeiter 1955 A) oder auch dadurch, daß man den schallerzeugenden Kristall in Form einer Kugelkalotte ausführt. Näheres über solche „Hohlschwinger“ findet sich bei Bergmann (1954).

## III. Bisherige Versuche.

Schon frühzeitig wurde von verschiedener Seite festgestellt (Lynn und Mitarbeiter 1942, 1944, Peters 1949; vgl. auch die Zusammenfassung bei Bergmann 1954), daß das zentrale Nervensystem besonders empfindlich für Ultraschall ist. Es wurden deshalb von verschiedener Seite Versuche an Ratten, Meerschweinchen und Fröschen aufgenommen (ALLEGRANZA 1950, GREGG 1944, LEONHARDT 1949, HEYCK und Mitarbeiter 1952, PETERS 1951). Ausführliche Versuche hierüber machten insbesondere FRY und Mitarbeiter (1953A, 1954, 1955A, 1955B, WALL und Mitarbeiter 1953) an Versuchstieren mit hohen Schallintensitäten (einigen 100 W/cm²), welche sie durch Fokussierung des Ultraschalles mit einer Linse erhielten. Nach ursprünglich anderen Befunden (WALL und Mitarbeiter 1953) wurde nachgewiesen, daß Ultraschall hoher Intensität besonders leicht die Nervfibern zerstört (FRY und Mitarbeiter 1955B), während die Nervzellen weniger, Blutgefäße und andere Gewebe wesentlich weniger empfindlich für Ultraschall sind (WALL und Mitarbeiter 1953). Nach FRY und Mitarbeitern ist dies auf eine bisher nicht erklärte spezifische Wirkung des Ultraschalles auf die Nervfibern zurückzuführen und nicht auf die Temperaturerhöhung, die durch den Ultraschall im Gewebe hervorgerufen wird (FRY 1953A, WALL und Mitarbeiter 1953). Diese spezifische Wirkung kann auch nicht durch Auftreten von Kavitationserscheinungen erklärt werden (FRY 1953A, WALL und Mitarbeiter 1953). Als Grund für diese Annahme gibt FRY (1953A) Versuche am Zentralnervensystem von unterkühlten Fröschen an, in denen nach einer Beschallung von wenigen Sekunden mit fokussiertem Ultraschall hoher Intensität (1 MHz, etwa 50 W/cm²) eine vollständige Zerstörung der Nervzellen eintrat, obwohl die während der Bestrahlung mit dem Thermoelement an der Operationsstelle gemessenen Temperaturen 25° C nicht überstiegen.

Im Gegensatz hierzu führt HERRICK (1953) die spezifische Wirkung des Ultraschalles auf Nervenfibern auf die Wärmewirkung des Ultraschalles zurück. HERRICK untersuchte insbesondere die Einwirkung von fokussiertem Ultraschall (980 kHz) auf den Ischiasnerven von Hunden und Fröschen, da durch Ultraschallbehandlung dieses Nerven an Menschen gute Heilresultate erreicht worden sind. HERRICK untersuchte das Aktionspotential, welches in einem Nerven auftritt, wenn er an einem anderen Punkt künstlich stimuliert wird, vor und nach Ultraschallbehandlung des Teiles des Nerven, der zwischen dem Stimulator und der Empfangselektrode lag. Er fand dabei, daß eine totale irreversible Blockierung des Nerven eintritt, sobald die Temperatur des Nerven 45° C überschreitet, und zwar unabhängig davon, ob die Erwärmung des Nerven mit Ultraschall oder mit einer Wärmemanschette geschieht. Diese Resultate stimmen mit LEHMANNs Versuchen (1953) überein, welcher mit relativ geringen Ultraschallintensitäten von 4 W/cm² (1 MHz) die Wirkung des Ultraschalles auf Nerven untersucht. Auch er findet, daß sich diese ganz auf die Wärmewirkung des Ultraschalles zurückführen läßt, und nimmt an, daß die spezielle Wirkung des Ultraschalles auf Nerven auf der erhöhten Erwärmung der Grenzschichten zwischen den Nervzellen bzw. Nervfibern beruht (HERRICK 1953, LEHMANN 1953).

FRY und Mitarbeiter (1953A) stellten weiterhin bei Beschallung des Zentralnervensystems von Fröschen fest, daß bei langsamer Erhöhung der Ultraschallsintensität zunächst reversible Schädigungen des Nervensystems eintreten, was durch Lähmungen bestimmter Gliedmaßen zum Ausdruck kommt. Eine relativ unbedeutende Erhöhung der Ultraschallintensität über diesen Wert erzeugt dann irreversible Schäden, welche histologisch durch die vollständige Zerstörung aller Nervenzellen nachgewiesen werden kann. Die Differenz zwischen den Ultraschallintensitäten, welche zu reversiblen bzw. irreversiblen Schädigungen führen, ist jedoch zu klein, um mit Ultraschall eine temporäre Blockierung bestimmter Nerven unter kontrollierbaren Bedingungen zu erzielen.

FRY und Mitarbeiter haben weiterhin ausführliche Versuche angestellt, um mit fokussiertem Ultraschall kleine, gut abgegrenzte Läsionen im Gehirn von Tieren (Ratten und Katzen) zu erzeugen und so ohne direkten operativen Eingriff bestimmte Nervenbahnen abzuschneiden (FRY und Mitarbeiter 1954, 1955A, 1955B, BARNARD 1956, WALL und Mitarbeiter 1953). Bei diesen Versuchen kam Ultraschall mit der Frequenz von 1 MHz zur Anwendung, der von vier separaten Quarzkristallen mit je einer Linse zur Fokussierung des Schalles erzeugt wurde. Diese waren in einer Halterung so befestigt, daß ihre Brennpunkte alle an derselben Stelle lagen, so daß mit dieser Anordnung im gemeinsamen Brennpunkt Schallintensitäten bis zu 400 W/cm² erzeugt werden konnten. Auch hier mußte das Schädelbein des Versuchstieres wegen der oben genannten starken Erwärmung durch den Ultraschall entfernt werden.

Wurde nach diesen Vorbereitungen etwa 4 sec mit einer Schallintensität im Brennpunkt von etwa 200 W/cm² beschallt, so konnte nach Abtötung des Tieres 12 Tage später eine etwa 1 mm große Läsion tief im Gehirn des Versuchstieres gefunden werden (FRY und Mitarbeiter 1955A). Zur Herstellung ausgedehnterer Läsionen mußte der Schallgeber schrittweise bewegt werden, so daß viele kleine Läsionen nebeneinander entstanden. Nach der Beschallung wiesen die Versuchstiere motorische Defekte auf, die selbst nach 8 Wochen nicht verschwanden, d. h. die so hervorgerufenen Schäden sind irreversibel.

Die einzigen Versuche, mit Ultraschalläsionen im Gehirn an Menschen hervorzurufen, hat LINDSTRÖM (1954) mit nichtfokussiertem Ultraschall gemacht. Nach anfänglichen Tierversuchen hat er in insgesamt 20 Fällen präfrontale Lobotomie durch Bestrahlung mit unfokussiertem Ultraschall ersetzt (7 W/cm², 1 MHz, Bestrahlungsdauer etwa 10 min). Obduktionsbefunde zeigten relativ ausgebreitete Läsionen in der weißen Gehirnsubstanz direkt unter den Schalleintrittstellen.

Zusammenfassend muß also festgestellt werden, daß es besonders mit Hilfe von fokussiertem Ultraschall möglich ist, an streng begrenzten Stellen des Gehirnes Läsionen zu erzeugen. Eine genaue Messung der Dosis am Operationsort ist dabei schwierig. Weiterhin ist es bisher nicht möglich gewesen, die Beschallung ohne Entfernung des Schädelbeines durch dieses hindurch vorzunehmen. Neuere Versuche von LEKSELL (1956) zeigten jedoch, daß der Brennpunkt des fokussierten Ultraschallstrahles recht wenig durch den Durchgang durch das menschliche Schläfenbein gestört wird, und daß es vielleicht möglich ist, auch die Erwärmung desselben in ertragbaren Grenzen zu halten. Es ist deshalb deutlich, daß die Anwendung fokussierten Ultraschalles schon jetzt ein wertvolles Instrument für die experimentelle Neurochirurgie ist und in Zukunft eventuell auch für gezielte Gehirnoperationen in der Klinik benutzt werden kann, was besonders auch deshalb wünschenswert wäre, da nach bisherigen Erfahrungen bei Ultraschallbehandlungen mit Spätschäden nicht gerechnet werden muß.

## Literatur.

### Gezielte Hirnoperationen.

AJURIAGUERRA, J. DE, PH. BENDA, J. CONSTANS, M. DAVID et M. TUBIANA: Étude expérimentale des lésions provoquées par l'implantation intracérébrale de fragments d'or radioactif; Incidences thérapeutiques. Revue neur. **91**, 260—285 (1954).

ALLEGRANZA, A.: Accessi epilettiformi in animali da esperimento, provocati dall'applicazione di energia ultrasonora sul cervello a teca integra. Arch. Psicol. neurol. **13**, 46—57 (1952).

AMADOR, L., u. P. BAILEY: Persönliche Mitteilung 1953.

ANDERSON, T. P., K. G. WAKIM, J. F. HERRICK, N. A. BENNET and F. H. KRUSEN: An experimental study of the effects of ultrasonic energy on the lower part of the spinal cord and peripheral nerves. Arch. Physic. Med. **32**, 71—79 (1951).

ARNOLD, A., P. BAILEY, R. A. HARVEY, L. L. HAAS and J. S. LAUGHLIN: Changes in the central nervous system following irradiation with 23 MeV X-rays from the betatron. Radiology **62**, 37—44 (1954).

— — — Intolerance of the primate brainstem and hypothalamus to conventional and high energy radiations. Neurology **4**, 575—585 (1954).

— — and J. S. LAUGHLIN: Effects of betatron radiations on the brain of primates. Neurology **4**, 165—178 (1954).

BAILEY, P., and S. N. STEIN: A stereotaxic apparatus for use on the human brain. Scientific Exhibit. A.M.A. Atlantic City 1951. Zit. nach SPIEGEL und WYCIS 1952.

BAIRD, H., B. GUIDETTI, V. REYES, H. T. WYCIS and E. A. SPIEGEL: Stimulation and elimination of anterior thalamic nuclei in man and cat. Federat. Proc. **10**, 8—9 (1951).

BARONE, A.: Aspects of the concentration of ultrasonic energy. Acustica **2**, 221—225 (1952).

BAUDOIN, A., et A. REMOND: Sur un appareil stéréotactique applicable à l'homme. IV. Congr. Neurol. Internat. Paris 1949, Bd. II, S. 132. Paris: Masson & Cie. 1949.

BAUDOIN, A., et A. REMOND: Nouveaux perfectionnements à l'appareillage stéréotactique humain. Revue neur. **85**, 573—576 (1951).

BORISON, H. L., and S. W. WANG: Quantitative effects of radon implanted in the medulla oblongata: A technique for producing discrete lesions. J. Comp. Neur. **94**, 35—55 (1951).

BUSNEL, R. G., J. GLIGORIEVIC, P. CHAUCHARD et H. MAZOUE: Mise en evidence des effets specifiques non thermiques dans l'action nerveuse des ultrasons. C. r. Acad. Sci. Paris **236**, 1684—1685 (1953).

CAMPBELL, B., and R. NOVICK: Effects of beta rays on central nervous tissues. Proc. Soc. Exper. Biol. a. Med. **72**, 34—38 (1949).

CARPENTER, B., and J. R. WHITTIER: Study of methods for pro-ducing experimental lesions of the central nervous system with special reference to stereotaxic tech- nique. J. Comp. Neur. **97**, 73—133 (1952).

CICARDO, V. H.: Effets des ultra-sons sur le diencéphale. C. r. Soc. Biol. Paris **145**, 1708—1709 (1951).

CLARKE, R. H.: Investigation of the central nervous system. Johns Hopkins Hosp. Rep. 1920, Spec. Bd. I, S. 1—160. Baltimore: The Lord Baltimore Press 1920.

DAVID, M., J. TALAIRACH et H. HECAEN: Perspectives therapeutiques issues de la méthode de repérage et de coagulation localisée des structures cérébrales souscorticales. Bull. Soc. méd. Hôp. Paris **35**, 459—464 (1949).

DELGADO, J. M. R., H. HAMLIN and D. J. NALEBUFF: Some innovations in human stereoencephalotomy. Neurology **4**, 14—18 (1954).

DELMAS, A., et B. PERTUISET: La topométrie encéphalique chez l'homme (noyau rouge, centre médian, noyau amygdalien). Presse méd. **60**, 1784 — 1787 (1952).

DUSSER DE BARENNE, J. G., and H. M. ZIMMERMAN: Changes in the cerebral cortex produced by thermocoagulation. Arch. of Neur. **33**, 123—131 (1935).

FISCHER, A. W., u. H. HOHLFELDER: Lokales Amyloid im Gehirn. Eine Spätfolge von Röntgenbestrahlungen. Dtsch. Z. Chir. **227**, 475—483 (1930).

FOLTZ, E. L., J. B. HOLYOKE and L. H. HENRY: Brain necrosis following X-ray therapy. J. of Neurosurg. **10**, 423—429 (1953).

FREED, H., E. A. SPIEGEL and H. T. WYCIS: Somatic procedures for the relief of anxiety. Psychiatr. Quart. **23**, 227—230 (1949).

FRY, W. J.: Action of ultrasound on nerve tissue — a review. J. Acoust. Soc. Amer. **25**, 1—5 (1953).

— J. W. BARNARD, F. J. FRY and J. F. BRENNAN: Ultrasonically produced localized selective lesions in the central nervous system. Amer. J. Physic. Med. **34**, 413—423 (1955).

— — — R. F. KRUMINS and J. F. BRENNAN: Ultrasonic lesions in the mammalian nervous system. Science (Lancaster, Pa.) **122**, 517—518 (1955).

— W. H. MOSBERG, J. W. BARNARD and F. J. FRY: Production of focal destructive lesions in the central nervous system with ultrasound. J. of Neurosurg. **11**, 471—478 (1954).

—, and V. J. WULFF: Effect of ultrasound on nervous tissues. Federat. Proc. **9**, 45 (1950).

GUIOT, G., et S. BRION: Traitement des mouvements anormaux par la coagulation pallidale. Technique et résultats. Revue neur. **89**, 578—580 (1953).

GÜTTNER, W., G. FIEDLER u. J. PÄTZOLD: Über Ultraschallabbildungen am menschlichen Schädel. Acustica **2**, 148—156 (1952).

GULEKE, N.: Die Eingriffe am N. trigeminus. In Allgemeine und spezielle chirurgische Operationslehre von M. KIRSCHNER, 2. Aufl., herausgeg. von GULEKE u. ZENKER, Bd. II, S. 359—426. Heidelberg: Springer 1950.

HASSLER, R., u. T. RIECHERT: Indikationen und Lokalisationsmethode der gezielten Hirnoperationen. Nervenarzt **25**, 441—447 (1954).

HAYNE, R. A., and R. MEYERS: An improved model of a human stereotaxic instrument. J. of Neurosurg. **7**, 463—466 (1950).

— A. STOWELL and J. B. DARROUGH: The use of the human HORSLEY CLARKE stereotaxic apparatus. Selective section of the thalamo-frontal tracts. Surgical Forum Clin. Congr. Amer. Coll. Surg.1951, S. 380—385. Philadelphia: W. B. Saunders Company 1952.

HECAEN, H., J. TALAIRACH, M. DAVID et M. B. DELL: Coagulations limitées du thalamus dans les algies du syndrome thalamique. Resultats thérapeutiques et physiologiques. Revue neur. **81**, 917—931 (1949).

HEYCK, H.: Ultraschall und Zentralnervensystem. Ergebnisse experimental-pathologischer, elektroencephalographischer und klinischer Untersuchungen. Schweiz. med. Wschr. **1952**, 97—99.

HICKS, S. P., and P. O. B. MONTGOMERY: Effects of acute radiation on the adult mammalian central nervous system. Proc. Soc. Exper. Biol. a. Med. **80**, 15—18 (1953).

HORNBERGER, W.: JACKSON-Epilepsie nach hochdosierter CHAOUL-Nahbestrahlung eines Schläfenmelanoms. Strahlenther. **85**, 459—477 (1951).

HORSLEY, V., and R. H. CLARKE: The structure and functions of the cerebellum examined by a new method. Brain **31**, 45—124 (1908).

HÜTER, T. F.: Messung der Ultraschallabsorption im menschlichen Schädelknochen und ihre Abhängigkeit von der Frequenz. Naturwiss. **39**, 21—22 (1952).

JASPER, H., and J. HUNTER: A stereotaxic instrument for man. Scientific Exhibit. Amer. EEG. Soc. Atlantic City 1949. Zit. nach SPIEGEL u. WYCIS 1952.

JEPPSSON, S., u. L. LEKSELL: Unveröffentlichte Beobachtungen. Vortrag von S. JEPPSSON: An experimental study of stereotaxic thermolesions in the brain. Nordisk Neurokir. Fören. 10. Tagg Göteborg 1954.

KIRSCHNER, M.: Die Punktionstechnik und die Elektrokoagulation des Ganglion Gasseri. Über „gezielte“ Operationen. Arch. klin. Chir. **176**, 581—620 (1933).

KÖBCKE, H.: Gezielte Hirnoperationen. Dtsch. med. Wschr. **1954**, 294—297.

LARSSON, B., B. REXED, P. SOURANDER u. L. LEKSELL: Unveröffentlichte Beobachtungen.

LEKSELL, L.: A stereotaxic apparatus for intracerebral surgery. Acta chir. scand. (Stockh.) **99**, 229—233 (1949).

— The stereotaxic method and radiosurgery of the brain. Acta chir. scand. (Stockh.) **102**, 316—319 (1951).

— A localization technique for intracerebral surgery. Kgl. fysiogr. Sällsk. Lund Förh. **25**, 130—137 (1955).

— Further note on a stereotaxic instrument for man. Kgl. fysiogr. Sällsk. Lund Förh. **25**, 138—141 (1955).

— Echo-encephalography. I. Detection of intracranial complications following head injury. Acta chir. scand. (Stockh.) **110**, 301—315 (1955/56).

— T. HERNER and K. LIDÉN: Stereotaxic radiosurgery of the brain. Report of a case. Kgl. fysiogr. Sällsk. Lund Förh. **25**, 142—151 (1955).

—, and K. LIDÉN: A therapeutic trial with radioactive isotopes in cystic brain tumor. In Radioisotope Techniques. Proc. Isotope Techniques Conf. Oxford 1951, Bd. I, S. 76 bis78. London: H. M. Stationery Off. 1953.

LINDGREN, E.: Some aspects on the technique of encephalography. Acta radiol. (Stockh.) **31**, 161—177 (1949).

LINDSTRÖM, P. A.: Prefrontal ultrasonic irradiation — a substitute for lobotomy. Arch. of Neur. **72**, 399—425 (1954).

LISTER, W. C., and S. L. SHERWOOD: A lightweight stereotaxic instrument. Electroencephalogr. Clin. Neurophysiol. **7**, 311—314 (1955).

LYNN, J. G., and T. PUTNAM: Histology of cerebral lesions producad by focused ultrasound. Amer. J. Path. **20**, 637—649 (1944).

— R. L. ZWEMER, A. J. CHICK and A. E. MILLER: A new method for the generation and use of focused ultrasound in experimental biology. J. Gen. Physiol. **26**, 179—193 (1942).

MALAMUD, N., E. B. BOLDREY, W. K. WELCH and E. J. FADELL: Necrosis of brain and spinal cord following X-ray therapy. J. of Neurosurg. **11**, 353—362 (1954).

MARK, V. H., P. M. MCPHERSON and W. H. SWEET: A new method for correcting distortion in cranial roentgenograms; with special reference to a new human stereotaxic instrument. Amer. J. Roentgenol. **71**, 435—444 (1954).

MARKIEWICZ, T.: Über Spätschädigungen des menschlichen Gehirns durch Röntgenstrahlen. Z. Neur. **152**, 548—568 (1935).

MCCLURE jr., C. C., E. L. CAROTHERS and P. F. HAHN: Distribution and pathology following intracerebral and intraventricular radio gold. Federat. Proc. **12**, 396 (1953).

MEYERS, R., and R. HAYNE: Tridimensional analysis of deep and superficial structures of human brain. Trans. Amer. Neur. Assoc. **1948**, 175.

MONNIER, M.: Contributions expérimentales à la physiologie du tronc cérébral chez l'homme. I. Technique de repérage, stimulation et coagulation des structures sous-corticales. Helvet. physiol. Acta **8**, 54—55 (1950).

— Contributions techniques à l'exploration de thalamus chez le singe et chez l'homme. IV. Congr. Neurol. Internat. Paris 1949, Bd. III, S. 188—191. Paris: Masson & Cie. 1951.

— Repérage, stimulation et coagulation thérapeutique des centres sous-corticaux chez le singe et chez l'homme. Schweiz. Arch. Neur. **67**, 217—221 (1951).

— Appareil stéréotaxique et technique de repérage pour la coagulation du relais thalamique de la douleur chez l'homme. Schweiz. med. Wschr. **1952**, 1031—1034.

—, u. R. FISCHER: Contributions expérimentales à la physiologie du tronc cérébral chez l'homme. II. Stimulation et coagulation des noyau látero-ventral, ventro-postéro-latéral et ventro-postéro-median du thalamus. Helvet. physiol. Acta **8**, 55—57 (1950).

— Contributions expérimentales à la physiologie du tronc cérébral chez l'homme. III. Stimulation et coagulation du Lemniscus médian. Helvet. physiol. Acta **9**, 1—12 (1951)

— Localisation, stimulation et coagulation du thalamus chez l'homme. J. de Physiol. **43**, 818 (1951).

— Stimulation électrique et coagulation thérapeutique du thalamus chez l'homme (névralgies faciales). Confinia neur. **11**, 282—286 (1951).

MURTAGH jr., F., H. T. WYCIS and E. A. SPIEGEL: Relief of thalamic pain by mesencephalotomy. Arch. of Neur. **65**, 255 (1951).

NARABAYASHI, H., and T. OKUMA: Procaine-oil blocking of the globus pallidus for the treatment of rigidity and tremor of parkinsonism. Proc. Japan Acad. **29**, 134—137 (1953).

O'CONNELL, J. E. A., and A. BRUNSCHWIG: Observations on the roentgen treatment of intracranial gliomata with especial reference to the effects of irradiation upon the surrounding brain. Brain **60**, 230—258 (1937).

ORCHINIK, C., R. KOCH, H. T. WYCIS, H. FREED and E. A. SPIEGEL: The effect of thalamic lesions upon the emotional reactivity (Rorschach and behavior studies). Proc. Assoc. Res. Nerv. Ment. Dis. **29**, 172—207 (1950).

PENNYBACKER, J., and D. S. RUSSEL: Necrosis of the brain due to radiation therapy. J. of Neur., N. S. **11**, 183—198 (1948).

PERTUISET, B.: Présentation d'un appareil stéreotaxique adapté à l'homme. 14. Congr. Soc. Internat. Chir. Paris 1951. Zit. nach SPIEGEL u. WYCIS 1952.

PETERS, G.: Die Wirkung der Ultraschallwellen auf das Zentralnervensystem. Strahlenther. **79**, 653—658 (1949).

— Ultraschallwirkung auf das Nervensystem. In Der Ultraschall in der Medizin. Kongr.-Ber. Erlanger Ultraschall-Tagg 1949, S. 166—169. Zürich: S. Hirzel 1949.

RIECHERT, T.: Die gezielten Hirnoperationen. In Handbuch der inneren Medizin von v. BERGMANN, FREY u. SCHWIEGK, Bd. V/1, Neurologie, S. 1514—1518. Heidelberg: Springer 1953.

—, u. M. WOLFF: Zielgerät zur intrakraniellen elektrischen Ableitung und Ausschaltung mit besonderer Berücksichtigung der Eingriffe am Trigeminus. Nervenarzt **22**, 437 (1951).

— — Über ein neues Zielgerät zur intrakraniellen elektrischen Ableitung und Ausschaltung. Arch. f. Psychiatr. u. Z. Neur. **186**, 225—230 (1951).

— — Die Entwicklung und klinische Bedeutung der gezielten Hirnoperationen. Med. Klin. **1951**, 609 bis 611.

— — Die technische Durchführung von gezielten Hirnoperationen. Arch. f. Psychiatr. u. Z. Neur. **190**, 297—316 (1953).

RONDEPIERRE, J. J., et J. TALAIRACH: Cinq cas de destruction de noyau ventral antérieur du thalamus chez des malades mentaux. Revue neur. **88**, 535—538 (1953).

ROSS, J., S. LEAVITT and E. A. HOLST: Neurological and EEG changes in monkeys following x-irradiation of the head. Federat. Proc. **12**, 120 (1953).

RUSSEL, D. S., C. W. WILSON and K. TANSLEY: Experimental radionecrosis of the brain in rabbits. J. of Neurol., Neurosurg. a. Psychiatry **12**, 187—195 (1949).

SCHALTENBRAND, G.: Ortoroentgenography. Amer. J. Roentgenol. **70**, 114—118 (1953).

SCHMIEDT, E.: Kraniozerebrale Lagebestimmung des Nucleus dorsomedialis im menschlichen Thalamus. Acta neurochir. (Wien) **3**, 17—37 (1952).

SILVER, M. L., and A. E. WALKER: Histopathology of thermocoagulation of the cerebral cortex. J. of Neuropath. **6**, 311—322 (1947).

SPIEGEL, E. A., and H. FREED: Evaluation of the results of thalamotomy and other surgical procedures for the relief of psychosis. Surg. etc. **92**, 615—617 (1951).

—, and H. T. WYCIS: The stereoencephalotome and its applications. IV. Congr. Neurol. Internat. Paris 1949, Bd. II, S. 136. Paris: Masson & Cie. 1949.

— — Mesencephalothalamotomy for relief of pain. (Principles of the method.) Festschrift OTTO PÖTZL, herausgeg. von H. J. Urban, S. 438—442. Insbruck: Wagner 1949.

— — Physiological and psychological results of thalamotomy. Proc. Roy. Soc. Med. **42**, Suppl. 84—92 (1949).

— — Principles and applications of stereoencephalotomy. J. Internat. Coll. Surg. **14**, 394—402 (1950).

— — Principes et applications de la stéréoencéphalotomie. Acta neurochir. **1**, 137—153 (1950).

— — Thalamic recordings in man with special reference to seizure discharges. Electroencephalogr. Clin. Neurophysiol. **2**, 23—27 (1950).

— — Stereoencephalotomy (Thalamotomy and related procedures). I. Methods and stereotaxic atlas of the human brain. New York: Grune & Stratton 1952. 176 S.

— — Mesencephalo tomy in treatment of „intractable" facial pain. Arch. of Neur. **69**, 1—13 (1953).

— — Thalamotomy and pallidotomy for treatment of choreic movements. Acta neurochir. (Wien) **2**, 417—422 (1952).

— — Ansotomy in paralysis agitans. Arch. of Neur. **71**, 598—614 (1954).

— — and H. K. FISCHER: Electrographic and neurovegetative studies in thalamotomy. Trans. Amer. Neur. Assoc. **1949**, 238—240.

— — and H. FREED: Thalamotomy: Neuropsychiatric Aspects. N. Y. State J. Med. **49**, 2273—2274 (1949).

— — — Stereoencephalotomy, thalamotomy and related procedures. J. Amer. Med. Assoc. **148**, 446—451 (1952).

— — — and A. J. LEE: Stereoencephalotomy. Proc. Soc. Exper. Biol. a. Med. **69**, 175—177 (1948).

— — — — Stereoencephalotomy. Trans. Amer. Neur. Assoc. **1948**, 160—162.

SPIEGEL, E. A., H. T. WYCIS, H. FREED and C. ORCHINIK: The central mechanism of the emotions. (Experiences with circumscribed thalamic lesions.) Amer. J. Psychiatr. **108**, 426—432 (1951).

— — M. KLETZKIN and C. THUR: Studies in stereoencephalotomy II: A new procedure for exploration and elimination of subcortical structures. Electroencephalogr. Clin. Neurophysiol. **5**, 309—311 (1953).

— — M. MARKS and A. J. LEE: Stereotaxic apparatus for operations on the human brain. Science (Lancaster, Pa.) **106**, 349—350 (1947).

— — and V. REYES: Diencephalic mechanisms in petit mal epilepsy. Electroencephalogr. Clin. Neurophysiol. **3**, 473—475 (1951).

— — and C. THUR: The stereoencephalotome. (Model III of our stereotaxic apparatus for operations on the human brain.) J. of Neurosurg. **8**, 452—453 (1951).

— — and C. W. UMLAUF: Electroencephalographic studies before and after thalamotomy. Monthly Rev. Psychiatr. a. Neur. **120**, 398—411 (1950).

STEIN, S. N., and E. W. PETERSON: The use of radon seeds to produce deep cerebral lesions. Proc. Soc. Exper. Biol. a. Med. **74**, 583—585 (1950).

SWEET, W. H., and V. H. MARK: Unipolar anodal electrolytic lesions in the brain of man and cat. Report of five human cases with electrically produced bulbar or mesencephalic tractotomies. Arch. of Neur. **70**, 224—234 (1953).

TALAIRACH, J.: Destruction du noyau ventral antérieur thalamique dans le traitement des maladies mentales. Revue neur. **87**, 352—357 (1952).

— Les explorations radiologiques stéréotaxiques. Revue neur. **90**, 556—584 (1954).

— P. ABOULKER, G. RUGGIERO et M. DAVID: Utilisation de la méthode radiostéréotaxique pour le traitement radioactif in situ des tumeurs cérébrales. Revue neur. **90**, 656—657 (1954).

— J. DE AJURIAGUERRA et M. DAVID: A propos des coagulations thérapeutiques sous-corticales. Presse méd. **58**, 697—701 (1950).

— — — Études stéréotaxiques des structures encéphaliques profondes chez l'homme. Technique. Intérêt physiopathologique et thérapeutique. Presse méd. **60**, 605—609 (1952).

— — et H. HECAÉN: Étude topographique du thalamus en fonction des images ventriculaires. IV. Congr. Neurol. Internat. Paris 1949, Bd. III, 138—142. Paris: Masson & Cie. 1951.

— — — Étude topographique du système ventriculaire en fonction des noyaux gris centraux. Ann. Méd. **51**, 83—100 (1950).

— — et M. DAVID: Lobotomie préfrontale limitée par électrocoagulation des fibres thalamo-frontales à leur émergence du bras antérieur de la capsule interne. IV. Congr. Neurol. Internat. Paris 1949, Bd. II, S. 141. Paris: Masson & Cie. 1949.

— — — et M. MONNIER: Traitement de certaines algies par électrocoagulation de la région postero-ventrale du thalam us. IV. Congr. Neurol. Internat Paris 1949, Bd. II, S. 45—46. Paris: Masson & Cie. 1949.

— H. HECAÉN, M. DAVID, M. MONNIER et J. DE AJURIAGUERRA: Recherches sur la coagulation thérapeutique des structures sous-corticales chez l'homme. Revue neur. **81**, 4—24 (1949).

— J. E. PAILLAS et M. DAVID: Dyskinésie de type hémiballique traitée par cortectomie frontale limité e, puis par coagulation de l'anse lenticulaire et de [a portion interne du globus pallidus. Amélioration importante depuis un an. Revue neur. **83**, 440—451 (1950).

— G. RUGGIERO, J. ABOULKER et M. DAVID: A new method of treatment of inoperable brain tumours by stereotaxic implantation of radio-active gold. A preliminary report. Brit. J. Radiol. **28**, 62—74 (1955).

TOBIAS, C. A., H. O. ANGER and J. H. LAWRENCE: Radiological use of high energy deuterons and alpha particles. Amer. J. Roentgenol. **68**, 1—27 (1952).

UCHIMURA, Y., u. H. NARABAYASHI: Stereoencephalotomy. 47. Japanese Neuropsychiatric. Conf. Kyoto 1950. Zit. nach SPIEGEL u. WYCIS 1952.

*U.S. Atomic Energy Commission:* Studies in methods in instruments to improve the localization of radioactive materials in the body with special reference to the diagnosis of brain tumors, and the use of ultrasonic techniques. Progress rep. AECU — 3012. Aug. 1955.

WACHOWSKI, T. J., u. H. CHENAULT: Degenerative effects of large doses of roentgen rays on the human brain. Radiology **45**, 227—246 (1945).

WALL, P. D., W. J. FRY, R. STEPHENS, D. TUCKER and J. Y. LETTVIN: Changes produced in the central nervous system by ultrasound. Science (Lancaster, Pa.) **114**, 686—687 (1951).

— D. TUCKER, F. J. FRY and W. H. MOSBERG: The use of high intensity ultrasound in experimental neurology. J. Acoust. Soc. Amer. **25**, 281—285 (1953).

WARREN, S.: Effects of radiation on normal tissue. IX. Effects on the nervous system. Arch. of Path. **35**, 127—139 (1943).

WOEBER, K.: Über das Auftreten von Schädigungen am Zentralnervensystem der Ratte durch Ultraschallwellen. Strahlenther. **79**, 643—652 (1949).

WOLFF, M.: Die Ausmessung von Röntgenaufnahmen des Schädels unter besonderer Berücksichtigung der gezielten Operationen und der Koagulation des Ganglion semilunare. Fortschr. Röntgenstr. **77**, 679—683 (1952).

WULFF, V. J., W. J. FRY, D. TUCKER, F. J. FRY and C. MELTON: Effects of ultrasonic vibrations on nerve tissue. Proc. Soc. Exper. Biol. a. Med. **76**, 361—366 (1951).
WYCIS, H. T., R. ROBBINS, M. SPIEGEL-ADOLF, J. MESZARES and E. A. SPIEGEL: Studies in stereoencephalotomy III; treatment of a cystic craniopharyngioma by injection of radioaktive $P^{32}$. Confinia neur. (Basel) **4**, 193—202 (1954).
— L. SOLOFF and E. A. SPIEGEL: Facial pain persisting after retrogasserian rhizotomy relieved by mesencephalothalamotomy. Surgery **27**, 115—121 (1950).
—, and E. A. SPIEGEL: Thalamotomy and mesencephalothalamotomy: neurosurgical aspects (including treatment of pain). N. Y. State J. Med. **49**, 2275—2277 (1949).
— — Thalamotomy: neurosurgical aspects. Proc. Roy. Soc. Med. **42**, Suppl., 12 (1949).
— — Mesencephalotomy and mesencephalothalamotomy for treatment of unbearable pain. IV. Congr. Neurol. Internat. 1949, Bd. III, S. 310—313. Paris: Masson & Cie. 1951.
— — The effect of thalamotomy and pallidotomy upon involuntary movements in chorea and athetosis. Surgical Forum. Clin. Congr. Amer. Coll. Surg. 1950, S. 329—332. Philadelphia: W. B. Saunders Company 1951.
— — Ansotomy in Paralysis Agitans. Confinia neur. (Basel) **12**, 245—246 (1952).
— — Stereoencephalotomy in extrapyramidal disorders. V. Internat. Neurol.-Congr. Lisbon 1953, Bd. II, S. 183—184. Lisboa 1953.
ZEMAN, W.: Zur Frage der Röntgenstrahlenwirkung am tumorkranken Gehirn. Arch. f. Psychiatr. u. Z. Neur. **182**, 713—730 (1949).
ZUBIANI, A.: Sull' applicazione della energia ultrasonora al sistema nervoso centrale. Minerva med. (Torino) **1951**, 431—436.

### Physikalische Grundlagen für die Verwendung von ionisierender Strahlung bei gezielter Hirnchirurgie.

BALZ, G.: Brit. J. Radiol. **1953**, Suppl. No 5: Central axis depth dose data.
— R. BIRKNER u. F. WACHSMANN: Experimentelle Untersuchungen über die Absorption von Röntgenstrahlen in verschiedenen Geweben. Strahlenther. **97**, 382—388 (1955).
CEDERLUND, J., K. LIDÉN u. M. LINDGREN: Depth dose measurements in human brain tissue. Acta radiol. **41**, 473—477 (1954).
GREBE, L., u. W. WIEBE: Tabellen zur Dosierung der Röntgenstrahlen, Sonderbd. 25 der Strahlenther. München u. Berlin 1950.
JOHNS, H. E.: The Physics of Radiation Therapy. Springfield, Ill.: Ch. C. Thomas 1954.
LAUGHLIN, J. S.: Physical aspects of Betatron Therapy. Springfield, Ill.: Ch. C. Thomas 1953.
—, J. OVADIA, J. W. BEATTIE, W. J. HENDERSON, R. A. HARVEY u. L. L. HAAS: Some physical aspects of electron beam therapy. Radiology **60**, 165—185 (1953).
MAYNEORD, W. V., u. L. F. LAMERTON: A survey of depth dose data. Brit. J. Radiol. **14**, 255 bis 264 (1941).
OLDENDORF, W. H.: Focal neurological lesions produced by microwave irradiation. Proc. Soc. Exper. Biol. a. Med. **72**, 432—434 (1949).
SPIERS, F. W.: Effective atomic number and energy absorption in tissues. Brit. J. Radiol. **19**, 52—63 (1946).
— The influence of energy absorption and electron range on dosage in irradiated bone. Brit. J. Radiol. **22**, 521—533 (1949).
TOBIAS, C. A., H. O. ANGER u. J. H. LAWRENCE: Radiological use of high energy deuterons and alpha particles. Amer. J. Roentgenol. **67**, 1—27 (1952).
—, J. E. ROBERTS, J. H. LAWRENCE, B. V. A. LOW-BEER, H. O. ANGER, J. L. BORN, R. MCCOMBS u. C. HUGGINS: Radiation hypophysectomy with high energy proton beams. A preliminary report. Univ. Calif. Radiation Lab. Rep. No. UCRL-3035, 1—50 (1955).
VETTERLEIN, K. TH.: Über die Ionisation von Roentgenstrahlungen in verschiedenen Geweben. Diss. Erlangen 1949.
WACHSMANN, F.: Ausblick auf die Anwendungsmöglichkeiten der Elektronenschleuder in der Medizin und bisherige Versuchsergebnisse mit ultraharten Strahlungen. Acta radiol. **32**, 145—158 (1949).

### Die Anwendung von Ultraschall für gezielte Hirnoperationen.

ALLEGRANZA, A.: Effetti distruttivi degli ultrasouni sul sistema nervosa centrale. Biol. Lat. (Milano) **3**, 454 (1950).
BARNARD, J. W., W. J. FRY, F. J. FRY and J. F. BRENNAN: Small localized ultrasonic lesions in the white and grey matter of cat brain. A. M. A. Arch. of Neur. **75**, 15 (1956).
BARONE, A.: Aspects of the concentration of ultrasonic energy. Acustica **2**, 221 (1952).
BERGMANN, L.: Der Ultraschall, 6. Aufl. 1954.
ESCHE, R.: Untersuchungen zur Ultraschallabsorption in tierischen Geweben und Kunststoffen. Akust. Beih. **71** (1952).

FRY, W. J.: Action of ultrasound on nerve tissue: A review. J. Acoust. Soc. Amer. **25**, 1 (1953A).

— J. W. BARNARD, F. J. FRY and J. F. BRENNAN: Ultrasonically produced localized selective lesions in the central nervous system. Amer. J. Phys. Med. **34**, 413 (1955A).

— — — R. F. KUMMINS and J. F. BRENNAN: Ultrasonic lesions in the mammalian central nervous system. Science (Lancaster, Pa.) **122**, 517 (1955B).

—, and R. B. FRY: Temperature changes produced in tissues during ultrasonic irradiation. J. Acoust. Soc. Amer. **25**, 6 (1953A).

— W. H. MOSBERG, J. W. BARNARD and F. J. FRY: Production of focal destructive lesions in the central nervous system with ultrasound. J. of Neurosurg. **11**, 471 (1954).

GREGG, E. C.: Ultrasonics; biological effects. Medical Physics, Bd. 1, S. 1591 (Editor O. GLASSER). 1944.

HERRICK, J. F.: Temperatures produced in tissues by ultrasound: experimental study using various techniques. J. Acoust. Soc. Amer. **25**, 12 (1953).

HEYCK, H.: Ultraschall und Zentralnervensystem. Schweiz. med. Wschr. **1952**, 97.

—, u. W. HÖPKER: Hirnveränderungen bei der Ratte durch Ultraschall. Mschr. Psychiatr. **123**, 42 (1952).

HÜTER, TH.: Messung der Ultraschallabsorption in tierischen Geweben und ihre Abhängigkeit von der Frequenz. Naturwiss. **35**, 285 (1948).

— Messung der Ultraschallabsorption im menschlichen Schädelknochen und ihre Abhängigkeit von der Frequenz. Naturwiss. **39**, 21 (1952).

LEHMANN, J., u. W. NITSCH: Über die Frequenzabhängigkeit biologischer Ultraschallreaktionen mit besonderer Berücksichtigung der spezifischen Temperaturverteilung im Organismus. Strahlenther. **85**, 606 (1951).

LEHMANN, J. F.: The biophysical mode of action of biologic and therapeutic ultrasonic reactions. J. Acoust. Soc. Amer. **25**, 17 (1953).

LEKSELL, L.: Private Mitteilung (1956).

LEONHARDT, H.: Untersuchungen über die Einwirkungen von Ultraschall auf das Gehirn. Med. Klin. **1949**, 1162.

LINDSTRÖM, P. A.: Prefrontal ultrasonic irradiation, — a substitute for lobotomy. A.M.A. Arch. of Neur. **72**, 399 (1954).

LUDWIG, G. D.: The velocity of sound through tissues and the acoustic impedance of tissues. J. Acoust. Soc. Amer. **22**, 862 (1950).

LYNN, J. G., and T. J. PUTNAM: Histology of cerebral lesions produced by focused ultrasound. Amer. J. Path. **20**, 637 (1944).

— R. L. ZWEMER and A. J. CHICK: Biological applications of focused ultrasonic waves. Science (Lancaster, Pa.) **96**, 119 (1942).

PÄTZOLD, J., u. H. BORN: Behandlung biologischer Gewebe mit gebündeltem Ultraschall. Strahlenther. **76**, 486 (1947).

PETERS, G.: Morphologische Untersuchungen über die Wirkung von Ultraschallwellen auf das Zentralnervensystem. Fortschr. Neur. **17**, 85 (1949). (Siehe auch Kongreßbericht der Erlanger Ultraschalltagung 1949, S. 166.)

— Experimentelle Ultraschallschäden am Gehirn. Ultraschall in Med. **4**, 60 (1951).

THEISMANN, H., u. F. PFANDER: Über die Durchlässigkeit des Knochens für Ultraschall. Strahlenther. **80**, 607 (1949).

WALL, P. D., D. TUCKER, F. J. FRY and W. H. MOSBERG: The use of high intensity ultrasound in experimental neurology. J. Acoust. Soc. Amer. **25**, 281 (1953).

# Namenverzeichnis.

Die *kursiv* gesetzten Seitenzahlen beziehen sich auf die Literatur.

# Sachverzeichnis.

# Subject Index.